Dietary Supplements in Cardiovascular and Metabolic Diseases

Dietary Supplements in Cardiovascular and Metabolic Diseases

Editors

Bruno Trimarco
Gaetano Santulli

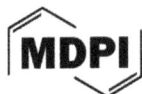

Basel • Beijing • Wuhan • Barcelona • Belgrade • Novi Sad • Cluj • Manchester

Editors

Bruno Trimarco
Università degli Studi di
Napoli Federico II
Naples
Italy

Gaetano Santulli
Department of Medicine,
Albert Einstein College of
Medicine
New York, NY
USA

Editorial Office
MDPI
St. Alban-Anlage 66
4052 Basel, Switzerland

This is a reprint of articles from the Special Issue published online in the open access journal *Nutrients* (ISSN 2072-6643) (available at: https://www.mdpi.com/journal/nutrients/special_issues/supplements_efficiency_cardiovascular).

For citation purposes, cite each article independently as indicated on the article page online and as indicated below:

Lastname, A.A.; Lastname, B.B. Article Title. *Journal Name* **Year**, *Volume Number*, Page Range.

ISBN 978-3-7258-1295-0 (Hbk)
ISBN 978-3-7258-1296-7 (PDF)
doi.org/10.3390/books978-3-7258-1296-7

Cover image courtesy of Gaetano Santulli

© 2024 by the authors. Articles in this book are Open Access and distributed under the Creative Commons Attribution (CC BY) license. The book as a whole is distributed by MDPI under the terms and conditions of the Creative Commons Attribution-NonCommercial-NoDerivs (CC BY-NC-ND) license.

Contents

Bruno Trimarco and Gaetano Santulli
Dietary Supplements in Cardiovascular and Metabolic Diseases
Reprinted from: *Nutrients* **2024**, *16*, 1418, doi:10.3390/nu16101418 1

Rosita Stanzione, Maurizio Forte, Maria Cotugno, Francesca Oppedisano, Cristina Carresi, Simona Marchitti, et al.
Beneficial Effects of Citrus Bergamia Polyphenolic Fraction on Saline Load-Induced Injury in Primary Cerebral Endothelial Cells from the Stroke-Prone Spontaneously Hypertensive Rat Model
Reprinted from: *Nutrients* **2023**, *15*, 1334, doi:10.3390/nu15061334 4

Rocco Mollace, Roberta Macrì, Annamaria Tavernese, Micaela Gliozzi, Vincenzo Musolino, Cristina Carresi, et al.
Comparative Effect of Bergamot Polyphenolic Fraction and Red Yeast Rice Extract in Rats Fed a Hyperlipidemic Diet: Role of Antioxidant Properties and PCSK9 Expression
Reprinted from: *Nutrients* **2022**, *14*, 477, doi:10.3390/nu14030477 16

Micaela Gliozzi, Roberta Macrì, Anna Rita Coppoletta, Vincenzo Musolino, Cristina Carresi, Miriam Scicchitano, et al.
From Diabetes Care to Heart Failure Management: A Potential Therapeutic Approach Combining SGLT2 Inhibitors and Plant Extracts
Reprinted from: *Nutrients* **2022**, *14*, 3737, doi:10.3390/nu14183737 25

María José Sánchez-Quintero, Josué Delgado, Dina Medina-Vera, Víctor M. Becerra-Muñoz, María Isabel Queipo-Ortuño, Mario Estéveγz, et al.
Beneficial Effects of Essential Oils from the Mediterranean Diet on Gut Microbiota and Their Metabolites in Ischemic Heart Disease and Type-2 Diabetes Mellitus
Reprinted from: *Nutrients* **2022**, *14*, 4650, doi:10.3390/nu14214650 41

Michał Majewski, Jerzy Juśkiewicz, Magdalena Krajewska-Włodarczyk, Leszek Gromadziński, Katarzyna Socha, Ewelina Cholewińska, et al.
The Role of 20-HETE, COX, Thromboxane Receptors, and Blood Plasma Antioxidant Status in Vascular Relaxation of Copper-Nanoparticle-Fed WKY Rats
Reprinted from: *Nutrients* **2021**, *13*, 3793, doi:10.3390/nu13113793 67

Agata Walkowiak-Bródka, Natalia Piekuś-Słomka, Kacper Wnuk and Bogumiła Kupcewicz
Analysis of White Mulberry Leaves and Dietary Supplements, ATR-FTIR Combined with Chemometrics for the Rapid Determination of 1-Deoxynojirimycin
Reprinted from: *Nutrients* **2022**, *14*, 5276, doi:10.3390/nu14245276 78

Leona Yuen-Ling Leung, Sidney Man-Ngai Chan, Hon-Lon Tam and Emily Sze-Wan Wong
Astaxanthin Influence on Health Outcomes of Adults at Risk of Metabolic Syndrome: A Systematic Review and Meta-Analysis
Reprinted from: *Nutrients* **2022**, *14*, 2050, doi:10.3390/nu14102050 92

Gaetano Santulli, Urna Kansakar, Fahimeh Varzideh, Pasquale Mone, Stanislovas S. Jankauskas and Angela Lombardi
Functional Role of Taurine in Aging and Cardiovascular Health: An Updated Overview
Reprinted from: *Nutrients* **2023**, *15*, 4236, doi:10.3390/nu15194236 108

Huan Yu, Junhui Wu, Hongbo Chen, Mengying Wang, Siyue Wang, Ruotong Yang, et al.
Glucosamine Use Is Associated with a Higher Risk of Cardiovascular Diseases in Patients with Osteoarthritis: Results from a Large Study in 685,778 Subjects
Reprinted from: *Nutrients* **2022**, *14*, 3694, doi:10.3390/nu14183694 . . . . **126**

Matteo Tosato, Riccardo Calvani, Anna Picca, Francesca Ciciarello, Vincenzo Galluzzo, Hélio José Coelho-Júnior, et al.
Effects of L-Arginine Plus Vitamin C Supplementation on Physical Performance, Endothelial Function, and Persistent Fatigue in Adults with Long COVID: A Single-Blind Randomized Controlled Trial
Reprinted from: *Nutrients* **2022**, *14*, 4984, doi:10.3390/nu14234984 . . . . **137**

Jesús Castro-Marrero, Maria Jose Segundo, Marcos Lacasa, Alba Martinez-Martinez, Ramon Sanmartin Sentañes and Jose Alegre-Martin
Effect of Dietary Coenzyme Q10 Plus NADH Supplementation on Fatigue Perception and Health-Related Quality of Life in Individuals with Myalgic Encephalomyelitis/Chronic Fatigue Syndrome: A Prospective, Randomized, Double-Blind, Placebo-Controlled Trial
Reprinted from: *Nutrients* **2021**, *13*, 2658, doi:10.3390/nu13082658 . . . . **150**

Zezhong Tian, Kongyao Li, Die Fan, Xiaoli Gao, Xilin Ma, Yimin Zhao, et al.
Water-Soluble Tomato Concentrate, a Potential Antioxidant Supplement, Can Attenuate Platelet Apoptosis and Oxidative Stress in Healthy Middle-Aged and Elderly Adults: A Randomized, Double-Blinded, Crossover Clinical Trial
Reprinted from: *Nutrients* **2022**, *14*, 3374, doi:10.3390/nu14163374 . . . . **166**

Federica Fogacci, Elisabetta Rizzoli, Marina Giovannini, Marilisa Bove, Sergio D'Addato, Claudio Borghi, et al.
Effect of Dietary Supplementation with Eufortyn® Colesterolo Plus on Serum Lipids, Endothelial Reactivity, Indexes of Non-Alcoholic Fatty Liver Disease and Systemic Inflammation in Healthy Subjects with Polygenic Hypercholesterolemia: The ANEMONE Study
Reprinted from: *Nutrients* **2022**, *14*, 2099, doi:10.3390/nu14102099 . . . . **182**

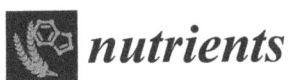

Editorial

Dietary Supplements in Cardiovascular and Metabolic Diseases

Bruno Trimarco [1,2] and Gaetano Santulli [1,2,3,4,*]

1. Department of Advanced Biomedical Sciences, Federico II University Hospital, 80131 Naples, Italy; bruno.trimarco@unina.it
2. International Translational Research and Medical Education (ITME) Consortium, Academic Research Unit, 80100 Naples, Italy
3. Department of Medicine, Fleischer Institute for Diabetes and Metabolism (FIDAM), Albert Einstein College of Medicine, New York, NY 10461, USA
4. Department of Molecular Pharmacology, Wilf Family Cardiovascular Research Institute, Einstein Institute for Aging Research, Einstein-Mount Sinai Diabetes Research Center (ES-DRC), Einstein Institute for Neuroimmunology and Inflammation (INI), Albert Einstein College of Medicine, New York, NY 10461, USA
* Correspondence: gsantulli001@gmail.com

Recent research has sparked increasing interest in the effects of dietary supplements on cardiovascular and metabolic disorders. The aim of this Special Issue was to compile top-tier research papers with a strong foundation in basic research and/or potential for translation in this area, to offer an up-to-date systematic examination of the functional role of dietary supplements in cardiovascular and metabolic disease. We included both clinical and pre-clinical studies on this compelling topic.

The Special Issue begins with two preclinical investigations studying the effects of the extract of the bergamot fruit (*Citrus bergamia*) in vitro [1] and in vivo [2], observing a reduction in oxidative stress (research led by Dr. Speranza Rubattu [1]) and dyslipidemia (research led by Vincenzo Mollace [2]). Dr. Mollace's group also contributed a review on the potential therapeutic approach of combining SGLT2 inhibitors and plant extracts [3].

In another in vivo study, led by Dr. Francisco Javier Pavón-Morón, humanized mice were supplemented with L-carnitine and orally administered essential oil emulsions derived from patients with ischemic heart disease and type 2 diabetes mellitus for 40 days [4]. The researchers evaluated the impact on the gut microbiota composition, microbial metabolites, and plasma markers related to cardiovascular disease, inflammation, and oxidative stress. The results indicated that essential oil emulsions, particularly those containing parsley and rosemary essential oils, exhibited prebiotic effects on beneficial commensal bacteria, primarily of the Lactobacillus genus; moreover, mice treated with these essential oils showed a decrease in plasma trimethylamine N-oxide (TMAO) levels and an increase in fecal short-chain fatty acids (SCFAs) levels [4]. An assay in Wistar–Kyoto rats demonstrated that increased oxidative stress accompanied the intake of copper nanoparticles, which further modulated vascular relaxation with the participation of 20-hydroxyeicosatetraenoic acid (20-HETE), through the thromboxane-A_2 receptors [5]. Another study evaluated the quality of 19 products, including herbal teas and dietary supplements, by assessing the content of 1-deoxynojirimycin (DNJ, known for its ability to inhibit α-glucosidase and regulate postprandial glucose levels), selected (poly)phenols, and antioxidant activity [6]. The results revealed subpar quality in many dietary supplements, potentially compromising their health benefits, due to the low nutraceutical content. Furthermore, a novel method utilizing ATR-FTIR spectroscopy combined with PLS regression for DNJ content determination was proposed, offering a rapid screening tool for assessing product quality without the need for complex chromatographic processes.

Two reviews are included in the Special Issue. The first one considered astaxanthin, a natural carotenoid commonly found in various aquatic animals, including salmon, shrimp, and crustaceans, which shows a very strong antioxidant effect that is 14, 65, and 54 times

Citation: Trimarco, B.; Santulli, G. Dietary Supplements in Cardiovascular and Metabolic Diseases. *Nutrients* 2024, *16*, 1418. https://doi.org/10.3390/nu16101418

Received: 18 April 2024
Accepted: 28 April 2024
Published: 8 May 2024

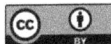

Copyright: © 2024 by the authors. Licensee MDPI, Basel, Switzerland. This article is an open access article distributed under the terms and conditions of the Creative Commons Attribution (CC BY) license (https://creativecommons.org/licenses/by/4.0/).

higher than that of vitamin E, C, and β-carotene, respectively [7]. The second one explored the role of taurine in aging and cardiovascular health [8].

Next, the Special Issue presents clinical studies. The first study was a retrospective analysis of 685,778 patients newly diagnosed with osteoarthritis, showing that the adherent usage of glucosamine was significantly associated with a higher risk for cardiovascular diseases in patients with osteoarthritis [9]. A single-blind randomized controlled trial, coordinated by Dr. Francesco Landi, demonstrated that L-Arginine plus vitamin C supplementation (an association that has been shown to be effective in long-COVID [10–13] by attenuating endothelial dysfunction and oxidative stress [13–16]) can improve walking performance, muscle strength, and fatigue in adults with long-COVID [17].

The Special Issue concludes with the presentation of three randomized, double-blind, and placebo-controlled trials. The first trial tested the effects of dietary Coenzyme Q10 plus NADH supplementation on the fatigue perception and health-related quality of life in patients with myalgic encephalomyelitis/chronic fatigue syndrome [18]. A 12-week clinical trial was conducted with 207 participants, showing significant reductions in cognitive fatigue perception and overall fatigue severity, as well as improvements in the health-related quality of life among those receiving CoQ10 and NADH; additionally, improvements in sleep duration and efficiency were observed in the experimental group [18].

The second trial aimed to assess the impact of water-soluble tomato concentrate (WSTC) from fresh tomatoes on platelet apoptosis and oxidative stress in a clinical trial lasting 10 weeks and involving 52 healthy middle-aged and elderly adults, revealing that WSTC supplementation for four weeks significantly increased the serum total antioxidant capacity levels and reduced the serum malondialdehyde levels [19].

The third trial demonstrated that dietary supplementation with standardized bergamot polyphenolic fraction phytosome, artichoke extracts, Q10 phytosome, and zinc safely exerted significant improvements in serum lipids, systemic inflammation, indexes of non-alcoholic fatty liver disease (NAFLD), and endothelial reactivity in healthy subjects with moderate hypercholesterolemia [20].

Author Contributions: Conceptualization, writing, supervision: G.S.; visualization, writing: B.T. All authors have read and agreed to the published version of the manuscript.

Conflicts of Interest: The authors declare no conflicts of interest.

References

1. Stanzione, R.; Forte, M.; Cotugno, M.; Oppedisano, F.; Carresi, C.; Marchitti, S.; Mollace, V.; Volpe, M.; Rubattu, S. Beneficial Effects of Citrus Bergamia Polyphenolic Fraction on Saline Load-Induced Injury in Primary Cerebral Endothelial Cells from the Stroke-Prone Spontaneously Hypertensive Rat Model. *Nutrients* 2023, 15, 1334. [CrossRef] [PubMed]
2. Mollace, R.; Macri, R.; Tavernese, A.; Gliozzi, M.; Musolino, V.; Carresi, C.; Maiuolo, J.; Fini, M.; Volterrani, M.; Mollace, V. Comparative Effect of Bergamot Polyphenolic Fraction and Red Yeast Rice Extract in Rats Fed a Hyperlipidemic Diet: Role of Antioxidant Properties and PCSK9 Expression. *Nutrients* 2022, 14, 477. [CrossRef] [PubMed]
3. Gliozzi, M.; Macri, R.; Coppoletta, A.R.; Musolino, V.; Carresi, C.; Scicchitano, M.; Bosco, F.; Guarnieri, L.; Cardamone, A.; Ruga, S.; et al. From Diabetes Care to Heart Failure Management: A Potential Therapeutic Approach Combining SGLT2 Inhibitors and Plant Extracts. *Nutrients* 2022, 14, 3737. [CrossRef] [PubMed]
4. Sanchez-Quintero, M.J.; Delgado, J.; Medina-Vera, D.; Becerra-Munoz, V.M.; Queipo-Ortuno, M.I.; Estevez, M.; Plaza-Andrades, I.; Rodriguez-Capitan, J.; Sanchez, P.L.; Crespo-Leiro, M.G.; et al. Beneficial Effects of Essential Oils from the Mediterranean Diet on Gut Microbiota and Their Metabolites in Ischemic Heart Disease and Type-2 Diabetes Mellitus. *Nutrients* 2022, 14, 4650. [CrossRef] [PubMed]
5. Majewski, M.; Juskiewicz, J.; Krajewska-Wlodarczyk, M.; Gromadzinski, L.; Socha, K.; Cholewinska, E.; Ognik, K. The Role of 20-HETE, COX, Thromboxane Receptors, and Blood Plasma Antioxidant Status in Vascular Relaxation of Copper-Nanoparticle-Fed WKY Rats. *Nutrients* 2021, 13, 3793. [CrossRef] [PubMed]
6. Walkowiak-Brodka, A.; Piekus-Slomka, N.; Wnuk, K.; Kupcewicz, B. Analysis of White Mulberry Leaves and Dietary Supplements, ATR-FTIR Combined with Chemometrics for the Rapid Determination of 1-Deoxynojirimycin. *Nutrients* 2022, 14, 5276. [CrossRef] [PubMed]
7. Leung, L.Y.; Chan, S.M.; Tam, H.L.; Wong, E.S. Astaxanthin Influence on Health Outcomes of Adults at Risk of Metabolic Syndrome: A Systematic Review and Meta-Analysis. *Nutrients* 2022, 14, 2050. [CrossRef] [PubMed]

8. Santulli, G.; Kansakar, U.; Varzideh, F.; Mone, P.; Jankauskas, S.S.; Lombardi, A. Functional Role of Taurine in Aging and Cardiovascular Health: An Updated Overview. *Nutrients* **2023**, *15*, 4236. [CrossRef] [PubMed]
9. Yu, H.; Wu, J.; Chen, H.; Wang, M.; Wang, S.; Yang, R.; Zhan, S.; Qin, X.; Wu, T.; Wu, Y.; et al. Glucosamine Use Is Associated with a Higher Risk of Cardiovascular Diseases in Patients with Osteoarthritis: Results from a Large Study in 685,778 Subjects. *Nutrients* **2022**, *14*, 3694. [CrossRef] [PubMed]
10. Trimarco, V.; Izzo, R.; Zanforlin, A.; Tursi, F.; Scarpelli, F.; Santus, P.; Pennisi, A.; Pelaia, G.; Mussi, C.; Mininni, S.; et al. Endothelial dysfunction in long-COVID: New insights from the nationwide multicenter LINCOLN Study. *Pharmacol. Res.* **2022**, *185*, 106486. [CrossRef] [PubMed]
11. Santulli, G.; Trimarco, V.; Trimarco, B.; Izzo, R. Beneficial effects of Vitamin C and L-Arginine in the treatment of post-acute sequelae of COVID-19. *Pharmacol. Res.* **2022**, *185*, 106479. [CrossRef] [PubMed]
12. Izzo, R.; Trimarco, V.; Mone, P.; Aloe, T.; Capra Marzani, M.; Diana, A.; Fazio, G.; Mallardo, M.; Maniscalco, M.; Marazzi, G.; et al. Combining L-Arginine with vitamin C improves long-COVID symptoms: The LINCOLN Survey. *Pharmacol. Res.* **2022**, *183*, 106360. [CrossRef] [PubMed]
13. Mone, P.; Izzo, R.; Marazzi, G.; Manzi, M.V.; Gallo, P.; Campolongo, G.; Cacciotti, L.; Tartaglia, D.; Caminiti, G.; Varzideh, F.; et al. L-Arginine Enhances the Effects of Cardiac Rehabilitation on Physical Performance: New Insights for Managing Cardiovascular Patients During the COVID-19 Pandemic. *J. Pharmacol. Exp. Ther.* **2022**, *381*, 197–203. [CrossRef] [PubMed]
14. Adebayo, A.; Varzideh, F.; Wilson, S.; Gambardella, J.; Eacobacci, M.; Jankauskas, S.S.; Donkor, K.; Kansakar, U.; Trimarco, V.; Mone, P.; et al. l-Arginine and COVID-19: An Update. *Nutrients* **2021**, *13*, 3951. [CrossRef] [PubMed]
15. Fiorentino, G.; Coppola, A.; Izzo, R.; Annunziata, A.; Bernardo, M.; Lombardi, A.; Trimarco, V.; Santulli, G.; Trimarco, B. Effects of adding L-arginine orally to standard therapy in patients with COVID-19: A randomized, double-blind, placebo-controlled, parallel-group trial. Results of the first interim analysis. *EClinicalMedicine* **2021**, *40*, 101125. [CrossRef] [PubMed]
16. Gambardella, J.; Khondkar, W.; Morelli, M.B.; Wang, X.; Santulli, G.; Trimarco, V. Arginine and Endothelial Function. *Biomedicines* **2020**, *8*, 277. [CrossRef] [PubMed]
17. Tosato, M.; Calvani, R.; Picca, A.; Ciciarello, F.; Galluzzo, V.; Coelho-Junior, H.J.; Di Giorgio, A.; Di Mario, C.; Gervasoni, J.; Gremese, E.; et al. Effects of l-Arginine Plus Vitamin C Supplementation on Physical Performance, Endothelial Function, and Persistent Fatigue in Adults with Long COVID: A Single-Blind Randomized Controlled Trial. *Nutrients* **2022**, *14*, 4984. [CrossRef] [PubMed]
18. Castro-Marrero, J.; Segundo, M.J.; Lacasa, M.; Martinez-Martinez, A.; Sentanes, R.S.; Alegre-Martin, J. Effect of Dietary Coenzyme Q10 Plus NADH Supplementation on Fatigue Perception and Health-Related Quality of Life in Individuals with Myalgic Encephalomyelitis/Chronic Fatigue Syndrome: A Prospective, Randomized, Double-Blind, Placebo-Controlled Trial. *Nutrients* **2021**, *13*, 2658. [CrossRef] [PubMed]
19. Tian, Z.; Li, K.; Fan, D.; Gao, X.; Ma, X.; Zhao, Y.; Zhao, D.; Liang, Y.; Ji, Q.; Chen, Y.; et al. Water-Soluble Tomato Concentrate, a Potential Antioxidant Supplement, Can Attenuate Platelet Apoptosis and Oxidative Stress in Healthy Middle-Aged and Elderly Adults: A Randomized, Double-Blinded, Crossover Clinical Trial. *Nutrients* **2022**, *14*, 3374. [CrossRef] [PubMed]
20. Fogacci, F.; Rizzoli, E.; Giovannini, M.; Bove, M.; D'Addato, S.; Borghi, C.; Cicero, A.F.G. Effect of Dietary Supplementation with Eufortyn((R)) Colesterolo Plus on Serum Lipids, Endothelial Reactivity, Indexes of Non-Alcoholic Fatty Liver Disease and Systemic Inflammation in Healthy Subjects with Polygenic Hypercholesterolemia: The ANEMONE Study. *Nutrients* **2022**, *14*, 2099. [CrossRef] [PubMed]

Disclaimer/Publisher's Note: The statements, opinions and data contained in all publications are solely those of the individual author(s) and contributor(s) and not of MDPI and/or the editor(s). MDPI and/or the editor(s) disclaim responsibility for any injury to people or property resulting from any ideas, methods, instructions or products referred to in the content.

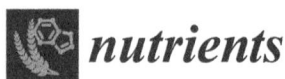

Article

Beneficial Effects of Citrus Bergamia Polyphenolic Fraction on Saline Load-Induced Injury in Primary Cerebral Endothelial Cells from the Stroke-Prone Spontaneously Hypertensive Rat Model

Rosita Stanzione [1,†], Maurizio Forte [1,†], Maria Cotugno [1], Francesca Oppedisano [2], Cristina Carresi [2], Simona Marchitti [1], Vincenzo Mollace [2,3], Massimo Volpe [3,4] and Speranza Rubattu [1,4,*]

1. IRCCS Neuromed, 86077 Pozzilli, Italy; stanzione@neuromed.it (R.S.); maurizio.forte@neuromed.it (M.F.); maria.cotugno@neuromed.it (M.C.); simona.marchitti@neuromed.it (S.M.)
2. Department of Health Science, Institute of Research for Food Safety & Health IRC-FSH, University Magna Graecia, 88100 Catanzaro, Italy; oppedisanof@libero.it (F.O.); carresi@unicz.it (C.C.); mollace@unicz.it (V.M.)
3. IRCCS San Raffaele, 00163 Rome, Italy; massimo.volpe@uniroma1.it
4. Department of Clinical and Molecular Medicine, School of Medicine and Psychology, Sapienza University of Rome, 00185 Rome, Italy
* Correspondence: speranzadonatella.rubattu@uniroma1.it
† These authors contributed equally to this work.

Abstract: High salt load is a known noxious stimulus for vascular cells and a risk factor for cardiovascular diseases in both animal models and humans. The stroke-prone spontaneously hypertensive rat (SHRSP) accelerates stroke predisposition upon high-salt dietary feeding. We previously demonstrated that high salt load causes severe injury in primary cerebral endothelial cells isolated from SHRSP. This cellular model offers a unique opportunity to test the impact of substances toward the mechanisms underlying high-salt-induced vascular damage. We tested the effects of a bergamot polyphenolic fraction (BPF) on high-salt-induced injury in SHRSP cerebral endothelial cells. Cells were exposed to 20 mM NaCl for 72 h either in the absence or the presence of BPF. As a result, we confirmed that high salt load increased cellular ROS level, reduced viability, impaired angiogenesis, and caused mitochondrial dysfunction with a significant increase in mitochondrial oxidative stress. The addition of BPF reduced oxidative stress, rescued cell viability and angiogenesis, and recovered mitochondrial function with a significant decrease in mitochondrial oxidative stress. In conclusion, BPF counteracts the key molecular mechanisms underlying high-salt-induced endothelial cell damage. This natural antioxidant substance may represent a valuable adjuvant to treat vascular disorders.

Keywords: salt loading; endothelial cell; oxidative stress; mitochondrial dysfunction; bergamot; polyphenols; stroke; SHRSP

Citation: Stanzione, R.; Forte, M.; Cotugno, M.; Oppedisano, F.; Carresi, C.; Marchitti, S.; Mollace, V.; Volpe, M.; Rubattu, S. Beneficial Effects of Citrus Bergamia Polyphenolic Fraction on Saline Load-Induced Injury in Primary Cerebral Endothelial Cells from the Stroke-Prone Spontaneously Hypertensive Rat Model. *Nutrients* 2023, 15, 1334. https://doi.org/10.3390/nu15061334

Academic Editor: Lindsay Brown

Received: 25 January 2023
Revised: 28 February 2023
Accepted: 8 March 2023
Published: 9 March 2023

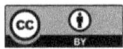

Copyright: © 2023 by the authors. Licensee MDPI, Basel, Switzerland. This article is an open access article distributed under the terms and conditions of the Creative Commons Attribution (CC BY) license (https://creativecommons.org/licenses/by/4.0/).

1. Introduction

The stroke-prone spontaneously hypertensive rat (SHRSP) represents a suitable animal model for the dissection of the pathogenetic basis of cerebrovascular damage associated with hypertension [1]. The stroke phenotype is accelerated in this model by feeding with a high-salt/low-potassium Japanese-style diet (JD) [2,3], with renal damage preceding stroke occurrence [4]. The stroke-resistant spontaneously hypertensive rat (SHRSR), which represents the strict control of the SHRSP strain, does not develop vascular damage upon same dietary treatment despite similar blood pressure levels [3]. A genetic linkage analysis demonstrated that few chromosomal loci contributed in a significant manner to the stroke phenotype variance between the two strains [3]. Subsequent investigations targeted to a chromosome 1 locus (*STR1*), explaining 20% of the stroke phenotype variance, highlighted a key role of mitochondrial dysfunction in mediating the high-salt-favored vascular damage of JD-fed SHRSP [5]. In fact, in this experimental condition, a mitochondrial complex I deficiency is induced by inhibition of the Ndufc2 subunit expression, whose gene maps are at the peak of linkage within *STR1*. Ndufc2 is a fundamental subunit to allow for regular assembly and function of the complex I, with consequent regular activity of the oxidative phosphorylation [5]. Subsequent studies revealed that this molecular mechanism also severely alters mitochondrial structure and function in peripheral blood mononuclear cells of healthy subjects once exposed to either high salt or lipopolysaccharides [6]. Most importantly, a decrease in the Ndufc2 subunit also contributes to both juvenile ischemic stroke and myocardial infarction occurrence in humans [5–8]. Interestingly, isolated primary cerebral endothelial cells (ECs) [6] from SHRSP, once exposed to saline load, show a significant degree of mitochondrial dysfunction, dependent from a decrease in Ndufc2 subunit expression, with a consequent increase in oxidative stress, reduced viability, and increased necrosis [9,10]. Therefore, this in vitro model mimics the in vivo condition quite well and represents a suitable experimental tool for testing the effects of protective molecules in vitro.

Vegetal substances are known for their beneficial vascular properties in both animal models and in humans due to their ability to counteract oxidative stress, inflammation, and mitochondrial dysfunction [11]. In this regard, our previous studies demonstrated the protective role of *Brassica oleracea* sprout extract, based on both anti-inflammatory and antioxidant actions, toward the high-salt-induced vascular injury of SHRSP [12,13]. The latter evidence, showing a remarkable decrease in both renal and cerebrovascular damage, further supported the significant adjuvant role of favorable nutritional components to combat cardiovascular and cerebrovascular diseases.

Among the emerging substances of natural origin provided of cardiovascular beneficial properties, the bergamot polyphenolic fraction (BPF), that is, the extract of the bergamot fruit (*Citrus bergamia*), is attracting much attention. BPF reduces serum lipid level (low-density lipoprotein cholesterol and triglycerides) and improves metabolic parameters and endothelial function in both animal models and in humans [14–21]. At the cellular level, BPF shows anti-inflammatory and antioxidant properties and can improve mitochondrial bioenergetics, mitochondrial function, and cell metabolism [16,22–24]. Interestingly, the protective action of BPF was also related to its ability to restore autophagy [25,26], a process with a fundamental role in cellular, tissue, and organismal homeostasis since it selectively targets dysfunctional organelles and pathogenic proteins [27]. Evidence that BPF can counteract high-salt-favored vascular injury in the context of arterial hypertension is still lacking.

On these premises, the goal of the present study was to test in vitro the potential beneficial impact of BPF toward high-salt-induced injury and the underlying molecular mechanisms in SHRSP cerebral ECs, as starting knowledge for subsequent in vivo investigations.

2. Materials and Methods

2.1. Preparation of the Bergamot Polyphenolic Fraction (BPF)

This step was performed through a standardized and previously reported procedure [14]. In particular, the cultivations of *Citrus bergamia* Risso & Poiteau are present along the Ionian coast of Calabria, in a geographical area of about 90 km between Bianco and Reggio Calabria, Italy. After harvesting, the peeled fruits were squeezed to obtain the bergamot juice, from which the oily fraction was removed by stripping. Furthermore, the juice was clarified by ultrafiltration. At the end of this process, the clarified juice was eluted through a polystyrene resin column, using a KOH solution, to retain the polyphenolic compounds with a molecular weight between 300 and 600 Da. Incubation of the basic eluate on a rocking platform allowed for a reduction in the furocoumarin content, on which the shaking time depended. In the next step, this phytocomplex was neutralized by filtration on cationic resin at acid pH, and after drying under vacuum and mincing, it was transformed into powdered BPF. Analysis of the BPF powder by UHPLC-HRMS/MS determined that it consisted of 40% flavonoids and 60% carbohydrates, fatty acids, pectins, and maltodextrins. The flavonoid profile analyzed by high-resolution mass spectrometry (Orbitrap spectrometer) and HRMSMS (ddMS2, data-dependent MS/MS) includes neoeriocitrin, naringin and neohesperidin. In addition, the entire HMG family is present with bruteridin and melitidin together with flavonoids such as 6.8-di-C-glycosides [24,28,29]. The BPF used in the present study was prepared and characterized by polyphenol content a month before performing the experiments.

2.2. Cell Isolation and Culture

Primary cerebral ECs were isolated from newborn SHRSP rat brains (1–3 days old) by enzymatic and mechanic digestions and subsequent positive selection using microbeads magnetically labeled with CD31 antibody (Miltenyi Biotec, Bergisch Gladbach, Germany). For the enzymatic and mechanic digestions, neural tissue from neonatal brains was dissociated into single-cell suspension by using the Neural Tissue Dissociation Kit (Miltenyi Biotec) and the gentle MACS Dissociator (Miltenyi) with a specific program for neonatal brain. Afterword, the positive selection of ECs with CD31 antibody (Endothelial Cell Isolation Kit, Miltenyi) was performed by a separation over a MACS column placed in the magnetic field of a MACS separator (Miltenyi). ECs were grown in DMEM/F12 medium (Thermo Fisher Scientific, Waltham, MA, USA) supplemented with 5% FBS (Euroclone Srl, Pero, Italy) and ECGS (Sigma Aldrich–Merck, Darmstadt, Germany) on gelatin-precoated dishes at 37 °C and 5% CO_2 in an humified incubator. Cells were used between passages 1–4 for all experiments, as previously reported [9]. Animal experiments for EC isolation were performed in accordance with the European Commission guidelines (Dlg 2010/63/EU) and the protocol was approved by Italian Ministry of Health (protocol n.: 448/2022-PR).

2.3. Immunostaining of Primary Cerebral ECs for CD31

The purity of ECs was confirmed by immunofluorescence for CD31, a transmembrane glycoprotein expressed by ECs. For this purpose, 2×10^4 cells were plated in an 8-chamber slide and fixed for 10 min with 4% PFA, washed in PBS, blocked with 5% goat normal horse serum (Vector Laboratories, Burlingame, CA, USA) and incubated overnight at 4 °C with anti-CD31 antibody (0AAF00819-Aviva System Biology, San Diego, CA, USA). Then, Alexa fluor 488 (Invitrogen Carlsbad, CA, USA) was used for detection in fluorescence. Cell nuclei were stained with Höechst reagent (Thermo Fisher Scientific). Images were randomly taken with a fluorescence microscope.

2.4. Cell Treatments

Preliminary experiments testing different BPF concentrations (from 50 to 500 µg/mL) on cell viability identified 250 µg/mL as the appropriate concentration to perform all studies in our cellular model exposed to salt loading. The latter is a noxious stimulus previously used in our studies to mimic the in vivo exposure of SHRSP to JD as a stroke-promoting diet [9,10,30]. Therefore, to test the effects of BPF on cell proliferation, viability, oxidative stress, angiogenesis, wound healing, and mitochondrial function, ECs were exposed for 72 h to the following treatments: NaCl 20 mM, BPF alone (250 µg/mL), and NaCl + BPF (20 mM and 250 µg/mL, respectively). Both NaCl and BPF were diluted in the cell medium. All experiments were performed at least in triplicate.

2.5. Cell Viability

To test cell proliferation and viability, we used the quantitative colorimetric MTT (3-(4,5-Dimethylthiazol-2-yl)-2,5-Diphenyltetrazolium Bromide) test (Sigma Aldrich–Merck). MTT is a yellow powder containing bromide, which in living cells is transformed, by an enzymatic scission, into an insoluble blue/purple precipitate, the formazan. To perform the assay, ECs were plated in a 96-multiwell plate at a density of 1×10^4 cells per well, and they were exposed to 20 mM NaCl for 72 h, as previously described [9,10]. After the treatment, ECs were incubated for 2–3 h with 10 µL of MTT reagent (5 mg/mL) in a 37 °C,

5% CO_2 incubator. Then, 100 µL of DMSO were added to each well, and the mixture was stirred well until the formazan was completely dissolved. Finally, the absorbance of the solubilized substrate was measured with a microplate reader (Biorad, Hercules, CA, USA) at a wavelength of 570 nm.

2.6. Cellular Reactive Oxygen Species (ROS) Measurement

Cellular ROS were evaluated using the fluorescent probe 2′,7′-Dichlorofluorescein diacetate (DCFH-DA Sigma Aldrich). DCHF-DA is an apolar molecule that diffuses easily in cells, where by two successive enzymatic reactions, it is transformed into DCF, a highly fluorescent molecule that is emitted at a wavelength of 532 nm. The oxidation of DCHF to DCF occurs mainly by H_2O_2. Therefore, the fluorescence intensity is considered directly proportional to the quantity of H_2O_2 produced by the cells. In our experiments, ECs were treated with 200 µL of 10 µM DCFH-DA for 30 min at 37 °C in the darkness. Production of ROS was measured by a microplate reader (Berthold, Bad Wildbad, Germany) at an excitation wavelength of 485 nm and an emission wavelength of 530 nm.

2.7. Angiogenesis Assay

The angiogenesis assay was performed by using a Matrigel matrix (Corning, by Sigma Aldrich–Merck). In the specific, 50 microliters of Matrigel matrix were added to each well of a 96-multiwell plate and allowed to solidify for 1 h at 37 °C. After treatment with NaCl and BPF, 1×10^4 ECs were plated on top of the Matrigel layer and incubated for 4 h. Images were taken with EVOS Cell Imaging Systems (Thermo Fisher Scientific) and the number of master junctions was quantified using a specific plugin "Angiogenesis analyzer" of ImageJ software (National Institutes of Health, Bethesda, MD, USA) [31].

2.8. Wound-Healing Assay

Cell migration was evaluated by conventional wound-healing assay. For this purpose, 5×10^5 cells were plated on each well of a 24-multiwell plate until confluence was reached. Then, ECs were incubated with 20 mM NaCl for 72 h either in the absence or in the presence of BPF, and the cell monolayers were damaged by manual scratching with a sterile yellow tip. Images were randomly collected at different time points using an inverted microscope (EVOS Cell Imaging Systems, Thermo Fisher Scientific). Percentage of wound closure was calculated according to the following formula:

$$\% \text{ wound closure} = [\text{Area of the original wound (t0)} - \text{Area of the actual wound (t 72 h)}]/\text{Area of original wound (t0)} \times 100.$$

Wound area was calculated by ImageJ software (version 1.53t).

2.9. Assessment of Mitochondrial Membrane Potential Using JC-1 Staining

To determine the mitochondrial membrane potential depolarization by JC-1 reagent (Thermo Fisher Scientific), 3×10^4 cells were plated on each well of a 24-multiwell plate, and later, they were exposed to 20 mM NaCl for 72 h, as previously described [9], either in the absence or in the presence of BPF in a humidified CO_2 incubator. After 72 h, ECs were incubated with 10 µg/mL JC-1 at 37 °C for 20 min. After incubation, cells were washed twice with ice-cold PBS 1X. Finally, the images were taken with EVOS Cell Imaging Systems (Thermo Fisher Scientific). JC-1 is a cationic dye that exhibits potential-dependent accumulation in mitochondria, indicated by a fluorescence emission shift from green to red. Mitochondrial depolarization is indicated by a decrease in the red/green fluorescence intensity. The red-to-green fluorescence intensity ratio (R:G) was calculated by ImageJ software.

2.10. Assessment of Mitochondrial Function

To assess mitochondrial function, we measured mitochondrial complex I activity (assessed as NAD^+:NADH ratio) and ATP levels with two commercially available kits. To investigate the redox status of the ECs after 72 h of treatment, the concentrations of NADH and NAD⁺ were determined using an NAD⁺/NADH Assay Kit (ABCAM) in accordance with the manufacturer's instructions. The absorbance values were acquired at 450 nm by a microplate reader (Berthold), and data were analyzed following the manufacturer's protocol.

ATP levels were assessed with an ATP colorimetric assay (ABCAM), which, by a series of enzymatic reactions, forms a product that is quantified at 570 nm using a microplate reader (Berthold). Finally, data were analyzed following the manufacturer's protocol.

Mitochondrial ROS level was evaluated by using the MitoSOX™ Mitochondrial Superoxide Indicators (Thermo Fisher Scientific) following the manufacturer's instructions. The MitoSOX Red reagent specifically reacts with superoxide, but not with ROS and reactive nitrogen species (RNS). To perform this experiment, ECs were plated onto 8-well chambered cell culture slides (Corning by Thermo Fisher Scientific) and treated as reported above. After 72 h of high salt exposure, ECs were treated with MitoSOX Red (5 µM) for 30 min at room temperature and then washed. Cell nuclei were stained by Höechst reagent (Thermo Fisher Scientific). MitoSOX Red fluorescence and Höechst were acquired by a fluorescence microscope Axiophot2 (Zeiss, Oberkochen, Germany), and MitoSOX fluorescent signal was determined with Image J.

2.11. Statistical Analysis

All values are expressed as mean ± standard error (SEM). Comparisons between the experimental groups were performed by one-way ANOVA followed by Bonferroni post hoc test. A p value of <0.05 was considered significant. GraphPad Prism (Ver 5.01 GraphPad Software, Inc., La Jolla, CA, USA) statistical software was used for the statistical analysis.

3. Results

First of all, we checked and confirmed the purity of ECs extracted from the brain of neonatal SHRSP by immunofluorescence for CD31, an established marker of ECs. Results are shown in Figure 1.

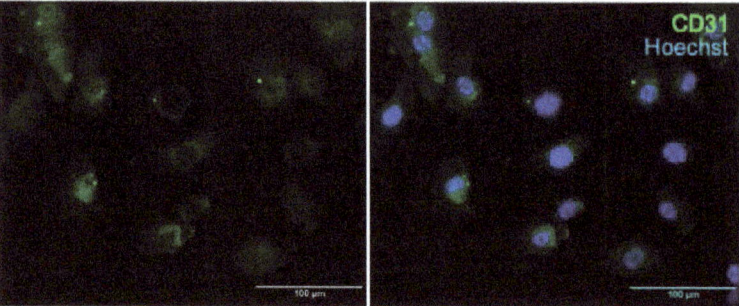

Figure 1. Homogeneity of ECs from brain of neonatal SHRSP. Representative images of immunofluorescence of the isolated cerebral ECs from SHRSP after incubation with CD31 antibody. Alexa Fluor 488 (green) was used as a secondary fluorescent antibody. Cell nuclei were stained with Höechst.

As previously shown [9,10,30], in the current set of studies, we confirmed that the saline load increased oxidative stress; reduced cell proliferation, viability, and migration; impaired angiogenesis, and induced mitochondrial dysfunction with an impairment of mitochondrial membrane potential, reduced complex I activity, and ATP synthesis in SHRSP primary cerebral ECs (Figures 2–4).

In the presence of BPF, cerebral ECs exposed to saline load for 72 h significantly reduced ROS production (Figure 2A) and rescued cell proliferation and viability (Figure 2B). Of note, BPF alone increased cell viability (Figure 2B).

BPF rescued the angiogenetic property of ECs, as shown by the increased number of master junctions in cells exposed to the high-salt treatment in the presence of BPF (Figure 3A,B). Moreover, BPF prompted wound healing by favoring EC migration

(Figure 3C,D). In fact, the wound appeared significantly covered by migrated cells upon the combined treatment with salt loading and BPF.

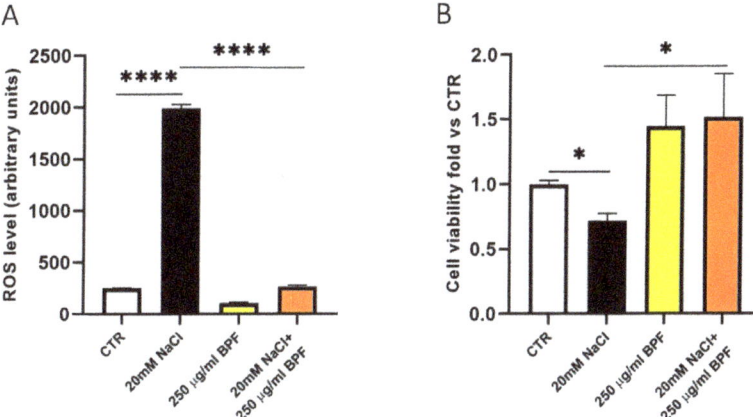

Figure 2. BPF reduces ROS level and rescues cell viability in SHRSP cerebral ECs exposed to high salt load. ECs were treated for 72 h with 20 mM NaCl either in the presence or in the absence of 250 µg/mL BPF. (**A**) Evaluation of total ROS level; (**B**) evaluation of cell viability; N = 3–4. CTR indicates nontreated cells. * $p < 0.05$ and **** $p < 0.0001$ obtained using one-way ANOVA followed by Bonferroni post hoc analysis. Data are reported as mean ± SEM.

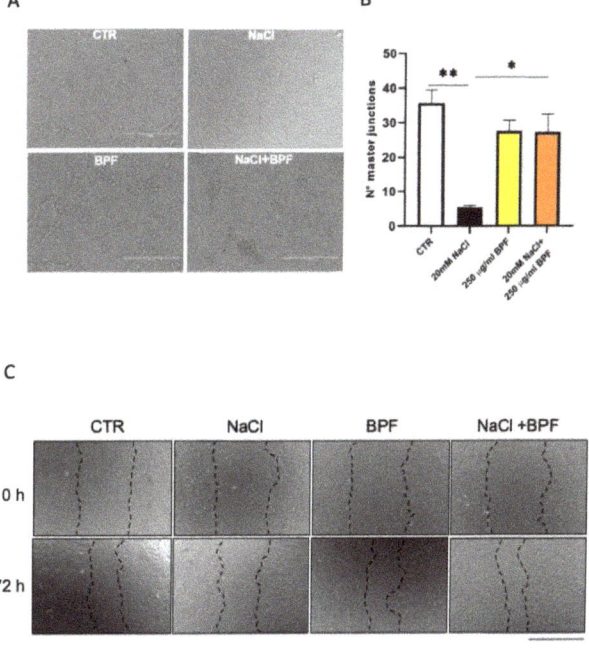

Figure 3. *Cont.*

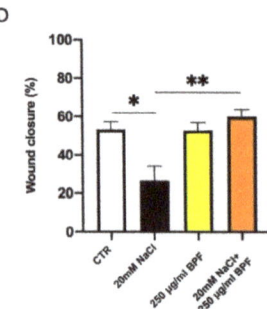

Figure 3. BPF rescues angiogenesis and promotes wound healing in SHRSP cerebral ECs exposed to high salt load. ECs were exposed to 20 mM NaCl for 72 h either in the presence or in the absence of 250 µg/mL BPF. CTR indicates nontreated cells. Representative images of Matrigel assay (**A**) and the quantification of master junctions (**B**); representative images of scratch wound-healing assay (**C**) and relative quantification of wound closure percentage (**D**). N = 3. * $p < 0.05$ and ** $p < 0.01$ obtained using one-way ANOVA followed by Bonferroni post hoc analysis. Data are reported as mean ± SEM.

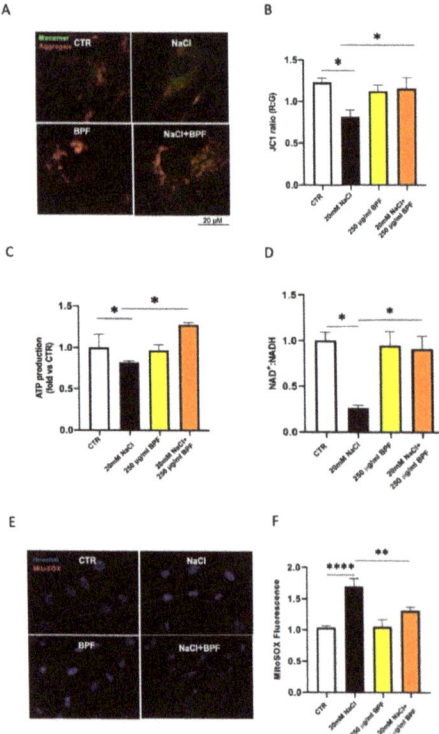

Figure 4. BPF exerts beneficial effect on mitochondrial function in SHRSP cerebral ECs exposed to high salt load. Fluorescence microscope analysis of mitochondrial membrane potential (ΔΨm) levels through JC1 dye; representative images (**A**) and corresponding quantification (**B**) are shown. (**C**) ATP levels, (**D**) NAD$^+$:NADH ratio (as a measure of Complex I activity), (**E**,**F**) mitochondrial ROS production detected by MitoSOX fluorescence and its graphical quantification. CTR indicates nontreated cells. N = 3–4. * $p < 0.05$, ** $p < 0.01$ and **** $p < 0.0001$ obtained using one-way ANOVA followed by Bonferroni post hoc analysis. Data are reported as mean ± SEM.

We also tested the impact of BPF on the saline load-induced mitochondrial dysfunction. First, we confirmed that salt loading caused a significant impairment of the mitochondrial membrane potential, which is fundamental to preserve cell integrity. Then, we observed that BPF rescued the mitochondrial membrane potential (Figure 4A,B), as documented by the increased JC1 red-to-green fluorescence ratio. BPF also rescued both ATP synthesis and complex I activity in cerebral ECs under saline load (Figure 4C,D). Consistently, the mitochondrial ROS production decreased in ECs treated with both saline load and BPF (Figure 4E,F).

The whole results of the present investigation indicate that BPF can antagonize the harmful effects induced by high salt load in cerebral ECs, obtained from the SHRSP rat model, on several parameters of cell survival and function.

4. Discussion

In the present study we demonstrate that BPF, a vegetal extract obtained from the *Citrus bergamia* fruit, exerts a significant protective effect toward the high-salt-induced injury in primary cerebral ECs isolated from the brain of newborn SHRSP rats. In fact, BPF treatment was able to rescue relevant cellular processes, including proliferation, viability, migration, angiogenesis, and mitochondrial function, which are all compromised upon saline load in the SHRSP experimental model. The latter represents a well-characterized animal model of human disease, particularly for its ability to accelerate cerebrovascular events upon high-salt dietary feeding, which is also based on a genetic predisposition [2–5,9,12,13,32]. The endothelial dysfunction precedes stroke occurrence in the JD-fed SHRSP as well as in humans [33–36], an observation that further supports the valuable role of this model for studies on the human disease. Interestingly, as shown in previous studies, the SHRSP primary cerebral ECs exposed to saline load quite closely mimic the in vivo condition and represent a unique experimental tool to test in vitro the effects of protective substances toward the molecular mechanisms involved in the higher predisposition to the vascular damage of the strain [9,10,30].

Herein, based on the available evidence supporting the beneficial properties of BPF in other experimental contexts [14,37–39], we aimed to test the potential protective effect of BPF on the cellular parameters known to be compromised upon saline load in the stroke predisposition of the SHRSP strain. We paid particular attention to the ability of BPF to rescue mitochondrial functional parameters (such as mitochondrial membrane potential, ATP synthesis, and complex I activity). A severe mitochondrial dysfunction, dependent on a complex I deficiency, has been previously identified as one of the main pathogenic molecular mechanisms underlying the higher predisposition of the JD-fed SHRSP to vascular damage and its dramatic consequences [5]. In fact, a significant reduction in complex I Ndufc2 subunit expression was observed in the JD-fed SHRSP. Importantly, we have already demonstrated that the recovery of the mitochondrial dysfunction through the correction in complex I deficiency with nicotinamide administration delayed both renal and cerebrovascular damage occurrence in JD-fed SHRSP [9].

The primary cerebral ECs also show an impaired mitochondrial function once exposed to the saline load [9,10,30].

As a result of our present study, BPF exposure led to a significant increase in cell survival, a reduction in oxidative stress and an increase in endothelial cell tubular formation. Remarkably, mitochondrial function was improved with a significant decrease in mitochondrial oxidative stress production.

Our current evidence is consistent with the results of previous investigations and strongly points to BPF as a valuable adjuvant substance to combat cardiovascular diseases. In this regard, an integrated therapeutic strategy, combining standard pharmacological treatments with natural protective substances of either vegetable or animal origin, can reduce the risk of common cardiovascular diseases such as stroke and ischemic heart disease. To support this concept and further validate the suitability of our rat model, we previously reported the significant protective effect of a *Brassica oleracea* sprout extract administration toward renal and cerebrovascular damage occurrence in JD-fed SHRSP [12]. Moreover, the administration of the natural disaccharide trehalose, present in different foods, led to a significant delay in renal damage and stroke occurrence in JD-fed SHRSP [40].

Among the natural available compounds, the bergamot polyphenolic fraction (BPF), extracted from the bergamot fruit (*Citrus bergamia*), a plant endemic to the Calabrian Ionian coast in Southern Italy, belongs to a class of molecules (the polyphenols) that are well known for their protective properties on human health. In particular, bergamot is rich in flavonoid glycosides, such as neoeriocitrin, neohesperidin, and naringin; and glycosylated polyphenols, such as bruteridin and melitidin [28]. Several studies have demonstrated the beneficial effects of polyphenols against widespread pathologies, including cardiovascular diseases, both in preclinical models and in humans [18]. Regarding stroke, a neuroprotective effect was reported even when polyphenols were administered after stroke induction, indicating that these molecules can also contribute to the recovery of patients suffering from stroke [18]. Contrasting effects were observed in schizophrenia [41,42]. The protective functions of BPF are mainly based on antioxidant, anti-inflammatory, lipid-lowering, and hypoglycemic effects of polyphenols [43]. Of note, polyphenols act as both reactive oxygen species scavengers and metal chelators [44]. Moreover, they activate transcription factors such as erythroid 2-related factor 2 (Nrf2), which are able to stimulate the expression of several antioxidant enzymes, including superoxide dismutase (SOD), heme oxygenase-1 (HO-1), catalase, glutathione reductase, and glutathione-S-transferase [45]. In addition, polyphenols exert an anti-inflammatory property that is based on their ability to modulate immune cell regulation, inflammatory gene expression, and the synthesis of inflammatory mediators [46].

In vitro studies revealed that BPF stimulated higher mitochondrial activity with increased ATP production from oxidative metabolism in both isolated mitochondria and porcine aortic endothelial cells [24]. In addition, BPF carried out its beneficial effect on the mitochondrial permeability transition pore (mPTP) phenomenon by desensitizing the pore opening [24], a known molecular mechanism causing cell damage [43]. In fact, BPF inhibited the Ca_2^+-activated F_1F_O-ATPase, therefore counteracting the opening and size of the mPTP with a final protective effect on mitochondrial dysfunction [24]. In the same cell line, the authors demonstrated that BPF counteracted the toxic effect of doxorubicin on cell viability and mitochondrial function [29]. Based on this in vitro study, BPF, by restoring the correct metabolic cellular functions, can behave as a positive agent toward the cardiovascular disorders resulting from the toxic action of doxorubicin.

Moreover, the protective effects of BPF were reported in a few models of cardiovascular diseases. For instance, consistently with the above-mentioned in vitro data, BPF exerted an antioxidant cardioprotective effect in a rat model of doxorubicin-induced cardiac damage [26]. Interestingly, in this work, the protective action of BPF was related to its ability to restore autophagy. BPF administration in the hyperlipidemic Wistar rat induced a significant reduction in malondialdehyde and glutathione peroxidase serum levels, two known markers of oxidative stress [47].

Furthermore, in a rat model of angioplasty, the pretreatment with bergamot essential oil reduced smooth muscle cell proliferation and neointima formation. This effect was associated with reduced free radical formation and reduced expression of LOX-1, the receptor for oxidized low-density lipoprotein [48].

A human study performed in subjects with moderate hypercholesterolemia evaluated the effects of a Bergamot extract on cardiometabolic parameters, including plasma lipids, atherogenic lipoproteins, and subclinical atherosclerosis, within a relatively short time frame of six months. As a result, the bergamot extracts reduced plasma lipids and improved the lipoprotein profile. Remarkably, a reduced subclinical atherosclerosis (assessed as carotid intimal media thickness) was observed [49].

Altogether, the available evidence, along with the results of the present study, strongly support the role of bergamot toward vascular protection and its potential role as an adjuvant for the treatment of vascular disorders and related acute events.

5. Conclusions

We provide the first evidence that BPF is a natural antioxidant able to counteract high-salt-induced injury in a suitable experimental tool, the primary cerebral endothelial cells obtained from the SHRSP model. The latter represents an optimal animal model of human disease, regarding the hypertensive target organ damage favored by high salt exposure. In our study, the treatment with BPF in the presence of high salt, a noxious stimulus, allowed for the recovery of all cellular vital parameters and turned off the key molecular mechanisms underlying endothelial cell damage and dysfunction. This in vitro study represents a fundamental basis for further in vivo investigations testing the impact of BPF toward cerebrovascular accidents. This vegetal substance, as part of the Mediterranean diet, may become an attractive and useful adjuvant to either prevent or treat vascular disorders, such as stroke, associated with hypertension.

Author Contributions: R.S., M.F. and S.R., conceptualization; M.F., R.S., C.C. and F.O., methodology; R.S., M.C. and M.F., software; V.M. and S.R., validation; R.S. and S.R., investigation; S.M., M.C., C.C. and F.O., resources; R.S., M.F. and S.R., writing—original draft; M.V. and S.R., supervision; S.R., funding acquisition. All authors have read and agreed to the published version of the manuscript.

Funding: The study was supported by a grant from the Italian Ministry of Health (Ricerca Corrente).

Institutional Review Board Statement: Not applicable.

Informed Consent Statement: Not applicable.

Data Availability Statement: Not applicable.

Conflicts of Interest: The authors declare no conflict of interest.

References

1. Rubattu, S.; Stanzione, R.; Volpe, M. Mitochondrial Dysfunction Contributes to Hypertensive Target Organ Damage: Lessons from an Animal Model of Human Disease. *Oxid. Med. Cell. Longev.* **2016**, *2016*, 1067801. [CrossRef] [PubMed]
2. Volpe, M.; Camargo, M.J.; Mueller, F.B.; Campbell, W.G., Jr.; Sealey, J.E.; Pecker, M.S.; Sosa, R.E.; Laragh, J.H. Relation of plasma renin to end organ damage and to protection of K+ feeding in stroke-prone hypertensive rats. *Hypertension* **1990**, *15*, 318–326. [CrossRef] [PubMed]
3. Rubattu, S.; Volpe, M.; Kreutz, R.; Ganten, U.; Ganten, D.; Lindpaintner, K. Chromosomal mapping of quantitative trait loci contributing to stroke in a rat model of complex human disease. *Nat. Genet.* **1996**, *13*, 429–434. [CrossRef] [PubMed]
4. Rubattu, S.; Hubner, N.; Ganten, U.; Evangelista, A.; Stanzione, R.; Di Angelantonio, E.; Plehm, R.; Langanki, R.; Gianazza, E.; Sironi, L.; et al. Reciprocal congenic lines for a major stroke QTL on rat chromosome 1. *Physiol. Genom.* **2006**, *27*, 108–113. [CrossRef]
5. Rubattu, S.; Di Castro, S.; Schulz, H.; Geurts, A.M.; Cotugno, M.; Bianchi, F.; Maatz, H.; Hummel, O.; Falak, S.; Stanzione, R.; et al. Ndufc2 Gene Inhibition Is Associated With Mitochondrial Dysfunction and Increased Stroke Susceptibility in an Animal Model of Complex Human Disease. *J. Am. Heart Assoc.* **2016**, *5*, e002701. [CrossRef]
6. Raffa, S.; Scrofani, C.; Valente, S.; Micaloni, A.; Forte, M.; Bianchi, F.; Coluccia, R.; Geurts, A.M.; Sciarretta, S.; Volpe, M.; et al. In vitro characterization of mitochondrial function and structure in rat and human cells with a deficiency of the NADH: Ubiquinone oxidoreductase Ndufc2 subunit. *Hum. Mol. Genet.* **2017**, *26*, 4541–4555. [CrossRef]
7. Raffa, S.; Chin, X.L.D.; Stanzione, R.; Forte, M.; Bianchi, F.; Cotugno, M.; Marchitti, S.; Micaloni, A.; Gallo, G.; Schirone, L.; et al. The reduction of NDUFC2 expression is associated with mitochondrial impairment in circulating mononuclear cells of patients with acute coronary syndrome. *Int. J. Cardiol.* **2019**, *286*, 127–133. [CrossRef]
8. Gallo, G.; Migliarino, S.; Cotugno, M.; Stanzione, R.; Burocchi, S.; Bianchi, F.; Marchitti, S.; Autore, C.; Volpe, M.; Rubattu, S. Impact of a NDUFC2 Variant on the Occurrence of Acute Coronary Syndromes. *Front. Cardiovasc. Med.* **2022**, *9*, 921244. [CrossRef]
9. Forte, M.; Bianchi, F.; Cotugno, M.; Marchitti, S.; De Falco, E.; Raffa, S.; Stanzione, R.; Di Nonno, F.; Chimenti, I.; Palmerio, S.; et al. Pharmacological restoration of autophagy reduces hypertension-related stroke occurrence. *Autophagy* **2020**, *16*, 1468–1481. [CrossRef]
10. Algieri, C.; Bernardini, C.; Marchi, S.; Forte, M.; Tallarida, M.A.; Bianchi, F.; La Mantia, D.; Algieri, V.; Stanzione, R.; Cotugno, M.; et al. 1,5-disubstituted-1,2,3-triazoles counteract mitochondrial dysfunction acting on F(1)F(O)-ATPase in models of cardiovascular diseases. *Pharmacol. Res.* **2022**, *187*, 106561. [CrossRef]
11. Pagliaro, B.; Santolamazza, C.; Simonelli, F.; Rubattu, S. Phytochemical Compounds and Protection from Cardiovascular Diseases: A State of the Art. *Biomed Res. Int.* **2015**, *2015*, 918069. [CrossRef] [PubMed]

12. Rubattu, S.; Di Castro, S.; Cotugno, M.; Bianchi, F.; Mattioli, R.; Baima, S.; Stanzione, R.; Madonna, M.; Bozzao, C.; Marchitti, S.; et al. Protective effects of Brassica oleracea sprouts extract toward renal damage in high-salt-fed SHRSP: Role of AMPK/PPARalpha/UCP2 axis. *J. Hypertens.* **2015**, *33*, 1465–1479. [CrossRef] [PubMed]
13. Rubattu, S.; Stanzione, R.; Bianchi, F.; Cotugno, M.; Forte, M.; Della Ragione, F.; Fioriniello, S.; D'Esposito, M.; Marchitti, S.; Madonna, M.; et al. Reduced brain UCP2 expression mediated by microRNA-503 contributes to increased stroke susceptibility in the high-salt fed stroke-prone spontaneously hypertensive rat. *Cell Death Dis.* **2017**, *8*, e2891. [CrossRef]
14. Mollace, V.; Sacco, I.; Janda, E.; Malara, C.; Ventrice, D.; Colica, C.; Visalli, V.; Muscoli, S.; Ragusa, S.; Muscoli, C.; et al. Hypolipemic and hypoglycaemic activity of bergamot polyphenols: From animal models to human studies. *Fitoterapia* **2011**, *82*, 309–316. [CrossRef]
15. Musolino, V.; Gliozzi, M.; Nucera, S.; Carresi, C.; Maiuolo, J.; Mollace, R.; Paone, S.; Bosco, F.; Scarano, F.; Scicchitano, M.; et al. The effect of bergamot polyphenolic fraction on lipid transfer protein system and vascular oxidative stress in a rat model of hyperlipemia. *Lipids Health Dis.* **2019**, *18*, 115. [CrossRef]
16. Maiuolo, J.; Carresi, C.; Gliozzi, M.; Musolino, V.; Scarano, F.; Coppoletta, A.R.; Guarnieri, L.; Nucera, S.; Scicchitano, M.; Bosco, F.; et al. Effects of Bergamot Polyphenols on Mitochondrial Dysfunction and Sarcoplasmic Reticulum Stress in Diabetic Cardiomyopathy. *Nutrients* **2021**, *13*, 2476. [CrossRef] [PubMed]
17. Carrizzo, A.; Izzo, C.; Forte, M.; Sommella, E.; Di Pietro, P.; Venturini, E.; Ciccarelli, M.; Galasso, G.; Rubattu, S.; Campiglia, P.; et al. A Novel Promising Frontier for Human Health: The Beneficial Effects of Nutraceuticals in Cardiovascular Diseases. *Int. J. Mol. Sci.* **2020**, *21*, 8706. [CrossRef] [PubMed]
18. Parrella, E.; Gussago, C.; Porrini, V.; Benarese, M.; Pizzi, M. From Preclinical Stroke Models to Humans: Polyphenols in the Prevention and Treatment of Stroke. *Nutrients* **2020**, *13*, 85. [CrossRef] [PubMed]
19. Gliozzi, M.; Walker, R.; Muscoli, S.; Vitale, C.; Gratteri, S.; Carresi, C.; Musolino, V.; Russo, V.; Janda, E.; Ragusa, S.; et al. Bergamot polyphenolic fraction enhances rosuvastatin-induced effect on LDL-cholesterol, LOX-1 expression and protein kinase B phosphorylation in patients with hyperlipidemia. *Int. J. Cardiol.* **2013**, *170*, 140–145. [CrossRef]
20. Carresi, C.; Gliozzi, M.; Musolino, V.; Scicchitano, M.; Scarano, F.; Bosco, F.; Nucera, S.; Maiuolo, J.; Macri, R.; Ruga, S.; et al. The Effect of Natural Antioxidants in the Development of Metabolic Syndrome: Focus on Bergamot Polyphenolic Fraction. *Nutrients* **2020**, *12*, 1504. [CrossRef]
21. Mirarchi, A.; Mare, R.; Musolino, V.; Nucera, S.; Mollace, V.; Pujia, A.; Montalcini, T.; Romeo, S.; Maurotti, S. Bergamot Polyphenol Extract Reduces Hepatocyte Neutral Fat by Increasing Beta-Oxidation. *Nutrients* **2022**, *14*, 3434. [CrossRef] [PubMed]
22. Impellizzeri, D.; Bruschetta, G.; Di Paola, R.; Ahmad, A.; Campolo, M.; Cuzzocrea, S.; Esposito, E.; Navarra, M. The anti-inflammatory and antioxidant effects of bergamot juice extract (BJe) in an experimental model of inflammatory bowel disease. *Clin. Nutr.* **2015**, *34*, 1146–1154. [CrossRef] [PubMed]
23. Ferlazzo, N.; Cirmi, S.; Calapai, G.; Ventura-Spagnolo, E.; Gangemi, S.; Navarra, M. Anti-Inflammatory Activity of Citrus bergamia Derivatives: Where Do We Stand? *Molecules* **2016**, *21*, 1273. [CrossRef]
24. Algieri, C.; Bernardini, C.; Oppedisano, F.; La Mantia, D.; Trombetti, F.; Palma, E.; Forni, M.; Mollace, V.; Romeo, G.; Nesci, S. Mitochondria Bioenergetic Functions and Cell Metabolism Are Modulated by the Bergamot Polyphenolic Fraction. *Cells* **2022**, *11*, 1401. [CrossRef] [PubMed]
25. Janda, E.; Salerno, R.; Martino, C.; Lascala, A.; La Russa, D.; Oliverio, M. Qualitative and quantitative analysis of the proautophagic activity of Citrus flavonoids from Bergamot Polyphenol Fraction. *Data Brief* **2018**, *19*, 1327–1334. [CrossRef]
26. Carresi, C.; Musolino, V.; Gliozzi, M.; Maiuolo, J.; Mollace, R.; Nucera, S.; Maretta, A.; Sergi, D.; Muscoli, S.; Gratteri, S.; et al. Anti-oxidant effect of bergamot polyphenolic fraction counteracts doxorubicin-induced cardiomyopathy: Role of autophagy and c-kit(pos)CD45(neg)CD31(neg) cardiac stem cell activation. *J. Mol. Cell. Cardiol.* **2018**, *119*, 10–18. [CrossRef] [PubMed]
27. Levine, B.; Kroemer, G. Biological Functions of Autophagy Genes: A Disease Perspective. *Cell* **2019**, *176*, 11–42. [CrossRef]
28. Salerno, R.; Casale, F.; Calandruccio, C.; Procopio, A. Characterization of flavonoids in Citrus bergamia (Bergamot) polyphenolic fraction by liquid chromatography–high resolution mass spectrometry (LC/HRMS). *Pharmanutrition* **2016**, *4*, S1–S7. [CrossRef]
29. Algieri, C.; Bernardini, C.; Oppedisano, F.; La Mantia, D.; Trombetti, F.; Palma, E.; Forni, M.; Mollace, V.; Romeo, G.; Troisio, I.; et al. The Impairment of Cell Metabolism by Cardiovascular Toxicity of Doxorubicin Is Reversed by Bergamot Polyphenolic Fraction Treatment in Endothelial Cells. *Int. J. Mol. Sci.* **2022**, *23*, 8977. [CrossRef]
30. Stanzione, R.; Forte, M.; Cotugno, M.; Bianchi, F.; Marchitti, S.; Rubattu, S. Relevance of stromal interaction molecule 1 (STIM1) in experimental and human stroke. *Pflugers Arch.* **2022**, *474*, 141–153. [CrossRef]
31. Carpentier, G.; Berndt, S.; Ferratge, S.; Rasband, W.; Cuendet, M.; Uzan, G.; Albanese, P. Angiogenesis Analyzer for ImageJ—A comparative morphometric analysis of "Endothelial Tube Formation Assay" and "Fibrin Bead Assay". *Sci. Rep.* **2020**, *10*, 11568. [CrossRef] [PubMed]
32. Rubattu, S.; Cotugno, M.; Bianchi, F.; Sironi, L.; Gelosa, P.; Stanzione, R.; Forte, M.; De Sanctis, C.; Madonna, M.; Marchitti, S.; et al. A differential expression of uncoupling protein-2 associates with renal damage in stroke-resistant spontaneously hypertensive rat/stroke-prone spontaneously hypertensive rat-derived stroke congenic lines. *J. Hypertens.* **2017**, *35*, 1857–1871. [CrossRef] [PubMed]
33. Cosentino, F.; Rubattu, S.; Savoia, C.; Venturelli, V.; Pagannonne, E.; Volpe, M. Endothelial dysfunction and stroke. *J. Cardiovasc. Pharmacol.* **2001**, *38* (Suppl. 2), S75–S78. [CrossRef] [PubMed]

34. Volpe, M.; Iaccarino, G.; Vecchione, C.; Rizzoni, D.; Russo, R.; Rubattu, S.; Condorelli, G.; Ganten, U.; Ganten, D.; Trimarco, B.; et al. Association and cosegregation of stroke with impaired endothelium-dependent vasorelaxation in stroke prone, spontaneously hypertensive rats. *J. Clin. Investig.* **1996**, *98*, 256–261. [CrossRef] [PubMed]
35. Cosentino, F.; Volpe, M. Hypertension, stroke, and endothelium. *Curr. Hypertens. Rep.* **2005**, *7*, 68–71. [CrossRef] [PubMed]
36. Tuttolomondo, A.; Daidone, M.; Pinto, A. Endothelial Dysfunction and Inflammation in Ischemic Stroke Pathogenesis. *Curr. Pharm. Des.* **2020**, *26*, 4209–4219. [CrossRef]
37. Mollace, V.; Sicchitano, M.; Paone, S.; Casale, F.; Calandruccio, C.; Gliozzi, M.; Musolino, V.; Carresi, C.; Maiuolo, J.; Nucera, S.; et al. Hypoglycemic and Hypolipemic Effects of a New Lecithin Formulation of Bergamot Polyphenolic Fraction: A Double Blind, Randomized, Placebo- Controlled Study. *Endocr. Metab. Immune Disord. Drug Targets* **2019**, *19*, 136–143. [CrossRef]
38. Nauman, M.C.; Johnson, J.J. Clinical application of bergamot (Citrus bergamia) for reducing high cholesterol and cardiovascular disease markers. *Integr. Food Nutr. Metab.* **2019**, *6*. [CrossRef]
39. Perna, S.; Spadaccini, D.; Botteri, L.; Girometta, C.; Riva, A.; Allegrini, P.; Petrangolini, G.; Infantino, V.; Rondanelli, M. Efficacy of bergamot: From anti-inflammatory and anti-oxidative mechanisms to clinical applications as preventive agent for cardiovascular morbidity, skin diseases, and mood alterations. *Food Sci. Nutr.* **2019**, *7*, 369–384. [CrossRef]
40. Forte, M.; Marchitti, S.; Cotugno, M.; Di Nonno, F.; Stanzione, R.; Bianchi, F.; Schirone, L.; Schiavon, S.; Vecchio, D.; Sarto, G.; et al. Trehalose, a natural disaccharide, reduces stroke occurrence in the stroke-prone spontaneously hypertensive rat. *Pharmacol. Res.* **2021**, *173*, 105875. [CrossRef]
41. Bruno, A.; Pandolfo, G.; Crucitti, M.; Cedro, C.; Zoccali, R.A.; Muscatello, M.R.A. Bergamot Polyphenolic Fraction Supplementation Improves Cognitive Functioning in Schizophrenia: Data From an 8-Week, Open-Label Pilot Study. *J. Clin. Psychopharmacol.* **2017**, *37*, 468–471. [CrossRef] [PubMed]
42. Bruno, A.; Pandolfo, G.; Crucitti, M.; Cacciola, M.; Santoro, V.; Spina, E.; Zoccali, R.A.; Muscatello, M.R.A. Low-Dose of Bergamot-Derived Polyphenolic Fraction (BPF) Did Not Improve Metabolic Parameters in Second Generation Antipsychotics-Treated Patients: Results from a 60-days Open-Label Study. *Front. Pharmacol.* **2017**, *8*, 197. [CrossRef] [PubMed]
43. Bernardi, P.; Rasola, A.; Forte, M.; Lippe, G. The Mitochondrial Permeability Transition Pore: Channel Formation by F-ATP Synthase, Integration in Signal Transduction, and Role in Pathophysiology. *Physiol. Rev.* **2015**, *95*, 1111–1155. [CrossRef] [PubMed]
44. Tressera-Rimbau, A.; Arranz, S.; Eder, M.; Vallverdu-Queralt, A. Dietary Polyphenols in the Prevention of Stroke. *Oxid. Med. Cell. Longev.* **2017**, *2017*, 7467962. [CrossRef]
45. Scapagnini, G.; Vasto, S.; Abraham, N.G.; Caruso, C.; Zella, D.; Fabio, G. Modulation of Nrf2/ARE pathway by food polyphenols: A nutritional neuroprotective strategy for cognitive and neurodegenerative disorders. *Mol. Neurobiol.* **2011**, *44*, 192–201. [CrossRef]
46. Yahfoufi, N.; Alsadi, N.; Jambi, M.; Matar, C. The Immunomodulatory and Anti-Inflammatory Role of Polyphenols. *Nutrients* **2018**, *10*, 1618. [CrossRef]
47. Mollace, R.; Macri, R.; Tavernese, A.; Gliozzi, M.; Musolino, V.; Carresi, C.; Maiuolo, J.; Fini, M.; Volterrani, M.; Mollace, V. Comparative Effect of Bergamot Polyphenolic Fraction and Red Yeast Rice Extract in Rats Fed a Hyperlipidemic Diet: Role of Antioxidant Properties and PCSK9 Expression. *Nutrients* **2022**, *14*, 477. [CrossRef]
48. Mollace, V.; Ragusa, S.; Sacco, I.; Muscoli, C.; Sculco, F.; Visalli, V.; Palma, E.; Muscoli, S.; Mondello, L.; Dugo, P.; et al. The protective effect of bergamot oil extract on lecitine-like oxyLDL receptor-1 expression in balloon injury-related neointima formation. *J. Cardiovasc. Pharmacol. Ther.* **2008**, *13*, 120–129. [CrossRef]
49. Toth, P.P.; Patti, A.M.; Nikolic, D.; Giglio, R.V.; Castellino, G.; Biancucci, T.; Geraci, F.; David, S.; Montalto, G.; Rizvi, A.; et al. Bergamot Reduces Plasma Lipids, Atherogenic Small Dense LDL, and Subclinical Atherosclerosis in Subjects with Moderate Hypercholesterolemia: A 6 Months Prospective Study. *Front. Pharmacol.* **2015**, *6*, 299. [CrossRef]

Disclaimer/Publisher's Note: The statements, opinions and data contained in all publications are solely those of the individual author(s) and contributor(s) and not of MDPI and/or the editor(s). MDPI and/or the editor(s) disclaim responsibility for any injury to people or property resulting from any ideas, methods, instructions or products referred to in the content.

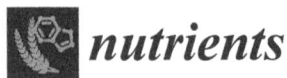

Article

Comparative Effect of Bergamot Polyphenolic Fraction and Red Yeast Rice Extract in Rats Fed a Hyperlipidemic Diet: Role of Antioxidant Properties and PCSK9 Expression

Rocco Mollace [1,2,†], Roberta Macrì [1,†], Annamaria Tavernese [1], Micaela Gliozzi [1], Vincenzo Musolino [1], Cristina Carresi [1], Jessica Maiuolo [1], Massimo Fini [1,2], Maurizio Volterrani [1,2] and Vincenzo Mollace [1,2,*]

[1] Institute of Research for Food Safety & Health (IRC-FSH), Department of Health Science, University Magna Graecia, 88100 Catanzaro, Italy; rocco.mollace@gmail.com (R.M.); robertamacri85@gmail.com (R.M.); an.tavernese@gmail.com (A.T.); micaela.gliozzi@gmail.com (M.G.); xabaras3@hotmail.com (V.M.); carresi@unicz.it (C.C.); jessicamaiuolo@virgilio.it (J.M.); massimo.fini@sanraffaele.it (M.F.); maurizio.volterrani@sanraffaele.it (M.V.)

[2] IRCCS San Raffaele Pisana, Via di Valcannuta, 88163 Rome, Italy

* Correspondence: mollace@libero.it

† These authors contributed equally to this work.

Abstract: Elevated serum cholesterol levels, either associated or not with increased triglycerides, represent a risk of developing vascular injury, mostly leading to atherothrombosis-related diseases including myocardial infarction and stroke. Natural products have been investigated in the last few decades as they are seen to offer an alternative solution to counteract cardiometabolic risk, due to the occurrence of side effects with the use of statins, the leading drugs for treating hyperlipidemias. Red yeast rice (RYR), a monacolin K-rich natural extract, has been found to be effective in counteracting high cholesterol, being its use accompanied by consistent warnings by regulatory authorities based on the potential detrimental responses accompanying its statin-like chemical charcateristics. Here we compared the effects of RYR with those produced by bergamot polyphenolic fraction (BPF), a well-known natural extract proven to be effective in lowering both serum cholesterol and triglycerides in animals fed a hyperlipidemic diet. In particular, BPF at doses of 10 mg/Kg given orally for 30 consecutive days, counteracted the elevation of both serum LDL cholesterol (LDL-C) and triglycerides induced by the hyperlipidemic diet, an effect which was accompanied by significant reductions of malondialdehyde (MDA) and glutathione peroxidase serum levels, two biomarkers of oxidative stress. Furthermore, the activity of BPF was associated to increased HDL cholesterol (HDL-C) levels and to strong reduction of Proprotein convertase subtilisin/kexin type 9 (PCSK9) levels which were found increased in hyperlipidemic rats. In contrast, RYR at doses of 1 and 3 mg/Kg, produced only significant reduction of LDL-C with very poor effects on triglycerides, HDL-C, glutathione peroxidase, MDA and PCSK9 expression. This indicates that while BPF and RYR both produce serum cholesterol-lowering benefits, BPF produces additional effects on triglycerides and HDL cholesterol compared to RYR at the doses used throughout the study. These additional effects of BPF appear to be related to the reduction of PCSK9 expression and to the antioxidant properties of this extract compared to RYR, thereby suggesting a more complete protection from cardiometabolic risk.

Keywords: hypercholesterolemia; red yeast rice (RYR); bergamot polyphenolic fraction (BPF); malondialdehyde (MDA); oxidative stress; proprotein convertase subtilisin/kexin type 9 (PCSK9)

Citation: Mollace, R.; Macrì, R.; Tavernese, A.; Gliozzi, M.; Musolino, V.; Carresi, C.; Maiuolo, J.; Fini, M.; Volterrani, M.; Mollace, V. Comparative Effect of Bergamot Polyphenolic Fraction and Red Yeast Rice Extract in Rats Fed a Hyperlipidemic Diet: Role of Antioxidant Properties and PCSK9 Expression. *Nutrients* 2022, 14, 477. https://doi.org/10.3390/nu14030477

Academic Editors: Susanna Iossa, Bruno Trimarco and Gaetano Santulli

Received: 4 December 2021
Accepted: 20 January 2022
Published: 22 January 2022

Publisher's Note: MDPI stays neutral with regard to jurisdictional claims in published maps and institutional affiliations.

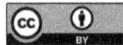

Copyright: © 2022 by the authors. Licensee MDPI, Basel, Switzerland. This article is an open access article distributed under the terms and conditions of the Creative Commons Attribution (CC BY) license (https://creativecommons.org/licenses/by/4.0/).

1. Introduction

Hypercholesterolemia, either associated or not to increased triglyceride serum levels, has been clearly shown to represent one of the key players in the development of atherosclerosis-associated vascular disorders including coronary artery disease and stroke [1,2]. On the other hand, a clear correlation exists suggesting that a significant reduction of low-density lipoprotein cholesterol (LDL-C) is required for both primary prevention of cardiovascular disorders and reduction of cardiovascular risk in patients with previous cardiovascular events, including myocardial infarction [3–5].

In the last decades, this was achieved by means of extensive use of very effective drugs such as the statins, which reduce endogenous biosynthesis of cholesterol, via inhibition of hydroxy-3-methylglutaryl-CoA reductase (HMGCoA reductase), the key enzyme of the pathway generating cholesterol from acetyl-CoA [6–8].

This class of drugs, due to their widespread activities in protecting vascular tissues, (anti-proliferative effects, atherosclerotic plaque stabilizing properties, reduction of vascular inflammatory biomarkers, etc.), has also been found able to reduce hospitalization and mortality in high-risk atherosclerotic patients [6,7].

Alongside their beneficial effect in the prevention and treatment of cardiovascular disorders, the use of statins is however associated to several side effects that include muscular pain, rhabdomyolysis and subsequent elevation of serum creatine phosphokinase (CPK) [9–11]. This seems to occur in nearly 5% of patients taking statins [12,13]. However, recent epidemiological studies revealed that nearly 30% of people stop statin treatment because of muscle aches [13,14]. Moreover, prolonged treatment with statins is also associated to increased risk of developing type 2 diabetes and neurological disorders, mostly characterized by memory loss [14]. Thus, based on the occurrence of these and other side effects, the use of statins in low-risk subjects is still controversial and alternative and more safe treatments for lowering serum cholesterol have been suggested in the last few decades, including nutraceutical supplementation by means of products able to inhibit HMGCoA reductase [15,16].

Red yeast rice (RYR) is a natural extract obtained via fermentation of white rice with the yeast *Monascus purpureus* mold that has widely been used to reduce serum cholesterol in patients [17,18]. The properties of RYR for lowering serum cholesterol remain to be clarified. However, evidence exists that RYR extract contains significant amounts of monacolin K, which is structurally identical to lovastatin, thereby suggesting a statin-like response in patients undergoing treatment with RYR [19]. To date, clinical data suggest an efficacy of RYR in lowering serum cholesterol which has been determined in a range from 14% to 24% with a satisfactory safety profile, though causality between therapy and side effects described in several studies remains to be confirmed [18–20]. However, a European Food Safety Authority (EFSA) Scientific Panel, in 2018, highlighted several warnings in vulnerable populations (e.g., pregnant women) and concluded *"to be unable to identify a dietary intake of monacolins from RYR, not giving rise to concerns about potentially harmful effects to health for the general population, and as appropriate, for vulnerable subgroups of the population"* [21].

Thus, based on this conclusion, it is necessary to identify better nutraceutical solutions to attenuate the potential risk of using RYR as a first line nutraceutical approach and to counteract potential side effects and uncertainties deriving from elevated amounts of monacolin K in final preparations.

Based on this preliminary evidence, the present study was addressed to evaluate the potential synergistic response in a formulation containing lower concentration of RYR either associated or not to bergamot polyphenolic fraction (BPF) a well characterized natural extract deriving from bergamot juice which has been found to produce consistent hypolipidemic response both in animal settings and in patients [15,16,22–26]. This was achieved in rats fed a hyperlipidemic diet.

2. Materials and Methods
2.1. Plant Material
2.1.1. Red Yeast Rice (RYR)

RyR extract (NLT 3% Monacolin K) was purchased from Giellepi S.p.A (Milano, Italy).

2.1.2. Preparation of BPF

C. bergamia Risso & Poiteau fruits were collected in the Calabrian region, from plantations that cover 90 km long costal area located between Reggio Calabria and Bianco. Bergamot juice (BJ) was obtained from peeled-off fruits by industrial pressing and squeezing. The depletion of oil fraction from juice was obtained through the stripping and the clarification by ultra-filtration; the subsequent loading on suitable polystyrene resin columns (Mitsubishi Chemical, Weekday, Japan Standard Time) that absorbed polyphenol compounds of MW between 300 and 600 Da [22]. The elution of polyphenol fractions was carried out through a mild KOH solution. Subsequently, the neutralization of phytocomplex was obtained through the filtration on cationic resin at acidic pH. Finally, it was vacuum dried and minced to the desired particle size to obtain BPF powder. The analysis of BPF powder was performed through HPLC to evaluate the flavonoid and other polyphenols content. Furthermore, in the toxicological analyses the presence of pesticides, heavy metals, phthalates and synephrine was not found (data not shown) [22]. Standard microbiological evaluation showed the absence of mycotoxins and bacteria. All procedures have been performed according to the European Community Guidelines concerning dietary supplements.

2.1.3. High-Pressure Liquid Chromatography (HPLC) Analysis

High-pressure liquid chromatography (HPLC) analysis was performed on Fast 1200 HPLC system (Agilent Technologies, 5301 Stevens Creek Blvd Santa Clara, USA) equipped with DAD detector and ZORBAX Eclipse XDB-C18 column—50 mm. Two µL of sample (BPF diluted in 50% ethanol and filtered through a 0.2 µm filter) was injected eluting with a two solvent gradient of water and acetonitrile. Different gradients were used for the determination of flavonoid content or possible fumocumarin contaminants. The flow-rate was 3 mL/min and the column was maintained at 35 °C. The detector was monitored at 280 nm. Flavonoid and furocumarin pure standards were purchased from Sigma-Aldrich (Burlington, MA, USA). Brutieridin and melitidin were identified according to Di Donna [22,23]. The estimated concentration of the five main flavonoids was: neoeriocitrin (77,700 ppm), naringin (63,011 ppm), neohesperidin (72,056 ppm), melitidin (15,606 ppm) and brutieridin (33,202 ppm) [22].

2.2. Animal Studies

Male Wistar rats (Harlan Laboratories Ltd., Fullinsdorf, Switzerland), weighing 180–200 g, were used for the experiments. The animals were kept under stable and controlled conditions (temperature, 22 °C; humidity, 60%) with water ad libitum. Animal care was in accordance with Italian regulations on protection of animals used for experimental and other scientific purposes (D.M. 116192), as well as with the European Community guidelines [23].

The effects of BPF, or RYR on total cholesterol, LDL-C, high density lipoprotein cholesterol (HDL-C), triglycerides, malondialdehyde (expressing peroxidative damage) and paraoxonase were evaluated in Wistar rats fed a hypercholesterolemic diet composed of a standard diet (Harlan Laboratories Ltd., Fullinsdorf, Switzerland), supplemented with cholesterol 2% (pur. 95%, Sigma-Aldrich, Burlington, MA, USA), 0.2% cholic acid (min. 98%, Sigma-Aldrich, Burlington, MA, USA) and 4.8% palm oil. Moreover, the effect of these treatments on proprotein convertase subtilisin/kexin type 9 (PCSK9) levels were also studied.

The rats were divided into five groups of 10 animals each:

Group 1 (normolipidemic controls) was kept on a standard diet (Harlan) for 30 days.
Group 2 (hyperlipidemic controls) received the hypercholesterolemic diet for 30 days.
Group 3 received the hypercholesterolemic diet for 30 days; from the 1st to the 30th day, each rat was administered by gavage with BPF (10 mg/kg/rat daily, same route).

Groups 4 and 5 received the hypercholesterolemic diet for 30 days; from the 1st to the 30th day, each rat was administered by gavage with RYR extract (3 and 1 mg/kg/rat daily, respectively, same route).

During the experiment, animals were weighed weekly, and 24 h food consumption was recorded daily. On day 29, rats were individually housed in metabolic cages. At the end of the study, the animals were fasted overnight; blood samples were collected from the penile vein of the rats and serum was separated and stored at $-20\,°C$ until analyzed. The analysis of serum T-CHOL, LDL-C and HDL-C, triglycerides, MDA and paraoxonase was performed as described below.

2.3. Blood Measurements

At the baseline and after 4 weeks of the experimental protocol, a 12 h fasting morning blood sample was collected, processed and stored at $-80\,°C$. All serum marker concentrations or activities were measured using classical methods and commercial assay kits, according to the manufacturers' instructions. Assay kits for total cholesterol, LDL-C, HDL-C, triglycerides, malondialdehyde (MDA), paraoxonase and glutathione peroxidase were purchased from Novamedical S.R.L. (Reggio Calabria, Italy). All the laboratory tests were performed in a blinded manner in respect to the assigned treatment.

2.4. PCSK9 Measurements

For proprotein convertase subtilisin/kexin type 9 (PCSK9) assay one serum aliquot from each rat was tested by colorimetric enzyme-linked immunosorbent assay from R&D Systems (Minneapolis, MN, USA). The minimal limit of detection was 125 pg/mL, the mean intra- and inter-assay coefficient of variation was at the accepted threshold of less than 8%.

2.5. Statistical Analysis

In case of homogenous set of data ANOVA was performed to determine the treatment effects, and Dunnett's test was employed as appropriate. In case of heterogeneous data, F test was carried out to determine which pairs of groups are heterogeneous. This was followed by Cochran's or Student's t tests, as appropriate. The analysis was performed by the Statistical analysis add-in component of Microsoft Excel 2007.

3. Results

Administration of hyperlipidemic diet in rats (Group 2) produced, compared to control group (Group 1) an elevation of serum levels of total cholesterol, LDL-C (Table 1) and an elevation of serum paraoxonase activity, MDA and PCSK9 expression, an effect accompanied by reduction of HDL-C levels and of glutathione peroxidase, an endogenous antioxidant enzyme. These effects were found significantly attenuated by treating rats with BPF 10 mg/Kg daily for 30 consecutive days (Group 3; Table 1, Figures 1 and 2). In fact BPF, according to previous evidence, significantly reduces the levels of serum total and LDL-C, an effect associated to reduced triglycerides, MDA, PCSK9 and paraoxonase activity. In addition, BPF increased HDL-C and glutathione peroxidase, as previously described.

Treatment of rats with RYR (3 and 1 mg/Kg for 30 consecutive days; Groups 4 and 5, respectively) reduced total cholesterol, LDL-C and paraoxonase (Table 1). However, when comparing the effect of RYR with BPF, we found BPF to better counteract diet-induced hyperlipidemia. Indeed, RYR produced no effect in triglycerides, HDL-C, MDA levels and glutathione peroxidase. In addition, RYR produced and very poor effects in PCSK9 when compared to BPF, thereby confirming that BPF is able to produce a better protection against diet-induced hyperlipidemia (Figures 1 and 2).

Table 1. The effect of BPF (10 mg/Kg daily; $n = 10$; Group 3) or RYR (3 and 1 mg/Kg daily; $n = 10$ for each group; Groups 4 and 5, respectively) on serum T-CHOL, LDL-C and HDL-C, triglycerides, malondialdehyde (MDA) paraoxonase and glutathione peroxidase in rats fed a hyperlipidemic diet. Groups 1 and 2 ($n = 10$ for each group represent animals receiving standard or hyperlipidemic diet, respectively. Data are expressed as mean ± SD. * $p < 0.05$ Control (Group 1) vs. Hyperlipidemic rats (Group 2); § $p < 0.05$ Hyperlipidemic (Group 2) vs. BPF, RYR 3 and 1 mg (Groups 3–5). Abbreviations. BPF: Bergamot Poliphenolic Fraction; RYR: Red yeast rice; T-CHOL: Total Cholesterol; LDL-C: Low density lipoprotein cholesterol; HDL-C: High density lipoprotein-cholesterol.

Study Groups	Serum T-CHOL (mg/dL)	Serum LDL-C (mg/dL)	Serum HDL-C (mg/dL)	Serum Triglycerides (mg/dL)	Serum Paraoxonase (nmol/mL/min)	Glutathione Peroxidase (U/mL)
Group 1 Standard diet ($n = 10$)	110 ± 12	34 ± 6	41 ± 6	145 ± 16	85 ± 6	186 ± 5
Group 2 Hyperlipidemic diet ($n = 10$)	196 ± 14 *	117 ± 10 *	32 ± 8 *	235 ± 18 *	132 ± 8 *	175 ± 4 *
Group 3 Hyperlipidemic diet + BPF 10 mg/Kg ($n = 10$)	154 ± 12 §	73 ± 8 §	46 ± 7 §	175 ± 15 §	102 ± 10 §	214 ± 4 §
Group 4 Hyperlipidemic diet + RYR (3 mg/Kg) ($n = 10$)	164 ± 14 §	83 ± 7 §	38 ± 5	215 ± 19	106 ± 9 §	192 ± 5
Group 5 Hyperlipidemic diet + RYR (1 mg/Kg) ($n = 10$)	176 ± 14 §	94 ± 11 §	36 ± 6	222 ± 16	116 ± 5 §	194 ± 6

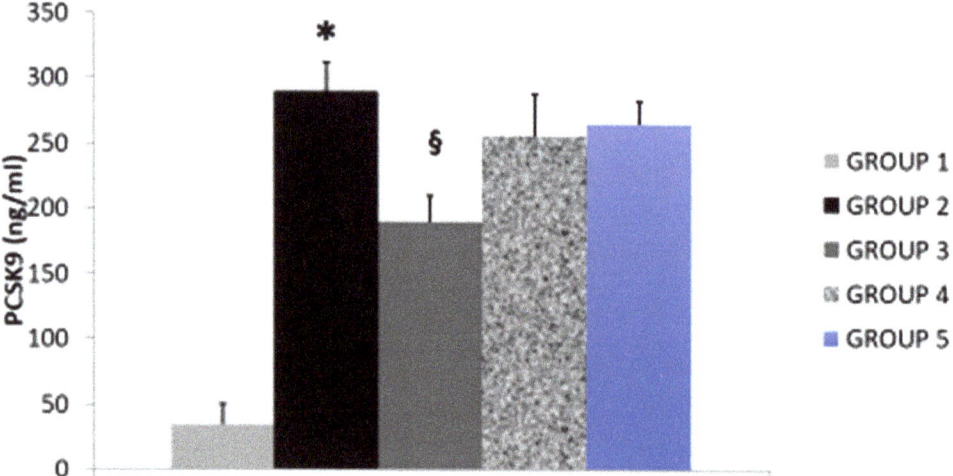

Figure 1. The effect of BPF (Group 3) or RYR (Groups 4 and 5) in PCSK9 serum levels in rats fed a hyperlipidemic diet (Group 2) compared to control rats (Group 1).*: $p < 0.05$ Control (Group 1) vs. Hyperlipidemic rats (Group 2); §: $p < 0.05$ Hyperlipidemic (Group 2) vs. BPF or RYR (Groups 3–5). Abbreviations. BPF: Bergamot Poliphenolic Fraction; RYR: Red yeast rice; PCSK9: Proprotein convertase subtilisin/kexin type 9.

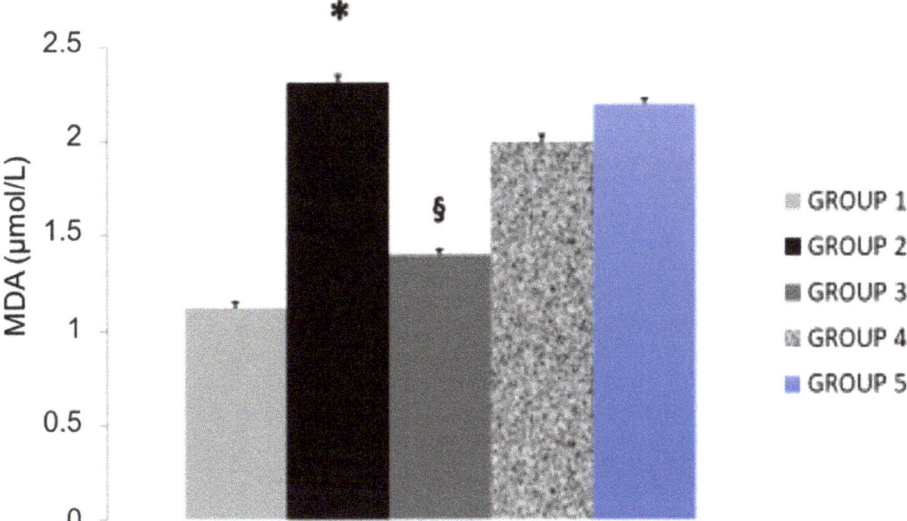

Figure 2. The effect of BPF (Group 3) or RYR (Groups 4 and 5) on MDA serum levels in rats fed a hyperlipidemic diet (Group 2) compared to control rats (Group 1). *: $p < 0.05$ Control (Group 1) vs. Hyperlipidemic rats (Group 2); §: $p < 0.05$ Hyperlipidemic (Group 2) vs. BPF or RYR (Groups 3–5), respectively. Abbreviations. BPF: Bergamot Poliphenolic Fraction; RYR: Red yeast rice; MDA: malondialdehyde.

4. Discussion

Our data show, for the first time, that BPF leads to a better hypolipidemic response when compared to RYR in rats fed a hyperlipidemic diet. In particular, our data demonstrate that BPF reduces both LDL-C and triglycerides, alongside with an elevation of HDL-C, as previously found in animal settings and patients with hyperlipidemia [15,16,24–27]. In contrast, the effect of RYR was limited to the reduction of LDL-C with no responses found in our model on triglycerides and HDL-C. On the other hand, the effect of BPF was higher to the one found in animals treated with RYR at doses used throughout the study.

The reason for a better performance of BPF when compared to RYR still remains to be better clarified. However, antioxidant properties of BPF and its subsequent activity against overexpression of PCSK9 seem to play a role.

Accumulated evidence has shown that BPF, a polyphenolic rich extract obtained from bergamot juice, produces consistent activities in regulating serum levels of cholesterol and triglycerides acting at different levels in the lipid metabolism [15,16,24–27]. In particular, data show that BPF reduces the activity of pancreatic cholesteryl ester hydrolase, a key enzyme in the absorption of cholesterol acting at the intestinal level [24]. In addition, the lipid transfer protein system in regulated by BPF, leading to better lipid transport into the bloodstream [25]. Furthermore, it was be found that the capability of the liver to release in blood vessel non-oxydized LDL occurs in patients with hyperlipidemia and liver steatosis, thereby playing a role in the regulation of the lipoprotein traffic in hepatic tissue [27]. Finally, BPF has been found to contain several glycosylated polyphenols such as bruteridine and melitidine which have been proven to antagonize the endogenous formation of HMGCoA reductase, the key enzyme which generate endogenous cholesterol [23–27], thereby contributing to serum cholesterol reduction. All these activities seem to involve the formation of free radical species, as also shown by data collected in our experiments here. In fact, the effect of BPF was associated to reduction of serum levels of MDA, a well recognized biomarker of oxidative stress. This effect did not occur in animals treated with RYR.

The effect of BPF was also associated to reduced expression of PCSK9 in animals fed an hyperlipidemic diet, thus suggesting that this effect may significantly contribute in the better reduction produced by this extract when compared to RYR.

The role of PCSK9 in the regulation of cholesterol metabolism and the relative cardioprotective action has been widely studied in the last few years [28–30]. In particular, evidence has been collected showing that PCSK9 modulates LDL-C concentrations by binding to hepatic LDL receptors, facilitating their catabolism [28–31], thereby increasing circulating LDL-C. This is also confirmed by the evidence that newly approved PCSK9 inhibitors reduce LDL receptor degradation and lower LDL-C by >50% [32–34], thus offering an additional therapeutic option for patients not meeting LDL-C treatment goals with diet and maximally tolerated lipid-lowering therapy. Several recent studies also showed the key role of natural derivatives and the importance of microbiota to inhibit the PCSK9, through its transcriptional and epigenetic regulation and the subsequent up-regulation of low-density lipoprotein receptor expression, thus increasing LDL metabolism [35–41]. Interestingly, statin therapy itself increases serum PCSK9 levels [42], a finding that may in part explain the nonlinear relationship between statin dose and LDL-C reduction and the intra-individual LDL-C response to statin therapy [43,44]. This could explain our data with BPF and RYR in PCSK9 expression in hyperlipidemic rats. In fact, hypelipidemia is accompanied by elevation of PCSK9 [28]. This effect, in our hands, is antagonized by BPF alone but not by RYR. The reason of this discrepancy is unclear. However, being the effect of RYR mainly due to the presence of lovastatin, it is likely that an overexpression of PCSK9 may attenuate the reduction of LDL-C seen in animals treated with RYR. On the other hand, elevation of PCSK9 occurs under conditions of increased oxidative stress and inflammation [45]. This also explains the better response found with BPF compared to RYR. In fact, being BPF a powerful antioxidant action in vivo, it is likely that this extract leads to a reduced formation of free radical species in liver tissue [26], an effect accompanied by reduced expression of PCSK9. This, in turn, leads to a better efficacy of BPF compared to RYR in modulating serum cholesterol and PCSK9.

5. Conclusions

Our data show that BPF produces consistent benefits in reducing serum cholesterol and triglycerides compared to RYR in animals fed a hyperlipidemic diet. This better performance seems to results from a better antioxidant profile, an effect associated to reduced expression of PCSK9, and this may represent a new perspective in nutraceutical supplementation in hyperlipidemic states. Obviously, the study takes into account the potential bias and imprecision of data collected in animal models that need to be confirmed in clinical studies to be carried out in patients.

Author Contributions: R.M. (Rocco Mollace), R.M. (Roberta Macrì), V.M. (Vincenzo Mollace), M.F. and M.V.: Conceptualization and supervision. R.M. (Rocco Mollace), R.M. (Roberta Macrì): Writing—original draft. A.T., V.M. (Vincenzo Musolino), M.G., C.C. and J.M.: Investigation, Methodology and Formal Analysis. All authors have read and agreed to the published version of the manuscript.

Funding: The work was supported by the public resources from the Italian Ministry of Research: PON-MIUR 03PE000_78_1 and PONMIUR 03PE000_78_2. POR Calabria FESR FSE 2014–2020 Asse 12-Azioni 10.5.6 e 10.5.12.

Institutional Review Board Statement: The study was conducted according to the guidelines of the Declaration of Helsinki, and approved by the the local Ethic Committee (Calabrian Region Prot. 185: 21 September 2018).

Data Availability Statement: The data presented in this study are available upon request from the corresponding author.

Conflicts of Interest: The authors declare no conflict of interest.

References

1. Michos, E.D.; McEvoy, J.W.; Blumenthal, R.S. Lipid Management for the Prevention of Atherosclerotic Cardiovascular Disease. *N. Engl. J. Med.* **2019**, *381*, 1557–1567. [CrossRef]
2. Trinder, M.; Francis, G.A.; Brunham, L.R. Association of Monogenic vs. Polygenic Hypercholesterolemia with Risk of Atherosclerotic Cardiovascular Disease. *JAMA Cardiol.* **2020**, *5*, 390–399. [CrossRef] [PubMed]
3. Silverman, M.G.; Ference, B.A.; Im, K.; Wiviott, S.D.; Giugliano, R.P.; Grundy, S.M.; Braunwald, E.; Sabatine, M.S. Association Between Lowering LDL-C and Cardiovascular Risk Reduction Among Different Therapeutic Interventions: A Systematic Review and Meta-analysis. *JAMA* **2016**, *316*, 1289–1297. [CrossRef] [PubMed]
4. Cholesterol Treatment Trialists' (CTT) Collaboration. Efficacy and safety of more intensive lowering of LDL cholesterol: A meta-analysis of data from 170,000 participants in 26 randomised trials. *Lancet* **2010**, *376*, 1670–1681. [CrossRef] [PubMed]
5. Gencer, B.; Marston, N.A.; Im, K.; Cannon, C.P.; Sever, P.; Keech, A.; Braunwald, E.; Giugliano, R.P.; Sabatine, M.S. Efficacy and safety of lowering LDL cholesterol in older patients: A systematic review and meta-analysis of randomised controlled trials. *Lancet* **2020**, *396*, 1637–1643. [CrossRef]
6. Lahera, V.; Goicoechea, M.; de Vinuesa, S.G.; Miana, M.; de las Heras, N.; Cachofeiro, V.; Luño, J. Endothelial dysfunction, oxidative stress and inflammation in atherosclerosis: Beneficial effects of statins. *Curr. Med. Chem.* **2007**, *14*, 243–248. [CrossRef]
7. Drexel, H.; Coats, A.J.S.; Spoletini, I.; Bilato, C.; Mollace, V.; Perrone Filardi, P.; Rosano, G.M.C. An expert opinion paper on statin adherence and implementation of new lipid-lowering medications by the ESC Working Group on Cardiovascular Pharmacotherapy: Barriers to be overcome. *Eur. Heart J. Cardiovasc. Pharmacother.* **2020**, *6*, 115–121. [CrossRef]
8. Sirtori, C.R. The pharmacology of statins. *Pharmacol. Res.* **2014**, *88*, 3–11. [CrossRef]
9. Castilla-Guerra, L.; Del Carmen Fernandez-Moreno, M.; Colmenero-Camacho, M.A. Statins in Stroke Prevention: Present and Future. *Curr. Pharm. Des.* **2016**, *22*, 4638–4644. [CrossRef]
10. Tomaszewski, M.; Stępień, K.M.; Tomaszewska, J.; Czuczwar, S.J. Statin-induced myopathies. *Pharmacol. Rep.* **2011**, *63*, 859–866. [CrossRef]
11. Sakamoto, K.; Kimura, J. Mechanism of statin-induced rhabdomyolysis. *J. Pharmacol. Sci.* **2013**, *123*, 289–294. [CrossRef] [PubMed]
12. Nissen, S.E.; Stroes, E.; Dent-Acosta, R.E.; Rosenson, R.S.; Lehman, S.J.; Sattar, N.; Preiss, D.; Bruckert, E.; Ceška, R.; Lepor, N.; et al. Efficacy and Tolerability of Evolocumab vs Ezetimibe in Patients with Muscle-Related Statin Intolerance: The GAUSS-3 Randomized Clinical Trial. *JAMA* **2016**, *315*, 1580–1590. [CrossRef]
13. Pohjola-Sintonen, S.; Julkunen, H. Muscle-related adverse effects of statins. *Duodecim* **2014**, *130*, 1622–1627.
14. Ward, N.C.; Watt, G.F.; Eckel, R.H. Statin Toxicity Mechanistic Insights and Clinical Implications. *Circ. Res.* **2019**, *124*, 328–350. [CrossRef]
15. Mollace, V.; Scicchitano, M.; Paone, S.; Casale, F.; Calandruccio, C.; Gliozzi, M.; Musolino, V.; Carresi, C.; Maiuolo, J.; Nucera, S.; et al. Hypoglycemic and Hypolipemic Effects of a New Lecithin Formulation of Bergamot Polyphenolic Fraction: A Double Blind, Randomized, Placebo-Controlled Study. *Endocr. Metab. Immune Disord. Drug Targets* **2019**, *19*, 136–143. [CrossRef]
16. Gliozzi, M.; Walker, R.; Muscoli, S.; Vitale, C.; Gratteri, S.; Carresi, C.; Musolino, V.; Russo, V.; Janda, E.; Ragusa, S.; et al. Bergamot polyphenolic fraction enhances rosuvastatin-induced effect on LDL-cholesterol, LOX-1 expression and protein kinase B phosphorylation in patients with hyperlipidemia. *Int. J. Cardiol.* **2013**, *170*, 140–145. [CrossRef]
17. Cicero, A.F.G.; Fogacci, F.; Banach, M. Red Yeast Rice for Hypercholesterolemia. *Methodist Debakey Cardiovasc. J.* **2019**, *15*, 192–199. [CrossRef]
18. Wang, T.J.; Lien, A.S.; Chen, J.L.; Lin, C.H.; Yang, Y.S.; Yang, S.H. A Randomized Clinical Efficacy Trial of Red Yeast Rice (*Monascus pilosus*) Against Hyperlipidemia. *Am. J. Chin. Med.* **2019**, *47*, 323–335. [CrossRef] [PubMed]
19. Nguyen, T.; Karl, M.; Santini, A. Red Yeast Rice. *Foods* **2017**, *6*, 19. [CrossRef]
20. Burke, F.M. Red yeast rice for the treatment of dyslipidemia. *Curr. Atheroscler. Rep.* **2015**, *17*, 22. [CrossRef] [PubMed]
21. Younes, M.; Aggett, P.; Aguilar, F.; Crebelli, R.; Dusemund, B.; Filipič, M.; Frutos, M.J.; Galtier, P.; Gott, D.; Gundert-Remy, U.; et al. Scientific opinion on the safety of monacolins in red yeast rice. *EFSA J.* **2018**, *16*, e05368. [CrossRef]
22. Mollace, V.; Sacco, I.; Janda, E.; Malara, C.; Ventrice, D.; Colica, C.; Visalli, V.; Muscoli, S.; Ragusa, S.; Muscoli, C.; et al. Hypolipemic and hypoglycaemic activity of bergamot polyphenols: From animal models to human studies. *Fitoterapia* **2011**, *82*, 309–316. [CrossRef] [PubMed]
23. European Communities (EC). Council Directive 86/609/EEC of 24 November 1986 on the approximation of laws, regulations and administrative provisions of the Member States regarding the protection of animals used for experimental and other scientific purposes. *Off. J. Eur. Communities* **1986**, *L358*, 1–28.
24. Musolino, V.; Gliozzi, M.; Carresi, C.; Maiuolo, J.; Mollace, R.; Bosco, F.; Scarano, F.; Scicchitano, M.; Maretta, A.; Palma, E.; et al. Lipid-lowering effect of bergamot polyphenolic fraction: Role of pancreatic cholesterol ester hydrolase. *J. Biol. Regul. Homeost. Agents* **2017**, *31*, 1087–1093. [PubMed]
25. Musolino, V.; Gliozzi, M.; Nucera, S.; Carresi, C.; Maiuolo, J.; Mollace, R.; Paone, S.; Bosco, F.; Scarano, F.; Scicchitano, M.; et al. The effect of bergamot polyphenolic fraction on lipid transfer protein system and vascular oxidative stress in a rat model of hyperlipemia. *Lipids Health Dis.* **2019**, *18*, 115. [CrossRef] [PubMed]
26. Musolino, V.; Gliozzi, M.; Bombardelli, E.; Nucera, S.; Carresi, C.; Maiuolo, J.; Mollace, R.; Paone, S.; Bosco, F.; Scarano, F.; et al. The synergistic effect of Citrus bergamia and Cynara cardunculus extracts on vascular inflammation and oxidative stress in non-alcoholic fatty liver disease. *J. Tradit. Complement. Med.* **2020**, *10*, 268–274. [CrossRef]

27. Musolino, V.; Gliozzi, M.; Scarano, F.; Bosco, F.; Scicchitano, M.; Nucera, S.; Carresi, C.; Ruga, S.; Zito, M.C.; Maiuolo, J.; et al. Bergamot Polyphenols Improve Dyslipidemia and Pathophysiological Features in a Mouse Model of Non-Alcoholic Fatty Liver Disease. *Sci. Rep.* **2020**, *10*, 2565. [CrossRef]
28. Di Donna, L.; De Luca, G.; Mazzotti, F.; Napoli, A.; Salerno, R.; Taverna, D.; Sindona, G. Statin-like principles of bergamot fruit (*Citrus bergamia*): Isolation of 3-hydroxymethylglutaryl flavonoid glycosides. *J. Nat. Prod.* **2009**, *72*, 1352–1354. [CrossRef]
29. Melendez, Q.M.; Krishnaji, S.T.; Wooten, C.J.; Lopez, D. Hypercholesterolemia: The role of PCSK9. *Arch. Biochem. Biophys.* **2017**, *625–626*, 39–53. [CrossRef] [PubMed]
30. Gliozzi, M.; Musolino, V.; Bosco, F.; Scicchitano, M.; Scarano, F.; Nucera, S.; Zito, M.C.; Ruga, S.; Carresi, C.; Macrì, R.; et al. Cholesterol homeostasis: Researching a dialogue between the brain and peripheral tissues. *Pharmacol. Res.* **2021**, *163*, 105215. [CrossRef]
31. Cammisotto, V.; Pastori, D.; Nocella, C.; Bartimoccia, S.; Castellani, V.; Marchese, C.; Scavalli, A.S.; Ettorre, E.; Viceconte, N.; Violi, F.; et al. PCSK9 Regulates Nox2-Mediated Platelet Activation via CD36 Receptor in Patients with Atrial Fibrillation. *Antioxidants* **2020**, *9*, 296. [CrossRef] [PubMed]
32. Seidah, N.G.; Awan, Z.; Chrétien, M.; Mbikay, M. PCSK9: A key modulator of cardiovascular health. *Circ. Res.* **2014**, *114*, 1022–1036. [CrossRef] [PubMed]
33. Giugliano, R.P.; Pedersen, T.R.; Park, J.G.; De Ferrari, G.M.; Gaciong, Z.A.; Ceska, R.; Toth, K.; Gouni-Berthold, I.; Lopez-Miranda, J.; Schiele, F.; et al. Clinical efficacy and safety of achieving very low LDL-cholesterol concentrations with the PCSK9 inhibitor evolocumab: A prespecified secondary analysis of the FOURIER trial. *Lancet* **2017**, *390*, 1962–1971. [CrossRef]
34. Rosenson, R.S.; Hegele, R.A.; Fazio, S.; Cannon, C.P. The Evolving Future of PCSK9 Inhibitors. *J. Am. Coll. Cardiol.* **2018**, *72*, 314–329. [CrossRef] [PubMed]
35. German, C.A.; Shapiro, M.D. Small Interfering RNA Therapeutic Inclisiran: A New Approach to Targeting PCSK9. *BioDrugs* **2020**, *34*, 1–9. [CrossRef] [PubMed]
36. Pirillo, A.; Catapano, A.L. Berberine, a plant alkaloid with lipid- and glucose-lowering properties: From in vitro evidence to clinical studies. *Atherosclerosis* **2015**, *243*, 449–461. [CrossRef] [PubMed]
37. Carrier, B.; Wen, S.; Zigouras, S.; Browne, R.W.; Li, Z.; Patel, M.S.; Williamson, D.L.; Rideout, T.C. Alpha-Lipoic Acid Reduces LDL-Particle Number and PCSK9 Concentrations in High-Fat Fed Obese Zucker Rats. *PLoS ONE* **2014**, *9*, e90863. [CrossRef]
38. Santulli, G.; Jankauskas, S.S.; Gambardella, J. Inclisiran: A new milestone on the PCSK9 road to tackle cardiovascular risk. *Eur. Heart J. Cardiovasc. Pharmacother.* **2021**, *7*, 11–12. [CrossRef]
39. Lin, Y.K.; Yeh, C.T.; Kuo, K.T.; Yadav, V.K.; Fong, I.K.; Kounis, N.J.; Hu, P.; Hung, M.Y. Pterostilbene Increases LDL Metabolism in HL-1 Cardiomyocytes by Modulating the PCSK9/HNF1α/SREBP2/LDLR Signaling Cascade, Upregulating Epigenetic hsa-miR-335 and hsa-miR-6825, and LDL Receptor Expression. *Antioxidants* **2021**, *10*, 1280. [CrossRef]
40. Wang, D.; Yang, X.; Chen, Y.; Gong, K.; Yu, M.; Gao, Y.; Wu, X.; Hu, H.; Liao, C.; Han, J.; et al. Ascorbic acid enhances low-density lipoprotein receptor expression by suppressing proprotein convertase subtilisin/kexin 9 expression. *J. Biol. Chem.* **2020**, *295*, 15870–15882. [CrossRef] [PubMed]
41. Morelli, M.B.; Wang, X.; Santulli, G. Functional role of gut microbiota and PCSK9 in the pathogenesis of diabetes mellitus and cardiovascular disease. *Atherosclerosis* **2019**, *289*, 176–178. [CrossRef] [PubMed]
42. Lammi, C.; Mulinacci, N.; Cecchi, L.; Bellumori, M.; Bollati, C.; Bartolomei, M.; Franchini, C.; Clodoveo, M.L.; Corbo, F.; Arnoldi, A. Virgin Olive Oil Extracts Reduce Oxidative Stress and Modulate Cholesterol Metabolism: Comparison between Oils Obtained with Traditional and Innovative Processes. *Antioxidants* **2020**, *9*, 798. [CrossRef]
43. Taylor, B.A.; Thompson, P.D. Statins and Their Effect on PCSK9-Impact and Clinical Relevance. *Curr. Atheroscler. Rep.* **2016**, *18*, 46. [CrossRef] [PubMed]
44. Pisciotta, L.; Fasano, T.; Bellocchio, A.; Bocchi, L.; Sallo, R.; Fresa, R.; Colangeli, I.; Cantafora, A.; Calandra, S.; Bertolini, S. Effect of ezetimibe coadministered with statins in genotype-confirmed heterozygous FH patients. *Atherosclerosis* **2007**, *194*, e116–e122. [CrossRef] [PubMed]
45. Dounousi, E.; Tellis, C.; Pavlakou, P.; Duni, A.; Liakopoulos, V.; Mark, P.B.; Papagianni, A.; Tselepis, A.D. Association between PCSK9 Levels and Markers of Inflammation, Oxidative Stress, and Endothelial Dysfunction in a Population of Nondialysis Chronic Kidney Disease Patients. *Oxid. Med. Cell. Longev.* **2021**, *2021*, 6677012. [CrossRef] [PubMed]

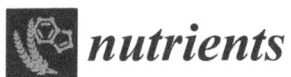

Review

From Diabetes Care to Heart Failure Management: A Potential Therapeutic Approach Combining SGLT2 Inhibitors and Plant Extracts

Micaela Gliozzi [1,†], Roberta Macrì [1,†], Anna Rita Coppoletta [1], Vincenzo Musolino [2,*], Cristina Carresi [3,*], Miriam Scicchitano [1], Francesca Bosco [1], Lorenza Guarnieri [1], Antonio Cardamone [1], Stefano Ruga [1], Federica Scarano [1], Saverio Nucera [1], Rocco Mollace [1], Irene Bava [1], Rosamaria Caminiti [1], Maria Serra [1], Jessica Maiuolo [2], Ernesto Palma [3] and Vincenzo Mollace [1,4]

[1] Pharmacology Laboratory, Institute of Research for Food Safety and Health IRC-FSH, Department of Health Sciences, University Magna Graecia of Catanzaro, 88100 Catanzaro, Italy
[2] Pharmaceutical Biology Laboratory, Institute of Research for Food Safety and Health IRC-FSH, Department of Health Sciences, University Magna Graecia of Catanzaro, 88100 Catanzaro, Italy
[3] Veterinary Pharmacology Laboratory, Institute of Research for Food Safety and Health IRC-FSH, Department of Health Sciences, University Magna Graecia of Catanzaro, 88100 Catanzaro, Italy
[4] Renato Dulbecco Institute, Lamezia Terme, 88046 Catanzaro, Italy
* Correspondence: v.musolino@unicz.it (V.M.); carresi@unicz.it (C.C.); Tel./Fax: +39-0961-3694301 (V.M. & C.C.)
† These authors contributed equally to this work.

Abstract: Diabetes is a complex chronic disease, and among the affected patients, cardiovascular disease (CVD)is the most common cause of death. Consequently, the evidence for the cardiovascular benefit of glycaemic control may reduce long-term CVD rates. Over the years, multiple pharmacological approaches aimed at controlling blood glucose levels were unable to significantly reduce diabetes-related cardiovascular events. In this view, a therapeutic strategy combining SGLT2 inhibitors and plant extracts might represent a promising solution. Indeed, countering the main cardiometabolic risk factor using plant extracts could potentiate the cardioprotective action of SGLT2 inhibitors. This review highlights the main molecular mechanisms underlying these beneficial effects that could contribute to the better management of diabetic patients.

Keywords: diabetes; insulin resistance; lipid accumulation; inflammation; reactive oxygen species (ROS); SGLT2 inhibitors; nutraceutical supplementation; cardiovascular risk

Citation: Gliozzi, M.; Macrì, R.; Coppoletta, A.R.; Musolino, V.; Carresi, C.; Scicchitano, M.; Bosco, F.; Guarnieri, L.; Cardamone, A.; Ruga, S.; et al. From Diabetes Care to Heart Failure Management: A Potential Therapeutic Approach Combining SGLT2 Inhibitors and Plant Extracts. *Nutrients* 2022, 14, 3737. https://doi.org/10.3390/nu14183737

Academic Editors: Bruno Trimarco and Gaetano Santulli

Received: 9 May 2022
Accepted: 7 September 2022
Published: 10 September 2022

Publisher's Note: MDPI stays neutral with regard to jurisdictional claims in published maps and institutional affiliations.

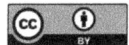

Copyright: © 2022 by the authors. Licensee MDPI, Basel, Switzerland. This article is an open access article distributed under the terms and conditions of the Creative Commons Attribution (CC BY) license (https://creativecommons.org/licenses/by/4.0/).

1. Introduction

Diabetes is a complex disease, characterised by chronic hyperglycaemia, which includes different subtypes of heterogeneous metabolic disorders, such as type 1 diabetes mellitus (T1DM) and type 2 diabetes mellitus (T2DM), gestational diabetes and monogenic diabetes syndromes [1].

In some forms of T1DM, the pathogenesis of the disease depends on the destruction of autoimmune β-cell that causes an absolute insulin deficiency, whereas a progressive loss of β-cell insulin secretion, frequently on the background of insulin resistance, leads to T2DM [1,2].

Clinically, the progressive loss of β-cell mass or function due to several genetic and environmental factors manifests as hyperglycaemia. In all subtypes of diabetes, it represents a risk for the development of chronic complications, although their progression may differ, as in the presence of different comorbidities (i.e., hyperlipidaemia) [1,3].

Among populations suffering from diabetes, cardiovascular disease (CVD) represents one of the most common causes of death. On the other hand, in the early stages of diabetes subtypes, glycaemic control and countering cardiovascular risk factors can reduce the CVD mortality rate [4].

Over the years, multiple pharmacological approaches aimed at controlling blood glucose concentrations in diabetic patients have been used. Starting from the use of insulin, the research progress in improving the pharmacotherapy of diabetes, through the discovery of metformin, sulfonylureas, and thiazolidinediones, failed to reduce cardiovascular events despite the beneficial effects on blood glucose regulation [5]. Differently, novel classes of antihyperglycaemic drugs, such as sodium-glucose cotransporter-2 (SGLT2) inhibitors (SGLT2i) and glucagon-like peptide-1 receptor agonist (GLP-1 RA), appeared more effective in preventing CV complications [6]. Starting from this evidence, some SGLT2i have even been approved to treat heart failure (HF) independently from the presence of diabetes [6–8]. Indeed, beyond the mechanisms underlying the benefit of SGLT2i on the cardio–renal axis [9], a recent study has shown that SGLT2i improve cardiovascular outcomes, affecting a small group of circulating intracellular proteins (e.g., IGFBP1 and TSMB10, implicated in cardioprotection and nephroprotection, respectively) which promote autophagic flux, reduce oxidative stress and inflammation, and stimulate repair and renewal in the heart and kidneys [10].

The purpose of this review is to focus on the molecular mechanisms underlying the therapeutic properties of SGLT2i in countering the detrimental effects of hyperglycaemia on cardiac function. On this background, we will overview the possible use of natural polyphenols in the prevention and management of diabetic cardiomyopathy (DCM) beyond glycaemic control.

2. SGLT2 Inhibitors and Molecular Mechanisms of Cardioprotection

SGLT2i are strongly favoured in diabetic patients with diagnosed HF or at risk of HF [11–13]. The choice of this therapeutic approach—preserving heart function—suggests the existence of specific mechanisms underlying these favourable effects based on the modulation of metabolism [14], haemodynamic parameters, electrolyte levels and neuro-hormonal activation [15]. In addition, cardiac protection is also mediated by the restoration of calcium homeostasis, anti-inflammatory, and antifibrotic effects.

2.1. SGLT2 Inhibitors and Modulation of Metabolism in Heart Tissue

As mentioned above, heart failure is associated with alterations in myocardial metabolic substrate flexibility [16]. In diabetic patients, the lack of glucose and fatty acid utilization, in turn, is associated with the gradual use of ketone bodies as a fuel source aimed to ensure cardiac function [17,18]. At the molecular level, this implies the downregulation of the fatty acid transporter carnitine palmitoyltransferase 1-α (CPT1-α), the downregulation of the glucose transporter type 4 (GLUT4), and the inhibition of the pyruvate dehydrogenase complex (PDH), mediated by the upregulation of pyruvate dehydrogenase kinase 4 (PDK4) [16], physiologically responsible for the entrance of carbohydrate intermediates into the Krebs cycle [19] (Figure 1).

In the insulin-resistant heart, impaired cardiac metabolism, characterised by deficient ATP production, can be prevented by empagliflozin [20], which promotes increased glucose oxidation associated with unchanged or lower ketone body oxidation rate. This suggests that SGLT2i-induced rise of circulating ketone body levels can represent an additional source of energy to support heart contractile function. In pigs, this beneficial metabolic effect afforded by empagliflozin was associated with an amelioration of left ventricle remodelling, and in humans, it was also confirmed in the presence of T2DM and coronary artery disease [15].

Thus, the restoration of the complex metabolic equilibrium in heart tissue, which is impaired under diabetes, represents an additional therapeutic goal of disease treatment.

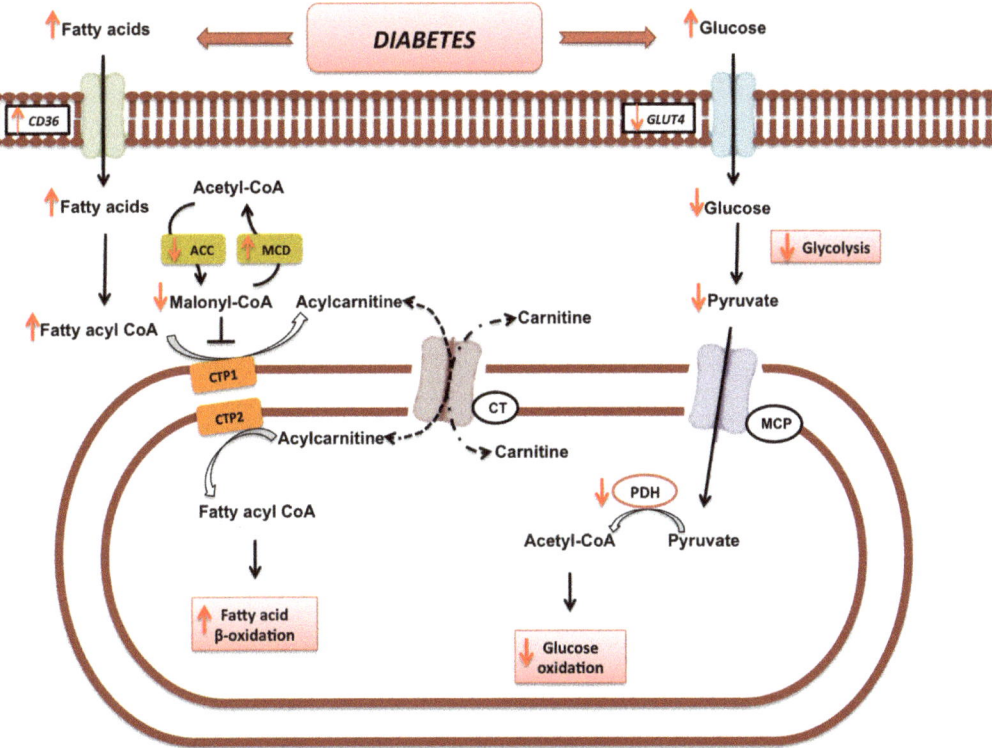

Figure 1. Metabolic alterations in diabetic patients. At the molecular level, insulin resistance causes an increase in both plasma glucose and serum insulin levels, which lead to a reduction in glucose transporter type 4 (GLUT4), and a decrease in glucose uptake. These events lead to a reduction in the glycolysis pathway and glucose oxidation caused by the downregulation of the pyruvate dehydrogenase complex (PDH). The hyperglycaemia is associated with the concomitant increase in hematic fatty acid concentration and the consequent upregulation of fatty acids uptake and oxidation due to the decreased levels of malonyl CoA and the consequent activation of carnitine palmitoyltransferase 1 (CPT1). CD36—cluster of differentiation 36; ACC—Acetyl-CoA carboxylase; MCD—Malonyl-CoA decarboxylase; CTP1—carnitine palmitoyltransferase 1; CTP2—carnitine palmitoyltransferase 2; MCP—mitochondrial pyruvate carrier; CT—carnitine translocase; PDH—pyruvate dehydrogenase complex; GLUT4—glucose transporter type 4.

2.2. SGLT2i-Mediated Anti-Inflammatory, Antifibrotic, and Antioxidant Effects on the Heart

Circulating leukocytes are involved in the development of a chronic low-grade inflammatory state, characterized by increased circulating leukocyte-produced proinflammatory cytokines and decreased anti-inflammatory IL-10, which represents the main cause of enhanced cardiovascular risk in T2DM patients [21,22]. In diabetes and heart failure, pathogenic inflammatory cytokines, specifically IL-1β, are promoted by the activation of the Nod-like receptor (NLR) family pyrin domain-containing 3 (NLRP3) inflammasome. Although empagliflozin was shown to possess an analogue glucose-lowering power compared with the sulfonylurea, it can reduce IL-1β secretion mostly with an enhancement of serum β-hydroxybutyrate (BHB) and decreased serum insulin. Chronic inflammation and persistent oxidative stress lead to the development and progression of vascular proliferative diseases. The proinflammatory cytokine interleukin IL-17A induces oxidative stress and increases inflammatory signalling in human aortic smooth muscle cells through TRAF3IP2-mediated NLRP3/caspase-1-dependent mitogenic and migratory proinflammatory cytokines IL-1β and IL-18. It has been shown that the inhibition of SGLT2 in smooth muscle cells by empagliflozin decreased IL-17A/TRAF3IP2-dependent oxidative stress, NLRP3 expression, caspase-1 activation, and IL-1β and IL-18 secretion [23]. Additionally, empagliflozin can lessen serum uric acid levels, which is a potent activator of NLRP3 inflammasome. Thus, the inhibition of NLRP3 inflammasome, caused by the mentioned mechanisms, might contribute to explaining SGLT2i cardioprotective effects [24].

As proinflammatory cytokines promote the accumulation of neutrophils and macrophages into the lesion site, it has been demonstrated that, in DCM, this inflammatory environment also determines the release of growth factors, triggering fibroblast activation and the consequent development of fibrosis [25]. The prevention of remodelling and fibrotic processes after early and late treatment with empagliflozin was highlighted by the reduced increase in left ventricle mass and by the diminished cardiomyocyte cross-sectional area of myocardial infarction (MI) in diabetic hearts. Furthermore, SGLT2i significantly reduce the inflammatory response and infarct size in type 2 diabetic patients with acute myocardial infarction through a mechanism independent of glucose-metabolic control [26]. Moreover, in noninfarcted areas, empagliflozin-induced myocardial protection was confirmed by the reduced expression of specific markers of fibrosis, such as collagen 1 and procollagen [19].

It has been demonstrated that the sodium hydrogen exchanger-1 (NHE-1) may play a fundamental role in HF and diabetes since cardiac NHE-1 is upregulated in both conditions [27,28]. In rodent and rabbit models of diabetes [29], the inhibition of NHE-1 by SGLT2i and modulation of intramyocardial Ca^{2+} and Na^+ fluxes seem to have a beneficial impact on diastolic myocardial function [29,30]. This effect can be connected to enhanced SERCA activity and to antifibrotic effects [31,32].

Although the NHE-1 inhibition affords cardioprotection in animal models, NHE-1 inhibitors failed in clinical practice, suggesting that the reduction in hyperactivation of the exchanger rather than the total inhibition of NHE-1 can represent the more appropriate therapeutic approach. In this view, the restoration of the basal activity might justify the cardioprotective effects of SGLT2i, similarly to other drugs modulating NHE1 activity through the control of its phosphorylation [33].

In turn, the reduced cytosolic Na^+ and Ca^{2+}, caused by the modification of NHE-1 activity by empagliflozin, can cause an increase in mitochondrial Ca^{2+} [29,30], favouring the maintenance of cellular calcium handling and the prevention of the oxidative stress. Then, calcium homeostasis preservation provokes the attenuation of oxidative Ca^{2+}/Calmodulin-dependent kinase IIδ (CaMKII) activity, downregulating NHE-1 and promoting the amelioration of diastolic and systolic functions [34] (Figure 2).

Further study indicated that oxidative stress and fibrosis development are suppressed by empagliflozin through the inhibition of TGF-beta, and the activation of Nrf2/ARE signalling [35].

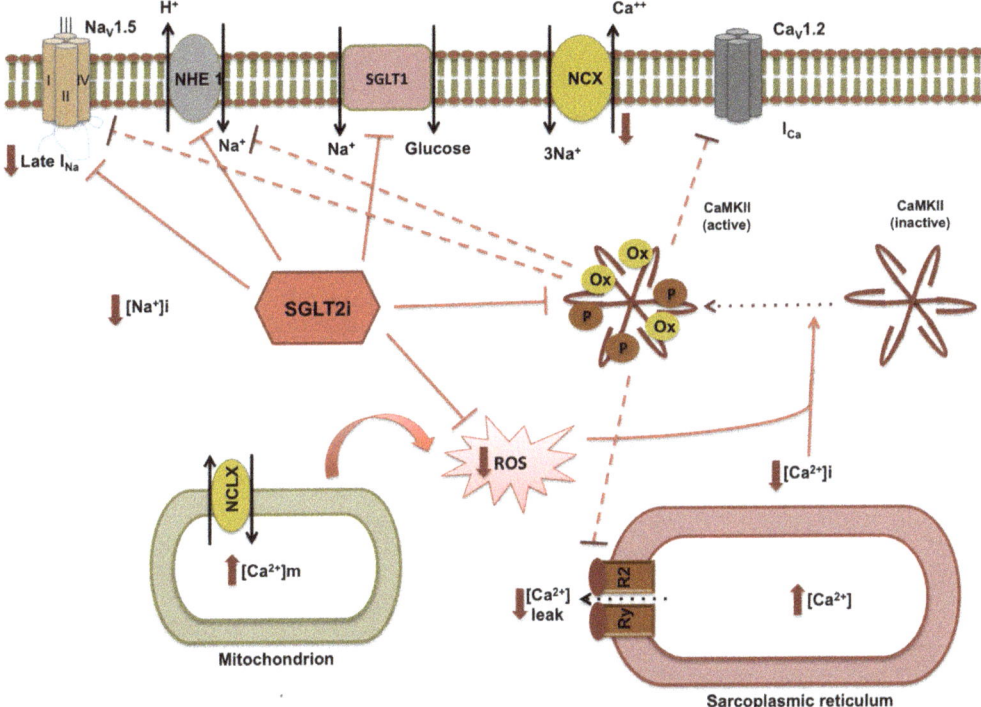

Figure 2. Downregulation of NHE-1, modulation of intramyocardial Ca^{2+} and Na^+ fluxes by SGLT-2 inhibitors. The sodium hydrogen exchanger-1 (NHE-1) is upregulated in heart failure (HF) and diabetes. SGLT2i have a key role in the inhibition of NHE-1, sodium-glucose co-transporter 1 (SGLT1), and Na^+/Ca^{2+} exchanger (NCX), preserving the calcium and sodium homeostasis and attenuating the oxidative Ca^{2+}/Calmodulin-dependent kinase IIδ (CaMKII) activity. The modulation of Ca^{2+} and Na^+ fluxes lead to a reduction in reactive oxygen species (ROS) and prevention of the cytosolic increase in calcium because of the mitochondrial and sarcoplasmic release caused by mitochondrial Na^+/Ca^{2+} exchanger (NCLX) and ryanodine receptor 2 S(RyR2).

3. SGLT2i and Cardiometabolic Risk Factors

It has been recognized that insulin resistance and atherogenic dyslipidaemia, characterised by the presence of low high-density lipoprotein (HDL)-cholesterol and high triglyceride levels [36,37], enhance the incidence of cardiovascular disease and diabetes mellitus. In this scenario, the positive impact of SGLT2i on cardiac tissue is due to counteracting the main cardiometabolic risk factors, which are also considered the cause of the metabolic activity dysregulation of other organs, such as liver and adipose tissue, which are directly involved in the control of lipid metabolism in the body.

Consequently, the modulation of specific molecular targets at those levels can also impact myocardial tissue function.

3.1. SGLT2i and Modulation of Lipid Metabolism

The most debated item related to the use of SGLT2i remains the effect on cholesterol low-density lipoprotein (cLDL) and triglycerides levels as, despite their proven cardioprotective effects, an increased level of cLDL emerged from several clinical studies. It has been hypothesised that the rise depends on the enhanced activity of lipoprotein lipase (LpL), independently of the turnover of circulating low-density lipoprotein (LDL), as confirmed by the lowered level of hepatic LDL receptors [38].

According to these discoveries, canagliflozin indirectly promotes LpL activity in the heart, white and brown adipose tissue, and skeletal muscle, also contributing to the decrease in triglycerides and very low levels of low-density lipoprotein (VLDL). On the other hand, the failed clearance of LDL is counterbalanced by a positive effect on LDL subclasses [39], further supporting the cardioprotective role of SGLT2i. In agreement with this evidence, canagliflozin administration contributed to very large high-density lipoprotein (VLHDL) and large high-density lipoprotein (LHDL) levels [40].

A meta-analysis of randomised clinical trials confirmed the amelioration of plasma lipid profile induced by SGLT2i in a dose-dependent manner [41]. In addition, although the most relevant effect concerns LDL subclass size and oxidation, canagliflozin [38] and dapagliflozin [42] have been shown to inhibit the hepatic synthesis of triglycerides through the downregulation of those enzymes responsible for the catabolism of fatty acids [43].

Among them, peroxisome proliferator-activated receptors (PPAR)-α and PPAR-γ appear to be interesting targets of SGLT2i because they might contribute to counteracting endothelial dysfunction too. Indeed, it has been demonstrated that their activation induces cholesterol removal from human macrophage foam cells [44]. Moreover, canagliflozin stimulates PPAR-α, promoting the uptake, utilization, and catabolism of fatty acids, whereas PPAR-γ activation ameliorates insulin sensitivity through the stimulation of fibroblast growth factor 21 (FGF21) and the cluster of differentiation 36 (CD36) enzyme [38].

In addition to the effects on plasma lipid profile and liver metabolism, SGLT2i therapy can exert its beneficial property by acting at the adipose tissue level. Indeed, although lower body weight in patients who have diabetes [45] has been correlated with the recovery of the caloric balance promoted by glucose excretion, it is also associated with the positive effects of SGLT2i on adipose tissue mass; indeed, its reduction is able to boost insulin sensitivity [46]. Moreover, SGLT2i-induced "visceral fat lowering" is associated with the reduction in inflammatory responses caused by dysfunctional adipocytes, which prevents lipotoxicity and energy imbalance.

Particularly, empagliflozin can ameliorate insulin sensitivity by counteracting inflammatory events promoted by M2 macrophage polarization through the browning of white adipose tissue, which promotes an increase in energy expenditure and thermogenesis [47,48]. Additionally, canagliflozin has been shown to improve insulin resistance by a reduction in visceral and ectopic fatty tissues [49], adipocytes number, and plasma lipids [47,48,50], whereas dapagliflozin improved adipocyte function by stimulating adiponectin production in obese patients with T2DM [51].

3.2. Haemodynamic and Vascular Effects

The origin of hypertension can be ascribed to the kidneys that are responsible for the control of haemodynamic parameters. As it occurs in diabetic patients, the injured kidneys determine an enhanced sympathetic activation and, consequently, vasoconstriction, sodium and water retention, and tachycardia, leading to a rise in blood pressure. The prolonged increase in sympathetic tone can ultimately lead to a decline in renal function and to an enhanced cardiac load contributing to the development of heart failure [52].

Thus, the favourable haemodynamic consequences of the SGLT2i action depend on the reduced preload and afterload at the ventricular level, and this final effect appears to be mediated by the regulation of several parameters, comprising osmotic diuresis, natriuresis, and plasma and interstitial fluid volume [53–55]. Overall, they contribute to relieving the renal load and reducing sympathetic nerve overactivation [50], lowering blood pressure [56,57]. Thus, the findings related to the action of SGLT2i on blood pressure highlight the dissociation of antihypertensive from antihyperglycemic effects [58]. Although some clinical studies suggest that SGLT2i do not directly affect haemodynamic parameters, it was highlighted that SGLT2i significantly reduce markers of tubular injury by certain mechanisms [59]. Indeed, at the molecular level, SGLT2i exert their beneficial effects also through the modulation of sodium hydrogen exchanger 3 (NH3), responsible for HCO_3^- absorption at proximal tubule level in the absence of luminal glucose. It has been demonstrated that

NH3 and SGLT2 can regulate each other; consequently, all those events characterizing diabetic conditions (i.e., low luminal glucose, the overactivation of the sympathetic nervous system, acidosis, oxidative stress, chronic kidney disease, and congestive heart failure (CHF)), contribute to inducing primarily NH3 and enhance SGLT2 expression [60]. Therefore, SGLT2 inhibition blocking sodium–hydrogen exchanger 3 (NHE3) may also prevent HCO_3^- absorption and metabolic acidosis [56].

It has been recognized that luminal glucose and uric acid compete to bind Urate transporter 1 (URAT-1) for reabsorption at the proximal tubule level [61]. Consequently, SGLT2i, increasing luminal glucose concentration, causes the inhibition of URAT-1 [62], favouring renal uric acid clearance [63] and, at the same time, counteracting the detrimental effects of high concentrations of plasma urate, such as reactive oxygen species overproduction, inflammation, vascular proliferation, and renal damage [64]. In turn, the reduction in vascular and renal ROS contributes to restoring the physiological level [65] and function [66] of endothelial nitric oxide (NO), counteracting aortic stiffness [67–69]. Additionally, the normalization of NO production, probably caused by the inhibition of sodium–hydrogen exchanger 1 (NHE1), further contributes to reducing blood pressure [56]. Moreover, SGLT2i improve macro- and microvascular endothelial function [70] through the modulation of AT1R/NADPH oxidase/SGLT1 and two pathways, providing a promising strategy to maintain physiological endothelial function [69,71].

Recently, Mone et al. have identified a signature of microRNA functionally involved in endothelial function. In frail patients with heart failure with preserved ejection fraction and diabetes, the treatment with the SGLT2i caused a modification of these microRNA signatures, indicating a maintained endothelial function [72].

Finally, SGLT2i reduce frailty in diabetic and hypertensive patients by a reduction in mitochondrial generation of ROS species in endothelial cells [73].

4. DCM and Cardiometabolic Risk: Can Plant Extract Supplementation Support SGLT2i Action?

Chemically, SGLT2 inhibitors are synthetic derivatives of phlorizin, the main phenolic glucoside in apple trees (roots, bark, shoots, and leaves) [74]. Despite its structural amelioration, aimed to selectively inhibit NHE-1 and promote renal glucose excretion, it has been proven that the phlorizin-rich extract can contribute to improving other aspects of diabetes as well as of other metabolic disorders, also ameliorating the most common cardiometabolic risk factors [75]. Recently, in accordance with this evidence, the peculiar value of several phytocomplexes in the prevention of CVD or as a supplement to most widespread therapies has emerged. This suggests a role for several plant extracts/nutraceuticals that, synergizing with SGLT2i or supporting their action through the modulation of glucose and lipid metabolism, might potentiate their cardioprotective effects under diabetes development (Figure 3).

4.1. Insulin Resistance

In vitro and in vivo studies demonstrated that several plant extracts can counteract insulin resistance through different mechanisms, such as the improvement of the glucose uptake process in tissues and the stimulation of pancreatic insulin secretion.

In particular, glucose uptake regulation occurs principally through the enhancement of GLUT-4 expression and translocation into the cells, which can be mediated by several signalling pathways, including the AMP-activated protein kinase (AMPK), phosphoinositide 3-PI3K/Akt, PKC, and G protein–phospholipase C (PLC)–PKC pathways.

Cassia angustifolia Vahl extract has been shown to improve GLUT-4 expression and turnover through the G protein–PLC–PKC signalling pathway and inositol 1,4,5-trisphosphate receptor (IP3R) [76].

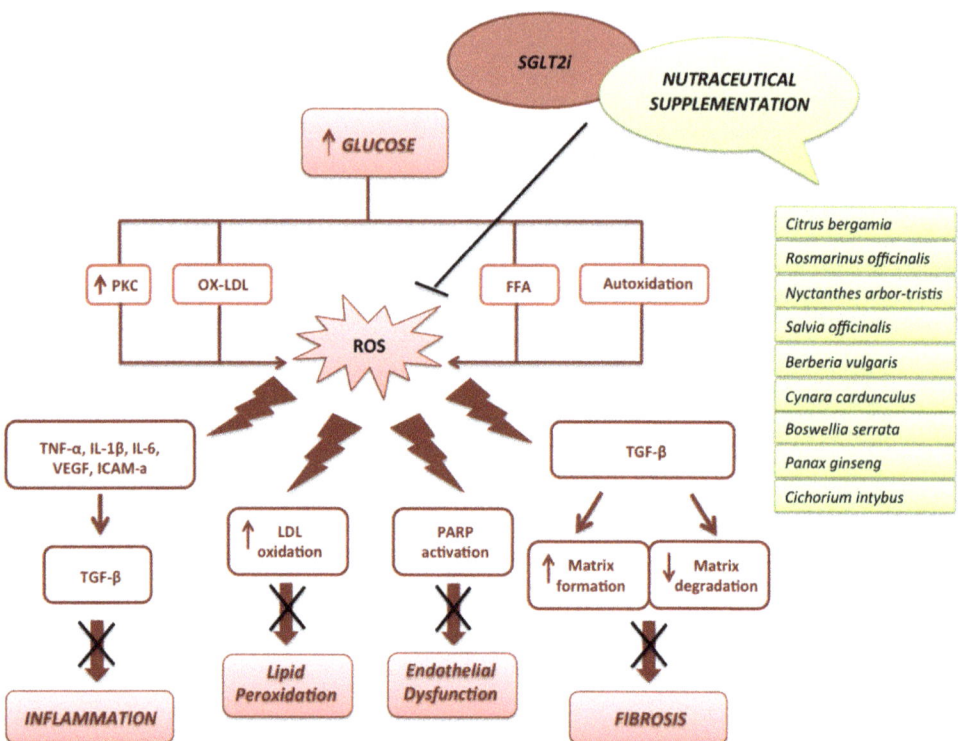

Figure 3. Common cardioprotective effects of the plant extract supplementation and SGLT2 inhibitors. The SGLT2i and several phytocomplexes show a similar action to counteract the ROS production caused by hyperglycemia. In particular, they play a key role in the inhibition of the inflammasome, leading to a reduction in inflammation and fibrosis. The downregulation of LDL oxidation and PARP activation lead to the reduction in lipid peroxidation and endothelial dysfunction. PKC—Protein kinase C; OX-LDL—Oxidized Low-Density Lipoprotein; FFA—Free fatty acids; ROS—reactive oxygen species; TNF-α—Tumour Necrosis Factor α; IL-1β—Interleukin 1 beta; IL-6—Interleukin 6; VEGF—Vascular-Endothelial Growth Factor; ICAM-a—intracellular adhesion molecule a, TGF-β—Transforming Growth Factor Beta; PARP—Poly (ADP-ribose) polymerase; LDL—Low-Density Lipoprotein.

Morus alba L. leaf extract counteracts insulin resistance and improves glucose metabolism through the activation of the IRS-1/PI3K/Glut4 signalling pathway at the muscular level. Additional mechanisms, due to anthocyanin extract of *Morus alba* L., are explicated by the activation of PI3K/Akt pathway [77] that regulates the basal expression of glucose-6-phosphatase (G6Pase) and phosphoenolpyruvate carboxyl kinase (PEPCK), two key rate-limiting enzymes of gluconeogenesis. Indeed, Akt activation inhibits gluconeogenesis through the phosphorylation of forkhead Box O1 (FOXO1) that renders the protein unable to translocate into the nucleus and to transcript G6Pase and PEPCK [78,79] proteins, thus blocking gluconeogenesis. In accordance with this evidence, FOXO1 downregulation has been shown to reverse hyperglycaemia in models of insulin resistance, and, in contrast, FOXO1 overactivation has been found to promote the insulin-resistant state [80–82].

Cinnamomum cassia extracts have also shown a significant improvement in glycaemic control in different animal models and patients with prediabetes dysfunction or diabetes [82]. The antidiabetic effect is due to different molecular mechanisms, including the control of insulin receptor (IR) phosphorylation, GLUT-4 expression and translocation, and the modulation of hepatic glucose metabolism, mediated by pyruvate kinase (PK) and phosphoenol pyruvate carboxykinase (PEPCK) activities [83].

Finally, *Rauwolfia serpentina* appears to counter insulin resistance, improving glucose metabolism, as proven by the reduction in total and glycosylated haemoglobin [76].

4.2. Antioxidant and Anti-Inflammatory Effects

Growing evidence shows that inflammation and oxidative stress can be counteracted by the active compounds of plant extracts.

Boswellia serrata extract [84], *Momordica charantia* L. fruit juice [85], and *Sclerocarya birrea* extract [86] have been shown to induce the overexpression of endogenous antioxidants, such as superoxide dismutase (SOD), catalase (CAT), and (glutathione) GSH, whereas *Nyctanthes arbor-tristis* L. leaf extract was able to suppress hyperglycaemia-induced oxidative stress and inflammation through the control of Nuclear factor kappa B (NF-kB) [87].

Boswellia serrata extract administration also reduced glucose, insulin, and cholesterol, in a T2DM rat model, preventing the hippocampal accumulation of Aβ 1-42 and glycogen synthase kinase-3β (GSK-3β) overexpression and counteracting excitotoxicity [84]. This beneficial response has been attributed to the downregulation of inflammatory mediators, such as TNF-α, IL-1β, and IL-6 and the amelioration of oxidative balance generated by the decrease in lipid peroxidation products and the upregulation of GSH and SOD levels [84].

Cichorium intybus L. extract improved insulin and glucose metabolism in high-fat diet-induced diabetic male C57BL/6 mice, and these effects were also mediated by the inhibition of NLRP3 inflammasome activation, leading to the decrease in IL-1β levels [88]. In adipose tissues, the inhibitory effect exerted on the NLRP3 inflammasome promoted the shift of M_1 proinflammatory macrophages towards the M_2 anti-inflammatory phenotype. In turn, this change was able to reduce the inducible nitric oxide synthase (iNOS) and TNF-α levels derived from M_1 macrophages and to increase the expression of Arg-1 and IL-10, which are typical M_2 markers [89].

Panax ginseng C.A. Meyer extract has been shown to ameliorate adipose inflammation in Ovariectomized female C57BL/6J mice through the reduction in the expression of proinflammatory cytokines CD68, TNF-α, and *Monocyte chemoattractant protein-1* (MCP-1) and the number of infiltrating inflammatory cells. In addition, it reduced MMP-2 and MMP-9 expression and activity, mRNA levels of *Vascular endothelial growth factor A* (VEGF-A), and Fibroblast growth factor 2 (FGF-2) [90].

Salvia officinalis extract has a strong antioxidant activity. Indeed, experimental studies have shown that it induced the activation of glutathione peroxidase [91], preventing DNA damage in hepatocytes, and improved cellular superoxide scavenging power, enhancing catalase, glutathione peroxidase, glutathione-S-transferase, and superoxide dismutase in the pancreas [92].

In in vivo models of different inflammatory stimuli than diabetes, *Rosmarinus officinalis* has shown anti-inflammatory activity. This effect depended on the inhibition of NF-kB, leading to a reduced expression of cyclooxygenase-2 (COX-2) and iNOS, suggesting an antioxidant effect, too [93,94].

4.3. Lipid Metabolism

The modulation of lipid metabolism operated by plant extracts can be exerted at the liver, adipose tissue, and skeletal muscle level, with a consequent beneficial impact on those tissues and on the oxidative state of circulating lipids.

Syzygium cumini (L.) Skeels. and *Zingiber officinale* Roscoe extracts can positively modulate lipid metabolism upregulating PPARα and PPARγ [83,95]. Differently, the hypolipidemic effects of *Morus alba* L. leaf extract in diabetic rats have manifested with reduced levels of triglycerides, total cholesterol, and LDL with consequent inhibition of lipid accumulation in skeletal muscles [76]. In an alternative way, *Rauwolfia serpentina* improved lipid metabolism through the inhibition of 3-hydroxy-3-methylglutaryl-coenzyme A (HMG-CoA) reductase activity, suggesting an improvement in liver function [76].

4.4. Pleiotropic Effects of Plant Extracts in Counteracting Cardiometabolic Risk Factors and Heart Failure: Berberia Vulgaris and Citrus Bergamia

Several phytocomplexes in plant extracts have interesting therapeutic potential in the treatment of patients in whom the main cardiovascular risk factors tend to cluster, impairing the whole metabolism.

Berberia vulgaris and *Citrus Bergamia* extracts can represent peculiar examples of natural compounds that might be candidate supplements in an SGLT2i-based therapy.

Berberia vulgaris, historically used in the treatment of inflammations and high blood pressure [96,97], has been shown to have antihyperglycemic, hypolipidemic, and antioxidant effects; consequently, different parts of this plant, including fruits, leaves, and roots, have been used in traditional medicine for a long time [97,98].

Most of these effects have been attributable to berberine, which is able to reduce serum levels of triglycerides and total cholesterol, to increase the expression of cardiac fatty acid transport protein-1, fatty acid transport proteins, fatty acid beta-oxidase, and PPAR-γ [99]. Moreover, it ameliorates plasma lipoprotein profile through the increase in hepatic low-density lipoprotein receptor (LDLR) expression [100]. An additional mechanism responsible for lowering blood cholesterol levels includes the inhibition of absorption at the intestinal level with a reduction in enterocyte cholesterol uptake and secretion and the interference with intraluminal cholesterol micellization. Moreover, the upregulation of thermogenesis mediated by Uncoupling protein 1 (UCP1) and phosphorylated signal transducer and activator of transcription 3 (p-STAT3) in adipose tissue determines the reduction in proinflammatory cytokines (IL-6, TNF-α and MCP1) and infiltrating macrophages [101], thus contributing to improving insulin sensitivity [89]. Finally, studies carried out in dogs have shown that berberine improves cardiac output and reduces left ventricular end-diastolic pressure and systemic vascular resistance caused by an ischemic injury [102]. The amelioration of hemodynamic parameters and the hypotensive effect was also confirmed in humans [103], suggesting the role of this extract in combination therapy to counteract high blood pressure.

Citrus bergamia Risso et Poiteau (Bergamot) is an endemic plant, growing in Calabria (Southern Italy), that is characterized by a unique composition of flavonoids and glycosides in the extracts derived from the different parts of the fruit (i.e., essential oil, hydro-alcoholic extract, and fruit juice). An additional distinctive feature is the concentration of these bioactive compounds that, in the juice, is more abundant than in other citrus fruits [103,104].

Growing evidence suggests a protective role for bergamot extracts in the management of the metabolic syndrome. Although bergamot polyphenols have been shown to improve insulin resistance and glucose tolerance through the molecular mechanisms that still need to be clarified, several beneficial effects can be imputed to the pleiotropic anti-oxidative, anti-inflammatory, and lipid-lowering effects of bergamot extracts. This peculiar action has been studied in different experimental models (in vitro and in vivo) of metabolic dysfunctions that are commonly considered the main cardiometabolic risk factors.

The antioxidant effect of bergamot was first discovered by testing the activity of the nonvolatile fraction of the bergamot essential oil (BEO-NVF) in an experimental model of neointima hyperplasia. The results showed that the antioxidant effect is mediated by the downregulation of Lectin-like oxidized low-density lipoprotein receptor-1 (LOX-1) receptor and ROS formation that led to a regression of artery injury [105]. The restoration of the total oxidative status has also been confirmed after oral administration of the bergamot polyphenol fraction (BPF), derived from juice and albedo, in an animal model of metabolic associated fatty liver disease (MAFLD). Specifically, it was associated with a reduction in specific markers of oxidative stress, such as c-Jun N-terminal kinase (JNK) and p38 MAP kinase activity, in the liver, and with the restoration of total antioxidant status, measured in the plasma [106]. The neutralization of free radical overproduction is further reflected by the amelioration of the oxidative status of the LDL profile detected in patients with metabolic syndrome. Particularly, BPF administration determined a significant re-arrangement of lipoproteins with a reduction in oxidated LDL small-size atherogenic particles and an increase in large-size antiatherogenic HDL [107]. In addition, in BPF-treated patients, a significant reduction in serum total cholesterol (TC) and LDL-C, probably due to the inhibition of HMG-CoA reductase and triglycerides (TG), was detected. Moreover, the amelioration of these parameters was associated with a significant decrease in serum glucose, transaminases, gamma-glutamyl-transferase, and inflammatory biomarkers, such as TNF-α and C-reactive protein [108]. The anti-inflammatory and lipid-lowering effects afforded by BPF were also confirmed in patients with isolated hypercholesterolemia, mixed hyperlipidaemia (hypercholesterolemia plus hypertriglyceridemia) as well as in patients with mixed hyperlipidaemia and hyperglycaemia [108], suggesting a potential use in the management of T2DM. In accordance with this hypothesis, BPF enriched with a *Cynara cardunculus* extract has shown a beneficial potentiated effect on vascular inflammation and oxidative stress in patients with T2DM and MAFLD [109], which also translated into an improvement of endothelial function and NO-mediated reactive vasodilation [109].

Finally, the BPF administration in rats revealed a very interesting effect; indeed, it can prevent heart failure through direct antioxidant action at the cardiac level, impeding myocyte apoptotic cell death. In addition, apoptosis was counterbalanced by the reduction in attrition in cardiac-resident stem cells with the consequent formation of new myocytes [110].

5. Conclusions

To date, the conjugation of therapies aimed to achieve the control of glucose plasma levels, and the prevention of cardiovascular disease occurring in diabetic patients, still represents a priority considering the growing incidence of hospitalization and death. In this view, a potential approach combining the use of SGLT2i and plant extracts might be considered a promising solution. Indeed, other than their hypoglycaemic effects, the molecular mechanisms underlying the cardioprotective action of SGLT2i could be potentiated through the combination with phytocomplexes able to prevent or limit the main cardiometabolic risk factors [76], thus contributing to better management of diabetic patients.

Author Contributions: M.G. and R.M. (Roberta Macrì) conceptualized, designed, and wrote the manuscript; V.M. (Vincenzo Musolino) and C.C. critically revised the manuscript; A.R.C. contributed to the collection of data and the design of figures; M.S. (Miriam Scicchitano), F.B., L.G., A.C., S.R., F.S., S.N., R.M. (Rocco Mollace), I.B., R.C., M.S. (Maria Serra), and J.M. collected the data; E.P. and V.M. (Vincenzo Mollace) contributed to drafting the article and revised it critically; V.M. (Vincenzo Mollace) supervised the manuscript. All authors have read and agreed to the published version of the manuscript.

Funding: The work was supported by public resources from the Italian Ministry of Research and POR Calabria FESR 2014–2020—PON-MIUR 03PE000_78_1 and PONMIUR 03PE000_78_2. PRIR Calabria Asse 1/Azione 1.5.1/FESR (Progetto AgrInfra Calabria).

Institutional Review Board Statement: Not applicable.

Informed Consent Statement: Not applicable.

Acknowledgments: This work has been supported by PON-MIUR 03PE000_78_1 and PONMIUR 03PE000_78_2. PRIR Calabria Asse 1/Azione 1.5.1/FESR (Progetto AgrInfra Calabria).

Conflicts of Interest: The authors declare no conflict of interest.

References

1. American Diabetes Association Professional Practice Committee. 2. Classification and Diagnosis of Diabetes: Standards of Medical Care in Diabetes-2022. *Diabetes Care* **2022**, *45* (Suppl. S1), S17–S38. [CrossRef]
2. Reid, J.B. Re: Registry. Can we talk. *Radiol. Technol.* **1990**, *61*, 307–308. [PubMed]
3. Silveira Rossi, J.L.; Barbalho, S.M.; Reverete de Araujo, R.; Bechara, M.D.; Sloan, K.P.; Sloan, L.A. Metabolic syndrome and cardiovascular diseases: Going beyond traditional risk factors. *Diabetes/Metab. Res. Rev.* **2022**, *38*, e3502. [CrossRef] [PubMed]
4. American Diabetes Association Professional Practice Committee. 6. Glycemic Targets: Standards of Medical Care in Diabetes-2022. *Diabetes Care* **2022**, *45* (Suppl. S1), S83–S96. [CrossRef] [PubMed]

5. Palmer, S.C.; Tendal, B.; Mustafa, R.A.; Vandvik, P.O.; Li, S.; Hao, Q.; Tunnicliffe, D.; Ruospo, M.; Natale, P.; Saglimbene, V.; et al. Sodium-glucose cotransporter protein-2 (SGLT-2) inhibitors and glucagon-like peptide-1 (GLP-1) receptor agonists for type 2 diabetes: Systematic review and network meta-analysis of randomised controlled trials. *BMJ* **2021**, *372*, m4573. [CrossRef] [PubMed]
6. Larkin, H.D. FDA Expands Empagliflozin Heart Failure Indication. *JAMA* **2022**, *327*, 1219. [CrossRef]
7. Zannad, F.; Ferreira, J.P.; Pocock, S.J.; Anker, S.D.; Butler, J.; Filippatos, G.; Brueckmann, M.; Ofstad, A.P.; Pfarr, E.; Jamal, W.; et al. SGLT2 inhibitors in patients with heart failure with reduced ejection fraction: A meta-analysis of the EMPEROR-Reduced and DAPA-HF trials. *Lancet* **2020**, *396*, 819–829. [CrossRef]
8. Thorvaldsen, T.; Ferrannini, G.; Mellbin, L.; Benson, L.; Cosentino, F.; McMurray, J.; Dahlström, U.; Lund, L.H.; Savarese, G. Eligibility for Dapagliflozin and Empagliflozin in a Real-world Heart Failure Population. *J. Card. Fail.* **2022**, *28*, 1050–1062. [CrossRef]
9. Prattichizzo, F.; de Candia, P.; Ceriello, A. Diabetes and kidney disease: Emphasis on treatment with SGLT-2 inhibitors and GLP-1 receptor agonists. *Metab. Clin. Exp.* **2021**, *120*, 154799. [CrossRef]
10. Zannad, F.; Ferreira, J.P.; Butler, J.; Filippatos, G.; Januzzi, J.L.; Sumin, M.; Zwick, M.; Saadati, M.; Pocock, S.J.; Sattar, N.; et al. Effect of Empagliflozin on Circulating Proteomics in Heart Failure: Mechanistic Insights from the EMPEROR Program. *Eur. Heart J.* **2022**; ehac495, Advance online publication. [CrossRef]
11. Seferovic, P.M.; Ponikowski, P.; Anker, S.D.; Bauersachs, J.; Chioncel, O.; Cleland, J.G.F.; de Boer, R.A.; Drexel, H.; Ben Gal, T.; Hill, L.; et al. Clinical practice update on heart failure 2019: Pharmacotherapy, procedures, devices and patient management. An expert consensus meeting report of the Heart Failure Association of the European Society of Cardiology. *Eur. J. Heart Fail.* **2019**, *21*, 1169–1186. [CrossRef]
12. Jiang, Y.; Yang, P.; Fu, L.; Sun, L.; Shen, W.; Wu, Q. Comparative Cardiovascular Outcomes of SGLT2 Inhibitors in Type 2 Diabetes Mellitus: A Network Meta-Analysis of Randomized Controlled Trials. *Front. Endocrinol.* **2022**, *13*, 802992. [CrossRef] [PubMed]
13. Hoong, C.; Chua, M. SGLT2 Inhibitors as Calorie Restriction Mimetics: Insights on Longevity Pathways and Age-Related Diseases. *Endocrinology* **2021**, *162*, bqab079. [CrossRef] [PubMed]
14. Xu, J.; Hirai, T.; Koya, D.; Kitada, M. Effects of SGLT2 Inhibitors on Atherosclerosis: Lessons from Cardiovascular Clinical Outcomes in Type 2 Diabetic Patients and Basic Researches. *J. Clin. Med.* **2021**, *11*, 137. [CrossRef] [PubMed]
15. Seferović, P.M.; Fragasso, G.; Petrie, M.; Mullens, W.; Ferrari, R.; Thum, T.; Bauersachs, J.; Anker, S.D.; Ray, R.; Çavuşoğlu, Y.; et al. Sodium-glucose co-transporter 2 inhibitors in heart failure: Beyond glycaemic control. A position paper of the Heart Failure Association of the European Society of Cardiology. *Eur. J. Heart Fail.* **2020**, *22*, 1495–1503. [CrossRef] [PubMed]
16. Booij, H.G.; Koning, A.M.; van Goor, H.; de Boer, R.A.; Westenbrink, B.D. Selecting heart failure patients for metabolic interventions. *Expert Rev. Mol. Diagn* **2017**, *17*, 141–152. [CrossRef]
17. Aubert, G.; Martin, O.J.; Horton, J.L.; Lai, L.; Vega, R.B.; Leone, T.C.; Koves, T.; Gardell, S.J.; Krüger, M.; Hoppel, C.L.; et al. The Failing Heart Relies on Ketone Bodies as a Fuel. *Circulation* **2016**, *133*, 698–705. [CrossRef]
18. Bedi, K.C.; Snyder, N.W.; Brandimarto, J.; Aziz, M.; Mesaros, C.; Worth, A.J.; Wang, L.L.; Javaheri, A.; Blair, I.A.; Margulies, K.B.; et al. Evidence for Intramyocardial Disruption of Lipid Metabolism and Increased Myocardial Ketone Utilization in Advanced Human Heart Failure. *Circulation* **2016**, *133*, 706–716. [CrossRef]
19. Yurista, S.R.; Silljé, H.H.W.; Oberdorf-Maass, S.U.; Schouten, E.M.; Pavez Giani, M.G.; Hillebrands, J.L.; van Goor, H.; van Veldhuisen, D.J.; de Boer, R.A.; Westenbrink, B.D. Sodium-glucose co-transporter 2 inhibition with empagliflozin improves cardiac function in non-diabetic rats with left ventricular dysfunction after myocardial infarction. *Eur. J. Heart Fail.* **2019**, *21*, 862–873. [CrossRef]
20. Verma, S.; Rawat, S.; Ho, K.L.; Wagg, C.S.; Zhang, L.; Teoh, H.; Dyck, J.E.; Uddin, G.M.; Oudit, G.Y.; Mayoux, E.; et al. Empagliflozin Increases Cardiac Energy Production in Diabetes: Novel Translational Insights Into the Heart Failure Benefits of SGLT2 Inhibitors. *JACC Basic Transl. Sci.* **2018**, *3*, 575–587. [CrossRef]
21. Levey, A.S.; Stevens, L.A.; Schmid, C.H.; Zhang, Y.L.; Castro, A.F.; Feldman, H.I.; Kusek, J.W.; Eggers, P.; Van Lente, F.; Greene, T.; et al. A new equation to estimate glomerular filtration rate. *Ann. Intern. Med.* **2009**, *150*, 604–612. [CrossRef]
22. Burhans, M.S.; Hagman, D.K.; Kuzma, J.N.; Schmidt, K.A.; Kratz, M. Contribution of Adipose Tissue Inflammation to the Development of Type 2 Diabetes Mellitus. *Compr. Physiol.* **2018**, *9*, 1–58. [CrossRef] [PubMed]
23. Sukhanov, S.; Higashi, Y.; Yoshida, T.; Mummidi, S.; Aroor, A.R.; Jeffrey Russell, J.; Bender, S.B.; DeMarco, V.G.; Chandrasekar, B. The SGLT2 inhibitor Empagliflozin attenuates interleukin-17A-induced human aortic smooth muscle cell proliferation and migration by targeting TRAF3IP2/ROS/NLRP3/Caspase-1-dependent IL-1β and IL-18 secretion. *Cell. Signal.* **2021**, *77*, 109825. [CrossRef] [PubMed]
24. Kim, S.R.; Lee, S.G.; Kim, S.H.; Kim, J.H.; Choi, E.; Cho, W.; Rim, J.H.; Hwang, I.; Lee, C.J.; Lee, M.; et al. SGLT2 inhibition modulates NLRP3 inflammasome activity via ketones and insulin in diabetes with cardiovascular disease. *Nat. Commun.* **2020**, *11*, 2127. [CrossRef] [PubMed]
25. Bajpai, A.; Tilley, D.G. The Role of Leukocytes in Diabetic Cardiomyopathy. *Front. Physiol.* **2018**, *9*, 1547. [CrossRef]
26. Paolisso, P.; Bergamaschi, L.; Santulli, G.; Gallinoro, E.; Cesaro, A.; Gragnano, F.; Sardu, C.; Mileva, N.; Foà, A.; Armillotta, M.; et al. Infarct size, inflammatory burden, and admission hyperglycemia in diabetic patients with acute myocardial infarction treated with SGLT2-inhibitors: A multicenter international registry. *Cardiovasc. Diabetol.* **2022**, *21*, 77. [CrossRef]

27. Packer, M. Activation and Inhibition of Sodium-Hydrogen Exchanger Is a Mechanism That Links the Pathophysiology and Treatment of Diabetes Mellitus With That of Heart Failure. *Circulation* 2017, *136*, 1548–1559. [CrossRef]
28. Chen, S.; Coronel, R.; Hollmann, M.W.; Weber, N.C.; Zuurbier, C.J. Direct cardiac effects of SGLT2 inhibitors. *Cardiovasc. Diabetol.* 2022, *21*, 45. [CrossRef]
29. Baartscheer, A.; Schumacher, C.A.; Wüst, R.C.; Fiolet, J.W.; Stienen, G.J.; Coronel, R.; Zuurbier, C.J. Empagliflozin decreases myocardial cytoplasmic Na+ through inhibition of the cardiac Na+/H+ exchanger in rats and rabbits. *Diabetologia* 2017, *60*, 568–573. [CrossRef]
30. Habibi, J.; Aroor, A.R.; Sowers, J.R.; Jia, G.; Hayden, M.R.; Garro, M.; Barron, B.; Mayoux, E.; Rector, R.S.; Whaley-Connell, A.; et al. Sodium glucose transporter 2 (SGLT2) inhibition with empagliflozin improves cardiac diastolic function in a female rodent model of diabetes. *Cardiovasc. Diabetol.* 2017, *16*, 9. [CrossRef]
31. Hammoudi, N.; Jeong, D.; Singh, R.; Farhat, A.; Komajda, M.; Mayoux, E.; Hajjar, R.; Lebeche, D. Empagliflozin Improves Left Ventricular Diastolic Dysfunction in a Genetic Model of Type 2 Diabetes. *Cardiovasc. Drugs* 2017, *31*, 233–246. [CrossRef]
32. Escudero, D.S.; Pérez, N.G.; Díaz, R.G. Myocardial Impact of NHE1 Regulation by Sildenafil. *Front. Cardiovasc. Med.* 2021, *8*, 617519. [CrossRef] [PubMed]
33. Valdivia, C.R.; Chu, W.W.; Pu, J.; Foell, J.D.; Haworth, R.A.; Wolff, M.R.; Kamp, T.J.; Makielski, J.C. Increased late sodium current in myocytes from a canine heart failure model and from failing human heart. *J. Mol. Cell. Cardiol.* 2005, *38*, 475–483. [CrossRef] [PubMed]
34. Trum, M.; Riechel, J.; Wagner, S. Cardioprotection by SGLT2 Inhibitors-Does It All Come Down to Na+. *Int. J. Mol. Sci.* 2021, *22*, 7976. [CrossRef]
35. Li, C.; Zhang, J.; Xue, M.; Li, X.; Han, F.; Liu, X.; Xu, L.; Lu, Y.; Cheng, Y.; Li, T.; et al. SGLT2 inhibition with empagliflozin attenuates myocardial oxidative stress and fibrosis in diabetic mice heart. *Cardiovasc. Diabetol.* 2019, *18*, 15. [CrossRef] [PubMed]
36. Cinti, F.; Moffa, S.; Impronta, F.; Cefalo, C.M.; Sun, V.A.; Sorice, G.P.; Mezza, T.; Giaccari, A. Spotlight on ertugliflozin and its potential in the treatment of type 2 diabetes: Evidence to date. *Drug Des. Devel.* 2017, *11*, 2905–2919. [CrossRef]
37. Zinman, B.; Inzucchi, S.E.; Lachin, J.M.; Wanner, C.; Ferrari, R.; Fitchett, D.; Bluhmki, E.; Hantel, S.; Kempthorne-Rawson, J.; Newman, J.; et al. Rationale, design, and baseline characteristics of a randomized, placebo-controlled cardiovascular outcome trial of empagliflozin (EMPA-REG OUTCOME™). *Cardiovasc. Diabetol.* 2014, *13*, 102. [CrossRef]
38. Szekeres, Z.; Toth, K.; Szabados, E. The Effects of SGLT2 Inhibitors on Lipid Metabolism. *Metabolites* 2021, *11*, 87. [CrossRef]
39. Hayashi, T.; Fukui, T.; Nakanishi, N.; Yamamoto, S.; Tomoyasu, M.; Osamura, A.; Ohara, M.; Yamamoto, T.; Ito, Y.; Hirano, T. Dapagliflozin decreases small dense low-density lipoprotein-cholesterol and increases high-density lipoprotein 2-cholesterol in patients with type 2 diabetes: Comparison with sitagliptin. *Cardiovasc. Diabetol.* 2017, *16*, 8. [CrossRef]
40. Kamijo, Y.; Ishii, H.; Yamamoto, T.; Kobayashi, K.; Asano, H.; Miake, S.; Kanda, E.; Urata, H.; Yoshida, M. Potential Impact on Lipoprotein Subfractions in Type 2 Diabetes. *Clin. Med. Insights Endocrinol. Diabetes* 2019, *12*, 1179551419866811. [CrossRef]
41. Shi, F.H.; Li, H.; Shen, L.; Fu, J.J.; Ma, J.; Gu, Z.C.; Lin, H.W. High-dose sodium-glucose co-transporter-2 inhibitors are superior in type 2 diabetes: A meta-analysis of randomized clinical trials. *Diabetes Obes. Metab.* 2021, *23*, 2125–2136. [CrossRef]
42. Li, L.; Li, Q.; Huang, W.; Han, Y.; Tan, H.; An, M.; Xiang, Q.; Zhou, R.; Yang, L.; Cheng, Y. Dapagliflozin Alleviates Hepatic Steatosis by Restoring Autophagy via the AMPK-mTOR Pathway. *Front. Pharm.* 2021, *12*, 589273. [CrossRef]
43. Ji, W.; Zhao, M.; Wang, M.; Yan, W.; Liu, Y.; Ren, S.; Lu, J.; Wang, B.; Chen, L. Effects of canagliflozin on weight loss in high-fat diet-induced obese mice. *PLoS ONE* 2017, *12*, e0179960. [CrossRef]
44. Chinetti, G.; Lestavel, S.; Bocher, V.; Remaley, A.T.; Neve, B.; Torra, I.P.; Teissier, E.; Minnich, A.; Jaye, M.; Duverger, N.; et al. PPAR-alpha and PPAR-gamma activators induce cholesterol removal from human macrophage foam cells through stimulation of the ABCA1 pathway. *Nat. Med.* 2001, *7*, 53–58. [CrossRef]
45. Cai, X.; Yang, W.; Gao, X.; Chen, Y.; Zhou, L.; Zhang, S.; Han, X.; Ji, L. The Association Between the Dosage of SGLT2 Inhibitor and Weight Reduction in Type 2 Diabetes Patients: A Meta-Analysis. *Obesity* 2018, *26*, 70–80. [CrossRef]
46. Clamp, L.D.; Hume, D.J.; Lambert, E.V.; Kroff, J. Enhanced insulin sensitivity in successful, long-term weight loss maintainers compared with matched controls with no weight loss history. *Nutr. Diabetes* 2017, *7*, e282. [CrossRef]
47. Xu, L.; Ota, T. Emerging roles of SGLT2 inhibitors in obesity and insulin resistance: Focus on fat browning and macrophage polarization. *Adipocyte* 2018, *7*, 121–128. [CrossRef]
48. Xu, L.; Nagata, N.; Nagashimada, M.; Zhuge, F.; Ni, Y.; Chen, G.; Mayoux, E.; Kaneko, S.; Ota, T. SGLT2 Inhibition by Empagliflozin Promotes Fat Utilization and Browning and Attenuates Inflammation and Insulin Resistance by Polarizing M2 Macrophages in Diet-induced Obese Mice. *EBioMedicine* 2017, *20*, 137–149. [CrossRef]
49. Koike, Y.; Shirabe, S.I.; Maeda, H.; Yoshimoto, A.; Arai, K.; Kumakura, A.; Hirao, K.; Terauchi, Y. Effect of canagliflozin on the overall clinical state including insulin resistance in Japanese patients with type 2 diabetes mellitus. *Diabetes Res. Clin. Pr.* 2019, *149*, 140–146. [CrossRef]
50. Singh, A.K.; Unnikrishnan, A.G.; Zargar, A.H.; Kumar, A.; Das, A.K.; Saboo, B.; Sinha, B.; Gangopadhyay, K.K.; Talwalkar, P.G.; Ghosal, S.; et al. Evidence-Based Consensus on Positioning of SGLT2i in Type 2 Diabetes Mellitus in Indians. *Diabetes* 2019, *10*, 393–428. [CrossRef]
51. Okamoto, A.; Yokokawa, H.; Sanada, H.; Naito, T. Changes in Levels of Biomarkers Associated with Adipocyte Function and Insulin and Glucagon Kinetics During Treatment with Dapagliflozin Among Obese Type 2 Diabetes Mellitus Patients. *Drugs R D* 2016, *16*, 255–261. [CrossRef]

52. Sano, M. Sodium glucose cotransporter (SGLT)-2 inhibitors alleviate the renal stress responsible for sympathetic activation. *Adv. Cardiovasc. Dis.* **2020**, *14*, 1753944720939383. [CrossRef]
53. Sasaki, T.; Sugawara, M.; Fukuda, M. Sodium-glucose cotransporter 2 inhibitor-induced changes in body composition and simultaneous changes in metabolic profile: 52-week prospective LIGHT (Luseogliflozin: The Components of Weight Loss in Japanese Patients with Type 2 Diabetes Mellitus) Study. *J. Diabetes Investig.* **2019**, *10*, 108–117. [CrossRef]
54. Cemerikić, D.; Wilcox, C.S.; Giebisch, G. Intracellular potential and K+ activity in rat kidney proximal tubular cells in acidosis and K+ depletion. *J. Membr. Biol.* **1982**, *69*, 159–165. [CrossRef]
55. Layton, A.T.; Vallon, V.; Edwards, A. Predicted consequences of diabetes and SGLT inhibition on transport and oxygen consumption along a rat nephron. *Am. J. Physiol. Ren. Physiol.* **2016**, *310*, F1269–F1283. [CrossRef]
56. Wilcox, C.S. Antihypertensive and Renal Mechanisms of SGLT2 (Sodium-Glucose Linked Transporter 2) Inhibitors. *Hypertension* **2020**, *75*, 894–901. [CrossRef]
57. Varzideh, F.; Kansakar, U.; Santulli, G. SGLT2 inhibitors in cardiovascular medicine. *Eur. Heart J. Cardiovasc. Pharmacother.* **2021**, *7*, e67–e68. [CrossRef]
58. Cherney, D.Z.I.; Cooper, M.E.; Tikkanen, I.; Pfarr, E.; Johansen, O.E.; Woerle, H.J.; Broedl, U.C.; Lund, S.S. Pooled analysis of Phase III trials indicate contrasting influences of renal function on blood pressure, body weight, and HbA1c reductions with empagliflozin. *Kidney Int.* **2018**, *93*, 231–244. [CrossRef]
59. Thiele, K.; Rau, M.; Hartmann, N.K.; Möller, M.; Möllmann, J.; Jankowski, J.; Keszei, A.P.; Böhm, M.; Floege, J.; Marx, N.; et al. Empagliflozin reduces markers of acute kidney injury in patients with acute decompensated heart failure. *ESC Heart Fail.* **2022**, *9*, 2233–2238. [CrossRef] [PubMed]
60. Onishi, A.; Fu, Y.; Patel, R.; Darshi, M.; Crespo-Masip, M.; Huang, W.; Song, P.; Freeman, B.; Kim, Y.C.; Soleimani, M.; et al. A role for tubular Na+/H+ exchanger NHE3 in the natriuretic effect of the SGLT2 inhibitor empagliflozin. *Am. J. Physiol.-Ren. Physiol.* **2020**, *319*, F712–F728. [CrossRef] [PubMed]
61. Lipkowitz, M.S. Regulation of uric acid excretion by the kidney. *Curr. Rheumatol. Rep.* **2012**, *14*, 179–188. [CrossRef]
62. Gisler, S.M.; Madjdpour, C.; Bacic, D.; Pribanic, S.; Taylor, S.S.; Biber, J.; Murer, H. PDZK1: II. an anchoring site for the PKA-binding protein D-AKAP2 in renal proximal tubular cells. *Kidney Int.* **2003**, *64*, 1746–1754. [CrossRef]
63. Wilcox, C.S.; Shen, W.; Boulton, D.W.; Leslie, B.R.; Griffen, S.C. Interaction Between the Sodium-Glucose-Linked Transporter 2 Inhibitor Dapagliflozin and the Loop Diuretic Bumetanide in Normal Human Subjects. *J. Am. Heart Assoc.* **2018**, *7*, e007046. [CrossRef]
64. Cristóbal-García, M.; García-Arroyo, F.E.; Tapia, E.; Osorio, H.; Arellano-Buendía, A.S.; Madero, M.; Rodríguez-Iturbe, B.; Pedraza-Chaverrí, J.; Correa, F.; Zazueta, C.; et al. Renal oxidative stress induced by long-term hyperuricemia alters mitochondrial function and maintains systemic hypertension. *Oxid. Med. Cell. Longev.* **2015**, *2015*, 535686. [CrossRef]
65. Rahman, A.; Fujisawa, Y.; Nakano, D.; Hitomi, H.; Nishiyama, A. Effect of a selective SGLT2 inhibitor, luseogliflozin, on circadian rhythm of sympathetic nervous function and locomotor activities in metabolic syndrome rats. *Clin. Exp. Pharm. Physiol.* **2017**, *44*, 522–525. [CrossRef]
66. Li, C.Y.; Wang, L.X.; Dong, S.S.; Hong, Y.; Zhou, X.H.; Zheng, W.W.; Zheng, C. Phlorizin Exerts Direct Protective Effects on Palmitic Acid (PA)-Induced Endothelial Dysfunction by Activating the PI3K/AKT/eNOS Signaling Pathway and Increasing the Levels of Nitric Oxide (NO). *Med. Sci. Monit. Basic. Res.* **2018**, *24*, 1–9. [CrossRef]
67. Aroor, A.R.; Das, N.A.; Carpenter, A.J.; Habibi, J.; Jia, G.; Ramirez-Perez, F.I.; Martinez-Lemus, L.; Manrique-Acevedo, C.M.; Hayden, M.R.; Duta, C.; et al. Glycemic control by the SGLT2 inhibitor empagliflozin decreases aortic stiffness, renal resistivity index and kidney injury. *Cardiovasc. Diabetol.* **2018**, *17*, 108. [CrossRef]
68. Cherney, D.Z.; Perkins, B.A.; Soleymanlou, N.; Har, R.; Fagan, N.; Johansen, O.E.; Woerle, H.J.; von Eynatten, M.; Broedl, U.C. The effect of empagliflozin on arterial stiffness and heart rate variability in subjects with uncomplicated type 1 diabetes mellitus. *Cardiovasc. Diabetol.* **2014**, *13*, 28. [CrossRef]
69. Wei, R.; Wang, W.; Pan, Q.; Guo, L. Effects of SGLT-2 Inhibitors on Vascular Endothelial Function and Arterial Stiffness in Subjects With Type 2 Diabetes: A Systematic Review and Meta-Analysis of Randomized Controlled Trials. *Front. Endocrinol.* **2022**, *13*, 826640. [CrossRef]
70. Sposito, A.C.; Breder, I.; Soares, A.; Kimura-Medorima, S.T.; Munhoz, D.B.; Cintra, R.; Bonilha, I.; Oliveira, D.C.; Breder, J.C.; Cavalcante, P.; et al. Dapagliflozin effect on endothelial dysfunction in diabetic patients with atherosclerotic disease: A randomized active-controlled trial. *Cardiovasc. Diabetol.* **2021**, *20*, 74. [CrossRef]
71. Park, S.H.; Belcastro, E.; Hasan, H.; Matsushita, K.; Marchandot, B.; Abbas, M.; Toti, F.; Auger, C.; Jesel, L.; Ohlmann, P.; et al. Angiotensin II-induced upregulation of SGLT1 and 2 contributes to human microparticle-stimulated endothelial senescence and dysfunction: Protective effect of gliflozins. *Cardiovasc. Diabetol.* **2021**, *20*, 65. [CrossRef]
72. Mone, P.; Lombardi, A.; Kansakar, U.; Varzideh, F.; Jankauskas, S.S.; Pansini, A.; De Gennaro, S.; Famiglietti, M.; Macina, G.; Frullone, S.; et al. Empagliflozin improves the microRNA signature of endothelial dysfunction in patients with HFpEF and diabetes. *J. Pharmacol. Exp. Ther.* **2022**, *382*, JPET-AR-2022-001251. [CrossRef]
73. Mone, P.; Varzideh, F.; Jankauskas, S.S.; Pansini, A.; Lombardi, A.; Frullone, S.; Santulli, G. SGLT2 Inhibition via Empagliflozin Improves Endothelial Function and Reduces Mitochondrial Oxidative Stress: Insights From Frail Hypertensive and Diabetic Patients. *Hypertension* **2022**, *79*, 1633–1643. [CrossRef]

74. Zhang, X.Z.; Zhao, Y.B.; Li, C.M.; Chen, D.M.; Wang, G.P.; Chang, R.F.; Shu, H.R. Potential polyphenol markers of phase change in apple (Malus domestica). *J. Plant Physiol.* **2007**, *164*, 574–580. [CrossRef]
75. Mollace, V.; Rosano, G.M.C.; Anker, S.D.; Coats, A.J.S.; Seferovic, P.; Mollace, R.; Tavernese, A.; Gliozzi, M.; Musolino, V.; Carresi, C.; et al. Pathophysiological Basis for Nutraceutical Supplementation in Heart Failure: A Comprehensive Review. *Nutrients* **2021**, *13*, 257. [CrossRef]
76. Lee, J.; Noh, S.; Lim, S.; Kim, B. Plant Extracts for Type 2 Diabetes: From Traditional Medicine to Modern Drug Discovery. *Antioxidants* **2021**, *10*, 81. [CrossRef]
77. Cho, H.; Thorvaldsen, J.L.; Chu, Q.; Feng, F.; Birnbaum, M.J. Akt1/PKBalpha is required for normal growth but dispensable for maintenance of glucose homeostasis in mice. *J. Biol. Chem.* **2001**, *276*, 38349–38352. [CrossRef]
78. Dong, X.C.; Copps, K.D.; Guo, S.; Li, Y.; Kollipara, R.; DePinho, R.A.; White, M.F. Inactivation of hepatic Foxo1 by insulin signaling is required for adaptive nutrient homeostasis and endocrine growth regulation. *Cell Metab.* **2008**, *8*, 65–76. [CrossRef]
79. Schmoll, D.; Walker, K.S.; Alessi, D.R.; Grempler, R.; Burchell, A.; Guo, S.; Walther, R.; Unterman, T.G. Regulation of glucose-6-phosphatase gene expression by protein kinase Balpha and the forkhead transcription factor FKHR. Evidence for insulin response unit-dependent and -independent effects of insulin on promoter activity. *J. Biol. Chem.* **2000**, *275*, 36324–36333. [CrossRef]
80. Cook, J.R.; Langlet, F.; Kido, Y.; Accili, D. Pathogenesis of selective insulin resistance in isolated hepatocytes. *J. Biol. Chem.* **2015**, *290*, 13972–13980. [CrossRef]
81. Nakae, J.; Kitamura, T.; Silver, D.L.; Accili, D. The forkhead transcription factor Foxo1 (Fkhr) confers insulin sensitivity onto glucose-6-phosphatase expression. *J. Clin. Invest.* **2001**, *108*, 1359–1367. [CrossRef]
82. He, L.; Li, Y.; Zeng, N.; Stiles, B.L. Regulation of basal expression of hepatic PEPCK and G6Pase by AKT2. *Biochem. J.* **2020**, *477*, 1021–1031. [CrossRef]
83. De Las Heras, N.; Valero-Muñoz, M.; Martín-Fernández, B.; Ballesteros, S.; López-Farré, A.; Ruiz-Roso, B.; Lahera, V. Molecular factors involved in the hypolipidemic- and insulin-sensitizing effects of a ginger (Zingiber officinale Roscoe) extract in rats fed a high-fat diet. *Appl. Physiol. Nutr. Metab.* **2017**, *42*, 209–215. [CrossRef]
84. Gomaa, A.A.; Makboul, R.M.; Al-Mokhtar, M.A.; Nicola, M.A. Polyphenol-rich Boswellia serrata gum prevents cognitive impairment and insulin resistance of diabetic rats through inhibition of GSK3β activity, oxidative stress and pro-inflammatory cytokines. *Biomed. Pharm.* **2019**, *109*, 281–292. [CrossRef]
85. Mahmoud, M.F.; El Ashry, F.E.; El Maraghy, N.N.; Fahmy, A. Studies on the antidiabetic activities of Momordica charantia fruit juice in streptozotocin-induced diabetic rats. *Pharm. Biol.* **2017**, *55*, 758–765. [CrossRef]
86. Ngueguim, F.T.; Esse, E.C.; Dzeufiet, P.D.; Gounoue, R.K.; Bilanda, D.C.; Kamtchouing, P.; Dimo, T. Oxidised palm oil and sucrose induced hyperglycemia in normal rats: Effects of Sclerocarya birrea stem barks aqueous extract. *BMC Complement. Altern. Med.* **2016**, *16*, 47. [CrossRef]
87. Mousum, S.A.; Ahmed, S.; Gawali, B.; Kwatra, M.; Ahmed, A.; Lahkar, M. Nyctanthes arbor-tristis leaf extract ameliorates hyperlipidemia- and hyperglycemia-associated nephrotoxicity by improving anti-oxidant and anti-inflammatory status in high-fat diet-streptozotocin-induced diabetic rats. *Inflammopharmacology* **2018**, *26*, 1415–1428. [CrossRef]
88. Shim, D.W.; Han, J.W.; Ji, Y.E.; Shin, W.Y.; Koppula, S.; Kim, M.K.; Kim, T.K.; Park, P.J.; Kang, T.B.; Lee, K.H. Cichorium intybus Linn. Extract Prevents Type 2 Diabetes Through Inhibition of NLRP3 Inflammasome Activation. *J. Med. Food* **2016**, *19*, 310–317. [CrossRef]
89. Pellegrini, C.; Fornai, M.; Antonioli, L.; Blandizzi, C.; Calderone, V. Phytochemicals as Novel Therapeutic Strategies for NLRP3 Inflammasome-Related Neurological, Metabolic, and Inflammatory Diseases. *Int. J. Mol. Sci.* **2019**, *20*, 2876. [CrossRef]
90. Lee, H.; Choi, J.; Shin, S.S.; Yoon, M. Effects of Korean red ginseng (Panax ginseng) on obesity and adipose inflammation in ovariectomized mice. *J. Ethnopharmacol.* **2016**, *178*, 229–237. [CrossRef]
91. Kozics, K.; Klusová, V.; Srančíková, A.; Mučaji, P.; Slameňová, D.; Hunáková, L.; Kusznierewicz, B.; Horváthová, E. Effects of Salvia officinalis and Thymus vulgaris on oxidant-induced DNA damage and antioxidant status in HepG2 cells. *Food Chem.* **2013**, *141*, 2198–2206. [CrossRef]
92. Govindaraj, J.; Sorimuthu Pillai, S. Rosmarinic acid modulates the antioxidant status and protects pancreatic tissues from glucolipotoxicity mediated oxidative stress in high-fat diet: Streptozotocin-induced diabetic rats. *Mol. Cell. Biochem.* **2015**, *404*, 143–159. [CrossRef] [PubMed]
93. Gonçalves, C.; Fernandes, D.; Silva, I.; Mateus, V. Potential Anti-Inflammatory Effect of Rosmarinus officinalis in Preclinical In Vivo Models of Inflammation. *Molecules* **2022**, *27*, 609. [CrossRef] [PubMed]
94. Carresi, C.; Gliozzi, M.; Musolino, V.; Scicchitano, M.; Scarano, F.; Bosco, F.; Nucera, S.; Maiuolo, J.; Macrì, R.; Ruga, S.; et al. The Effect of Natural Antioxidants in the Development of Metabolic Syndrome: Focus on Bergamot Polyphenolic Fraction. *Nutrients* **2020**, *12*, 1504. [CrossRef] [PubMed]
95. Sharma, S.; Pathak, S.; Gupta, G.; Sharma, S.K.; Singh, L.; Sharma, R.K.; Mishra, A.; Dua, K. Pharmacological evaluation of aqueous extract of syzigium cumini for its antihyperglycemic and antidyslipidemic properties in diabetic rats fed a high cholesterol diet-Role of PPARγ and PPARα. *Biomed. Pharm.* **2017**, *89*, 447–453. [CrossRef]
96. Arayne, M.S.; Sultana, N.; Bahadur, S.S. The berberis story: Berberis vulgaris in therapeutics. *Pak. J. Pharm. Sci.* **2007**, *20*, 83–92.
97. Tomosaka, H.; Chin, Y.W.; Salim, A.A.; Keller, W.J.; Chai, H.; Kinghorn, A.D. Antioxidant and cytoprotective compounds from Berberis vulgaris (barberry). *Phytother. Res.* **2008**, *22*, 979–981. [CrossRef]

98. Imenshahidi, M.; Qaredashi, R.; Hashemzaei, M.; Hosseinzadeh, H. Inhibitory Effect of Berberis vulgaris Aqueous Extract on Acquisition and Reinstatement Effects of Morphine in Conditioned Place Preferences (CPP) in Mice. *Jundishapur. J. Nat. Pharm. Prod.* **2014**, *9*, e16145. [CrossRef]
99. Grundy, S.M.; Vega, G.L.; Yuan, Z.; Battisti, W.P.; Brady, W.E.; Palmisano, J. Effectiveness and tolerability of simvastatin plus fenofibrate for combined hyperlipidemia (the SAFARI trial). *Am. J. Cardiol.* **2005**, *95*, 462–468. [CrossRef]
100. Vergès, B. Fenofibrate therapy and cardiovascular protection in diabetes: Recommendations after FIELD. *Curr. Opin. Lipidol.* **2006**, *17*, 653–658. [CrossRef]
101. Lin, J.; Cai, Q.; Liang, B.; Wu, L.; Zhuang, Y.; He, Y.; Lin, W. Berberine, a Traditional Chinese Medicine, Reduces Inflammation in Adipose Tissue, Polarizes M2 Macrophages, and Increases Energy Expenditure in Mice Fed a High-Fat Diet. *Med. Sci. Monit.* **2019**, *25*, 87–97. [CrossRef]
102. Zhang, C.H.; Yu, R.Y.; Liu, Y.H.; Tu, X.Y.; Tu, J.; Wang, Y.S.; Xu, G.L. Interaction of baicalin with berberine for glucose uptake in 3T3-L1 adipocytes and HepG2 hepatocytes. *J. Ethnopharmacol.* **2014**, *151*, 864–872. [CrossRef] [PubMed]
103. Gardana, C.; Nalin, F.; Simonetti, P. Evaluation of flavonoids and furanocoumarins from Citrus bergamia (Bergamot) juice and identification of new compounds. *Molecules* **2008**, *13*, 2220–2228. [CrossRef] [PubMed]
104. Salerno, R.; Casale, F.; Calandruccio, C.; Procopio, A. Characterization of flavonoids in Citrus bergamia (Bergamot) polyphenolic fraction by liquid chromatography–high resolution mass spectrometry (LC/HRMS). *Pharma Nutr.* **2016**, *4*, S1–S7. [CrossRef]
105. Mollace, V.; Ragusa, S.; Sacco, I.; Muscoli, C.; Sculco, F.; Visalli, V.; Palma, E.; Muscoli, S.; Mondello, L.; Dugo, P.; et al. The protective effect of bergamot oil extract on lecitine-like oxyLDL receptor-1 expression in balloon injury-related neointima formation. *J. Cardiovasc. Pharm.* **2008**, *13*, 120–129. [CrossRef]
106. Musolino, V.; Gliozzi, M.; Scarano, F.; Bosco, F.; Scicchitano, M.; Nucera, S.; Carresi, C.; Ruga, S.; Zito, M.C.; Maiuolo, J.; et al. Bergamot Polyphenols Improve Dyslipidemia and Pathophysiological Features in a Mouse Model of Non-Alcoholic Fatty Liver Disease. *Sci. Rep.* **2020**, *10*, 2565. [CrossRef]
107. Gliozzi, M.; Carresi, C.; Musolino, V.; Palma, E.; Muscoli, C.; Vitale, C.; Gratteri, S.; Muscianisi, G.; Janda, E.; Muscoli, S.; et al. The effect of bergamot-derived polyphenolic fraction on LDL small dense particles and non-alcoholic fatty liver disease in patients with metabolic syndrome. *Adv. Biol. Chem.* **2014**, *4*, 129–137. [CrossRef]
108. Mollace, V.; Sacco, I.; Janda, E.; Malara, C.; Ventrice, D.; Colica, C.; Visalli, V.; Muscoli, S.; Ragusa, S.; Muscoli, C.; et al. Hypolipemic and hypoglycaemic activity of bergamot polyphenols: From animal models to human studies. *Fitoterapia* **2011**, *82*, 309–316. [CrossRef]
109. Musolino, V.; Gliozzi, M.; Bombardelli, E.; Nucera, S.; Carresi, C.; Maiuolo, J.; Mollace, R.; Paone, S.; Bosco, F.; Scarano, F.; et al. The synergistic effect of Citrus bergamia and Cynara cardunculus extracts on vascular inflammation and oxidative stress in non-alcoholic fatty liver disease. *J. Tradit. Complement. Med.* **2020**, *10*, 268–274. [CrossRef] [PubMed]
110. Carresi, C.; Scicchitano, M.; Scarano, F.; Macrì, R.; Bosco, F.; Nucera, S.; Ruga, S.; Zito, M.C.; Mollace, R.; Guarnieri, L.; et al. The Potential Properties of Natural Compounds in Cardiac Stem Cell Activation: Their Role in Myocardial Regeneration. *Nutrients* **2021**, *13*, 275. [CrossRef]

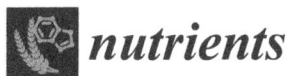

Article

Beneficial Effects of Essential Oils from the Mediterranean Diet on Gut Microbiota and Their Metabolites in Ischemic Heart Disease and Type-2 Diabetes Mellitus

María José Sánchez-Quintero [1,2,3], Josué Delgado [1,2,3,4,*], Dina Medina-Vera [1,2,5,6], Víctor M. Becerra-Muñoz [1,2,3], María Isabel Queipo-Ortuño [1,7,8], Mario Estévez [9], Isaac Plaza-Andrades [1,7], Jorge Rodríguez-Capitán [1,2,3], Pedro L. Sánchez [3,10], Maria G. Crespo-Leiro [3,11], Manuel F. Jiménez-Navarro [1,2,3,6,*] and Francisco Javier Pavón-Morón [1,2,3,5]

1. Instituto de Investigación Biomédica de Málaga y Plataforma en Nanomedicina (IBIMA-Plataforma BIONAND), 29590 Málaga, Spain
2. Unidad de Gestión Clínica Área del Corazón, Hospital Universitario Virgen de la Victoria, 29010 Málaga, Spain
3. Centro de Investigación Biomédica en Red de Enfermedades Cardiovasculares (CIBERCV), Instituto de Salud Carlos III, 28029 Madrid, Spain
4. Higiene y Seguridad Alimentaria, Facultad de Veterinaria, IPROCAR, Universidad de Extremadura, 10003 Cáceres, Spain
5. Unidad de Gestión Clínica de Salud Mental, Hospital Regional Universitario de Málaga, 29010 Málaga, Spain
6. Departamento de Dermatología y Medicina, Facultad de Medicina, Universidad de Málaga (UMA), 29010 Málaga, Spain
7. Unidad de Gestión Clínica Intercentros de Oncología Médica, Hospitales Universitarios Regional y Virgen de la Victoria y Centro de Investigaciones Médico Sanitarias (CIMES), 29010 Málaga, Spain
8. Departamento de Especialidades Quirúrgicas, Bioquímica e Inmunología, Facultad de Medicina, Universidad de Málaga (UMA), 29010 Málaga, Spain
9. Instituto Universitario de Investigación de Carne y Productos Cárnicos (IPROCAR), Universidad de Extremadura (UEX), 10003 Cáceres, Spain
10. Servicio de Cardiología, Hospital Universitario de Salamanca, Universidad de Salamanca, Instituto de Investigación Biomédica de Salamanca (IBSAL), 37007 Salamanca, Spain
11. Servicio de Cardiología, Complexo Hospitalario Universitario A Coruña (CHUAC), Universidade da Coruña (UDC), Instituto Investigación Biomédica A Coruña (INIBIC), 15006 A Coruña, Spain
* Correspondence: jdperon@unex.es (J.D.); mjimeneznavarro@uma.es (M.F.J.-N.); Tel.: +34-927251425 (J.D.)

Abstract: Ischemic heart disease (IHD) and type-2 diabetes mellitus (T2DM) remain major health problems worldwide and commonly coexist in individuals. Gut microbial metabolites, such as trimethylamine N-oxide (TMAO) and short-chain fatty acids (SCFAs), have been linked to cardiovascular and metabolic diseases. Previous studies have reported dysbiosis in the gut microbiota of these patients and the prebiotic effects of some components of the Mediterranean diet. Essential oil emulsions of savory (*Satureja hortensis*), parsley (*Petroselinum crispum*) and rosemary (*Rosmarinus officinalis*) were assessed as nutraceuticals and prebiotics in IHD and T2DM. Humanized mice harboring gut microbiota derived from that of patients with IHD and T2DM were supplemented with L-carnitine and orally treated with essential oil emulsions for 40 days. We assessed the effects on gut microbiota composition and abundance, microbial metabolites and plasma markers of cardiovascular disease, inflammation and oxidative stress. Our results showed that essential oil emulsions in mice supplemented with L-carnitine have prebiotic effects on beneficial commensal bacteria, mainly *Lactobacillus* genus. There was a decrease in plasma TMAO and an increase in fecal SCFAs levels in mice treated with parsley and rosemary essential oils. Thrombomodulin levels were increased in mice treated with savory and parsley essential oils. While mice treated with parsley and rosemary essential oils showed a decrease in plasma cytokines (INFγ, TNFα, IL-12p70 and IL-22); savory essential oil was associated with increased levels of chemokines (CXCL1, CCL2 and CCL11). Finally, there was a decrease in protein carbonyls and pentosidine according to the essential oil emulsion. These results suggest that changes in the gut microbiota induced by essential oils of parsley, savory and rosemary as prebiotics could differentially regulate cardiovascular and metabolic factors, which highlights the potential of these nutraceuticals for reducing IHD risk in patients affected by T2DM.

Citation: Sánchez-Quintero, M.J.; Delgado, J.; Medina-Vera, D.; Becerra-Muñoz, V.M.; Queipo-Ortuño, M.I.; Estévez, M.; Plaza-Andrades, I.; Rodríguez-Capitán, J.; Sánchez, P.L.; Crespo-Leiro, M.G.; et al. Beneficial Effects of Essential Oils from the Mediterranean Diet on Gut Microbiota and Their Metabolites in Ischemic Heart Disease and Type-2 Diabetes Mellitus. *Nutrients* 2022, *14*, 4650. https://doi.org/10.3390/nu14214650

Academic Editors: Bruno Trimarco and Gaetano Santulli

Received: 15 September 2022
Accepted: 29 October 2022
Published: 3 November 2022

Publisher's Note: MDPI stays neutral with regard to jurisdictional claims in published maps and institutional affiliations.

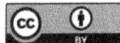

Copyright: © 2022 by the authors. Licensee MDPI, Basel, Switzerland. This article is an open access article distributed under the terms and conditions of the Creative Commons Attribution (CC BY) license (https://creativecommons.org/licenses/by/4.0/).

Keywords: carbonyl; cytokine; chemokine; nutraceutical; parsley; pentosidine; prebiotic; protein carbonyl; rosemary; savory; short-chain fatty acid; trimethylamine N-oxide

1. Introduction

Ischemic heart disease (IHD) is the most common form of cardiovascular disease and the leading cause of death in Europe in recent years in both men and women [1,2], excluding the emergence of COVID-19. In past decades, various strategies have been established to reduce the morbidity and mortality of patients with coronary disease, and important improvements have been achieved. Type-2 diabetes mellitus (T2DM) often leads to an increased risk of development of several forms of cardiovascular complications, such as IHD [3]. Previous studies in patients with IHD suggest that the presence of T2DM is linked to an impairment of the immune system mediated by the gut microbiota, finding significantly less beneficial or commensal bacteria in these patients [4]. In fact, it has been reported that T2DM can significantly alter intestinal microbial populations in patients with IHD [4]. Recently, there is a growing interest in replacing pharmaceutical therapies by dietary interventions based on natural bioactive food components, which has led to the development of new alternative therapies to extend and improve the quality of life of patients. On this line, plant-derived bioactive components, such as essential oils, have been studied as potential modulators of physiological processes related to IHD.

Growing evidence has demonstrated a link between gut dysbiosis and cardiovascular disease risk [5,6], and that the modulation of the gut microbiome may contribute to ameliorating these diseases. Inhibitory substances of non-beneficial microbiota can be present in spices or plants commonly used in the Mediterranean diet [7]. However, the consumption of usual levels from these plants within the diet would have a limited beneficial effect on bacteria population. Therefore, it would be necessary to use them as nutraceuticals, understanding this term as a food that provides health benefits, including the prevention and/or treatment of diseases. Furthermore, different studies have shown that essential oils affect both the microbial population composition and its activity, which have a direct effect on IHD [8]. Thus, these substances may be used to regulate the immune response and enhance the presence of beneficial microorganisms, such as *Lactobacillus* spp., to the detriment of those bacteria that do not provide benefits or produce unwanted metabolites [9].

One example of how gut microbiota has an impact on IHD is through the formation of trimethylamine N-oxide (TMAO). TMAO is a pro-atherogenic substance which has been associated with the development of adverse cardiovascular events in the general population over the last several years [10–13]. TMAO results from the oxidation of trimethylamine (TMA) in the liver, which is in turn produced by certain colonic microbial populations, such as some species of Bacteroidetes and Firmicutes [4]. These common microorganisms contribute to TMA formation in the colon through the precursors L-carnitine and phosphatidylcholine [14]. Previous studies have observed that plant origin substances can act as prebiotics and reduce the transformation of L-carnitine to TMA through their action on the colonic microbiota [15]. Considering this, the gut microbiota could be modulated to restore the balance between beneficial and detrimental microorganisms regarding TMA and TMAO production.

Another mechanism by which gut microbiota is related to IHD is through the formation of short-chain fatty acids (SCFAs). Dietary fibers, resistant starch and other polysaccharides that evade digestion by host enzymes in the upper gut are metabolized by the microbiota in the cecum and colon, through anaerobic fermentation [16,17]. Their major end-products are SCFAs, monocarboxylic acids with two to five carbons [18,19]. Acetic, propionic and butyric acids are the main SCFAs at the rate of 60:20:20, respectively, and are generated in the human gut daily, depending on the fiber content of the diet and microbiota structure [20–24]. The rate between these fatty acids has consequences in terms of gut health, adiposity and IHD. Butyric acid is used as an energy source by enterocytes and strengthens the intestinal epithelium; while acetic acid positively affects body weight control, insulin sensitivity and control of appetite; and propionic acid decreases liver lipogenesis, hepatic and serum cholesterol levels, preventing or hampering the IHD [23,25,26].

Besides the effects of essential oils on microbiota, these compounds may be related to IHD through many other mechanisms. For instance, the capacity of certain plant origin products to prevent the formation of free radicals that would interact with cellular DNA, confer antioxidant, antifungal, immunomodulatory, anticancer and anti-inflammatory activity in animal models [27,28]. In fact, higher inflammation levels are usually reported in patients suffering from cardiovascular disease and/or T2DM than those found in healthy ones [29]. Thus, extensive studies aiming to counteract these diseases have shown the potent therapeutic effects of plant-derived compounds against a series of chronic diseases, such as cardiovascular disease and T2DM, unraveling new anti-inflammatory and antioxidant molecules [30]. The accretion of oxidized proteins in tissues is a pathological hallmark of chronic diseases, such as those aforementioned, and hence, the protection of plant antioxidants against protein oxidation may be a plausible means to inhibit the biological consequences of protein oxidation: cell dysfunction and health disorders [31]. The formation of protein carbonyl and pentosidine is increased under a variety of stress conditions, especially oxidative stress and inflammation, contributing to severe vascular and cardiovascular complications [32]. Carbonyls are the result of a mechanism by which sensible alkaline amino acids (lysine, proline, arginine) undergo oxidative deamination to yield aldehydes (α-aminoadipic semialdehyde (AAS), also known as allysine, and γ-glutamic semialdehyde (GGS)) [33]. The formation of AAS in the presence of glucose and toxic diabetes metabolites suggests that it may be formed under pathological pro-diabetic conditions [34]. In fact, AAS and its final oxidation product, the α-aminoadipic acid, are commonly used as markers of many chronic diseases involving enduring oxidative stress, such as T2DM [31,35].

In this study, we generated a gnotobiotic murine model carrying colonic microbiota derived from patients with IHD and T2DM. The objective of this work was to evaluate the effect of the administration of essential oils from commonly used herbs in the Mediterranean diet on the gut microbial population, TMAO and SCFA levels, inflammation and oxidative stress, using this gnotobiotic murine model.

2. Materials and Methods

2.1. Ethical Statement and Animals

This study was designed in accordance with the European directive 2010/63/EU for the protection of animals used for scientific purposes and the Spanish regulations for the care and use of laboratory animals (RD53/2013 and RD118/2021). All protocols and experiments were approved by the "Animal Experimentation Ethics Committee of BIONAND", Málaga, Spain (23/10/2018/151). Randomly cycling female CD1 mice (Janvier Labs, Le Genest-Saint-Isle, France) were acclimated for 4 weeks and housed in a humidity and temperature-controlled vivarium and maintained on a 12-h light-dark cycle with food (Table S1) and water *ad libitum*.

2.2. Humanized Gnotobiotic Mouse Model

A humanized gnotobiotic mouse model was developed through the fecal microbiota transplantation of human feces into mice. Prior to the transplantation procedure, 18-week-old mice ($n = 40$) were treated with broad-spectrum antibiotics for 10 consecutive days to induce gut microbiota depletion, combining both oral gavage administration and drinking water supplementation. Thus, mice were orally treated by gavage every 12 h with an antibiotic cocktail (10 mL kg^{-1} body weight) consisting of vancomycin (5 mg mL^{-1}), neomycin (10 mg mL^{-1}) and metronidazole (10 mg mL^{-1}), and ampicillin was administered in drinking water (1 g L^{-1}) [36–38]. Then, mice received a fecal microbiota transplantation derived from a selection of patients to recolonize the gastrointestinal tract, as previously described [38]. Specifically, three patients with IHD, T2DM and high plasma levels of

TMAO were eligible for feces donation. Fresh fecal samples were suspended in sterile phosphate buffered saline (PBS), and glycerol was added at 10% (v/v) final concentration; then, samples were aliquoted into cryotubes and immediately stored at $-80\ °C$. At the moment of the transplantation, aliquot samples from these patients were thawed in ice and mixed in equal quantities as a sample pool to guarantee that every mouse received a similar microbiota load. The sample pool was centrifuged for 2 min at $2800\times g$, and the supernatant was transferred to mice by oral gavage for three consecutive days, according to previously published protocols [38–40]. Mice were moved to clean cages every two days to minimize the coprophagia and to prevent reinoculation from old feces.

2.3. Study Design and Treatments

2.3.1. Experimental Groups

Transplanted mice were randomly assigned to five experimental groups, with eight animals per group ($n = 8$), in a cage at the beginning of the study, based on a previous similar study [15]: (1) control group, mice without L-carnitine supplementation or essential oil administration; (2) carnitine group, mice with L-carnitine supplementation but not essential oil administration; (3) savory group, mice with L-carnitine supplementation and savory essential oil; (4) parsley group, mice with L-carnitine supplementation and parsley essential oil; and (5) rosemary group, mice with L-carnitine supplementation and rosemary essential oil. No criteria were used for including and excluding animals during the experiment.

2.3.2. Preparation of Essential Oil Emulsions

Three commercial essential oils derived from commonly used herbs in the Mediterranean diet were purchased from Farmacia Rico Néstares (Málaga, Spain): savory (*Satureja hortensis*), parsley (*Petroselinum crispum*) and rosemary (*Rosmarinus officinalis*). For oral administration, oil-in-water (O/W) emulsions were prepared with these essential oils at 3.38% (v/v) concentration in distilled water with lecithin (0.76%, w/v) and maltodextrin (21.47%, w/v) as emulsifiers to prevent the oil and water phases separation.

2.3.3. Treatment with Essential Oil Emulsions

During a total of 40 days, 20-week-old female mice from four groups (i.e., carnitine, savory, parsley and rosemary groups) were given drinking water supplemented with L-carnitine (0.02%, w/v), a precursor of TMA to stimulate the TMAO production, and treated with essential oil emulsions or vehicle emulsion (i.e., treatment with a vehicle solution containing distilled water, lecithin and maltodextrin in the same proportions but without essential oils). In contrast, mice from the control group were given drinking water without L-carnitine. The essential oils were administered daily by gavage at 100 mg kg^{-1} for 40 days after considering their spectrum of action and effective dose [41]. Following the same procedure, mice from the control and carnitine groups were administered daily by gavage with the vehicle emulsion. To avoid any confounder, treatments were always applied in the same order of groups, relocating the mice in a clean cage until the last mouse was treated. However, four mice died during the treatment period and the number of animals per group at the end of treatments was as follows: (1) control group, $n = 7$; (2) carnitine group, $n = 7$; (3) savory group, $n = 8$; (4) parsley group, $n = 8$; and (5) rosemary group, $n = 6$.

2.4. Collection of Fecal and Plasma Samples

Twenty-four hours after the last administration of essential oil emulsions or vehicle emulsion, mice were euthanized by decapitation, and trunk blood samples (0.8–1.0 mL) were collected in Microvette CB300 plasma/lithium heparin (Thermo Fisher Scientific, Waltham, MA, USA) tubes with volumes up to 300 µL. Blood samples were centrifuged at $3500\times g$ for 5 min and the supernatant plasmas were stored at $-80\ °C$ until determinations were performed. In addition, fresh fecal samples were collected directly into the small tubes and stored at $-80\ °C$ until.

2.5. Microbiota Analysis by 16S rRNA Gene Sequencing

Fecal microbiota was analyzed after essential oil treatments. Briefly, total DNA was isolated from feces using the QIAamp DNA Stool Mini Kit (Qiagen, Hilden, Germany). The Ion 16S Metagenomics Kit (Thermo Fisher Scientific, Waltham, MA, USA) was used to amplify the 16S rRNA gene region from stool DNA using two primer pools (V2-4-8 and V3-6, 7-9) covering hypervariable regions of the 16S rRNA region in bacteria. The Ion Plus Fragment Library Kit (Thermo Fisher Scientific, Waltham, MA, USA) was used to ligate barcoded adapters to the generated amplicons and create the barcoded libraries. Template preparation of the created amplicon libraries was performed on the automated Ion Chef System using the Ion 520^{TM}/530^{TM} Kit-Chef (Thermo Fisher Scientific, Waltham, MA, USA), according to the manufacturer's instructions. Sequencing was carried out on an Ion 520 chip using the Ion S5^{TM} System (Thermo Fisher Scientific, Waltham, MA, USA).

2.6. L-carnitine, TMA and TMAO Levels in Plasma

A total volume of 15 µL of plasma was incubated with 45 µL of cold methanol for 2 h at -80 °C. After incubation, samples were centrifuged at $18,200 \times g$ for 12 min at 4 °C, and supernatant was collected and stored at -80 °C for further analysis. L-carnitine, TMA and TMAO levels were quantified using a Dionex UltiMate 3000 RSLC system coupled to Q Exactive Hybrid Quadrupole-Orbitrap Mass Spectrometer (Thermo Fisher Scientific, Waltham, MA, USA). An Accucore HILIC 150 × 2.1 mm × 2.6 µm column was used as a stationary phase, while as a mobile phase we used a solvent (A: H_2O with 0.005 M ammonium formate pH 4.88; and B: acetonitrile and H_2O (9:1) with 0.005 M ammonium formate pH 4.9). The gradient was isocratic 70% (A/B), the injection volume was 5 µL and flow rate was set as 0.4 mL min^{-1}. Detection of L-carnitine, TMA and TMAO was performed with positive ionization in full scan with 70,000 full width at half maximum (FWHM), using the ions m/z 162.1125, 60.0808 and 76.0757 as targets, respectively, and setting 5 ppm of accuracy. Retention time was 2.08 ± 0.1 for L-carnitine, 2.3 ± 0.1 min for TMA and 2.03 ± 0.1 min for TMAO. Serial dilutions of commercial standards for both metabolites from Sigma-Aldrich (Merck KGaA, Darmstadt, Germany) were used to determine the linearity. Limit of detection (LOD) and limit of quantitation (LOQ) for TMA and TMAO were calculated at the lowest evaluable concentration level at which the qualifier ion signal exceeds the noise level by factor of 10 for LOD and 3.5 for LOQ: (1) L-carnitine, TMA: LOD = 0.2 ng mL^{-1} and LOQ = 0.6 ng mL^{-1}, LOD = 0.225 ng mL^{-1} and LOQ = 0.7 ng mL^{-1}; and (2) TMAO, LOD = 0.175 ng mL^{-1} and LOQ = 0.5 ng mL^{-1}.

2.7. SCFA Species in Feces

Acetic, propionic and butyric acids were determined in the feces of mice treated with essential oil emulsions or vehicle emulsion. Feces were weighted and treated with 3 mL of double deionized water and hexane 50% (v/v), vortexed and sonicated for 5 min in a bath. Finally, samples were centrifuged at $1400 \times g$ for 5 min. To measure acetic, butyric and propionic acid, a small volume from the upper phase was injected in a 6890 N Flame Ionization Detector Gas Chromatograph System equipped with a DB-WAX 60 × 0.32 mm × 0.25 µm column (Agilent, Santa Clara, CA, USA). The temperature of injector and detector was set starting at 100 °C and increasing up to 250 °C in 15 min. The retention time of these metabolites were 3.58 ± 0.05, 4.18 ± 0.05 and 4.93 ± 0.05 min for acetic, propionic and butyric acids, respectively. The standards used were purchased from Dr. Ehrenstorfer (LGC Standards, Middlesex, UK). SCFA species were expressed as mg g^{-1} feces.

2.8. Determination of Other Analytes in Plasma
2.8.1. Cardiovascular Markers-

Markers for cardiovascular disease were measured using the Mouse CVD Magnetic Bead Panel 1 (Merck Millipore, Burlington, MA, USA), according to manufacturer's instructions. A panel of seven cardiovascular markers was measured for this study using a 96-well plate: sE-Selectin, sICAM-1, Pecam-1, sP-Selectin, PAI-1 (total), proMMP-9 and

Thrombomodulin. All samples were prepared following the protocol and were run in duplicate in a 96-well plate. Briefly, a total volume of 25 mL of 1:20 diluted sample was mixed with 25 µL of Mixed Beads. The plate was incubated with agitation on a plate shaker overnight. After incubation, 25 µL of detection antibodies were added to wells, and the plate was incubated with agitation for 1 h at room temperature before adding 25 µL of Streptavidin-Phycoerythrin. Wells were incubated and washed and then mixed with 150 µL of sheath fluid to resuspend the beads. The plate was run on a Bio-Plex MAGPIX™ Multiplex Reader with Bio-Plex Manager™ MP Software (Luminex, Austin, TX, USA) and data were acquired. Cardiovascular markers were expressed as ng per mL of plasma.

2.8.2. Cytokines and Chemokines

The determination of inflammatory factors was performed using the ProcartaPlex™ Mouse Cytokine & Chemokine Convenience Panel 1 26-Plex (ThermoFisher Scientific, Waltham, MA, USA), following manufacturer's instructions. A panel of 26 cytokines and chemokines was measured for this study using a 96-well plate: (i) Th1/Th2 cytokines: GM-CSF, IFNγ, IL-1β, IL-2, IL-4, IL-5, IL-6, IL-12p70, IL-13, IL-18, TNFα; (ii) Th9/Th17/Th22/Treg cytokines: IL-9, IL-10, IL-17A (CTLA-8), IL-22, IL-23, IL-27; (iii) chemokines: Eotaxin (CCL11), GROα (CXCL1), IP-10 (CXCL10), MCP-1 (CCL2), MCP-3 (CCL7), MIP-1α (CCL3), MIP-1β (CCL4), MIP-2 and RANTES (CCL5). Briefly, 25 mL of non-diluted sample were mixed with an assay buffer and capture beads in a 96-well plate using duplicates. The plate was incubated with shaking at room temperature for 2 h to facilitate the reaction. After incubation, 25 mL of detection antibodies were added, and the plate was incubated with shaking at room temperature for 30 min. Following incubation, 50 µL of Streptavidin-PE were added to each well. After incubating and washing, 120 µL of reading buffer were added to wells, and the plate was incubated at room temperature for 5 min. Finally, the plate was run on a Bio-Plex MAGPIX™ Multiplex Reader with Bio-Plex Manager™ MP Software (Luminex, Austin, TX, USA), and data were acquired. Inflammatory markers were expressed as pg per mL of plasma.

2.8.3. Protein Carbonyls and Pentosidine

The AAS determination was carried out as previously described [42]. Briefly, 50 µL of plasma were treated with cold 10% trichloroacetic acid (TCA) solution, vortexed and centrifuged at $600\times g$ for 5 min at 4 °C. The supernatants were removed, and the pellets were incubated with freshly prepared solution composed of 0.5 mL of 250 mM 2-(N-morpholino) ethanesulfonic acid (MES) buffer, pH 6.0, containing 1 mM diethylenetriaminepentaacetic acid (DTPA); 0.5 mL of 50 mM 4-amino benzoic acid (ABA) in 250 mM of MES buffer pH 6.0 and 0.25 mL 100 mM sodium cyanoborohydride ($NaBH_3CN$) in 250 mM MES buffer pH 6.0. Samples were vortexed and incubated at 37 °C for 90 min, stirring them every 15 min. After derivatization, samples were treated with cold 50% TCA solution and centrifuged at $1200\times g$ for 10 min. Supernatants were removed and pellets were washed twice with 10% TCA and diethyl ether-ethanol (1:1). Finally, pellets were treated with 6N HCl and incubated at 110 °C for 18 h until completion of hydrolysis. The hydrolysates were dried in vacuo in a centrifugal evaporator. The generated residues were reconstituted with 200 µL of Milli-Q water and filtered through hydrophilic polypropylene GH Polypro (GHP) syringe filters with 0.45 µm pore size (Pall Corporation, Port Washington, NY, USA) for HPLC analysis. Samples were analyzed using a Shimadzu Prominence HPLC instrument equipped with a quaternary solvent delivery system (LC-20AD), DGU-20AS on-line degasser, SIL-20A auto-sampler, RF-10A XL fluorescence detector (FLD) and CBM-20A system controller (Shimadzu Corporation, Kyoto, Japan). An aliquot (1 µL) from the reconstituted protein was injected for the analysis. AAS-ABA, GGS-ABA and pentosidine were eluted in a Cosmosil $5C_{18}$-AR-II RP-HPLC column (150 × 4.6 mm × 5 µm) equipped with a guard column (10 × 4.6 mm). The flow rate was kept at 1 mL min^{-1}, and the temperature of the column was maintained constant at 30 °C. The eluate was monitored with excitation and emission wavelengths set at 283 and 350 nm, respectively. Standards (0.1 µL) were run and analyzed under the same conditions. Identification of both derivatized semialdehydes in the fluorescence detector chromatograms was carried out by comparing their retention times with those from the standard compounds. The peaks corresponding to analytes of interest (AAS-ABA, GGS-ABA and pentosidine) were manually integrated from fluorescence detector chromatograms and the resulting areas from derivatized semialdehydes plotted against an ABA standard curve with known concentrations, that ranged from 0.1 to 0.5 mM. Results were expressed as nmol of semialdehyde AAS per mg of protein. Pentosidine was not quantified and, hence, expressed as fluorescence intensity.

2.9. Bioinformatics and Statistical Analysis

Data in the graphs are expressed as bacterial composition (percentages), mean and standard error of the mean (mean ± SEM), and median and interquartile range. All determinations in mouse feces and plasmas were performed in five groups with six to eight animals per group (n = 6–8).

Regarding the bacterial diversity, the Chao1 and Shannon indices (i.e., alpha diversity) were used to measure the number and diversity of bacteria in the microbial community, and the Bray-Curtis dissimilarity index (i.e., beta diversity) was used to measure the dissimilarity in the microbial community composition of each group based on abundance data. Statistically, alpha diversity was assessed using the Kruskal-Wallis rank-sum test and the Benjamini-Hochberg procedure for multiple comparisons, and beta diversity was assessed using the analysis of similarity (ANOSIM). Principal coordinate analysis (PCoA) based on Bray-Curtis dissimilarity metrics was used to show the distance in the bacterial communities between the treatment groups.

The distribution of raw data from biochemical determinations was assessed using the D'Agostino-Pearson normality test in order to use parametric or non-parametric tests. Differences in normal variables were assessed using the Student's t test (two groups) or one-way analysis of variance (ANOVA) (more than two groups). In contrast, non-normal variables were assessed using the Mann-Whitney U test (two groups) or the Kruskal-Wallis rank-sum test (more than two groups) as non-parametric tests. When raw data were not normally distributed because of a positively skewed distribution, data were $\log_{10}$-transformed to approximate a normal distribution and to ensure statistical assumptions of the parametric tests. The Sidak's correction test was used as post hoc tests for multiple comparisons in the ANOVA and Kruskal-Wallis rank-sum test.

Correlation analyses were performed to examine the association between biochemical and/or microbial variables using the Spearman's correlation coefficient (rho) with categorical variables and the Pearson's correlation coefficient (r) with continuous variables.

Quantitative Insights into Microbial Ecology (QIIME2, version 2019.4) software [43] was used to analyze sequence quality and for diversity and taxonomic analysis, as previously described [44]. The statistical analysis of the microbiota sequencing was performed in R version 3.6.0., while the statistical analysis of biochemical data was performed using the Graph-Pad Prism version 5.04 software (GraphPad Software, San Diego, CA, USA). Test statistic values and degrees of freedom are indicated in the results. A p-value less than 0.05 was considered statistically significant.

3. Results

3.1. Mice from the Experimental Groups Showed Differences in the Composition and Bacterial Abundances of Gut Microbiota

To characterize and identify intestinal bacteria populations in the fecal samples of mice from the experimental groups, we assessed diversity indices and examined the gut microbiota at different taxa levels.

3.1.1. Alpha and Beta Diversity

Regarding the alpha diversity, the Chao1 (Figure 1A) and Shannon (Figure 1B) indices at genus level showed no significant differences in bacterial richness and diversity of samples from mice of the experimental groups (control, carnitine, savory, parsley and rosemary groups). In contrast, the Bray-Curtis dissimilarity index showed a significant dissimilarity in the microbial community composition of fecal samples comparing the mean of ranked dissimilarities between and within groups (R = 0.175, p = 0.001, ANOSIM) (Figure 1C). The PCoA of the Bray-Curtis distance matrix based at genus level abundances allowed for representation of the dissimilarities of each sample and showed the percentage of variation explained by the principal coordinates (PCoA1 = 32% and PCoA2 = 19%) (Figure 1D).

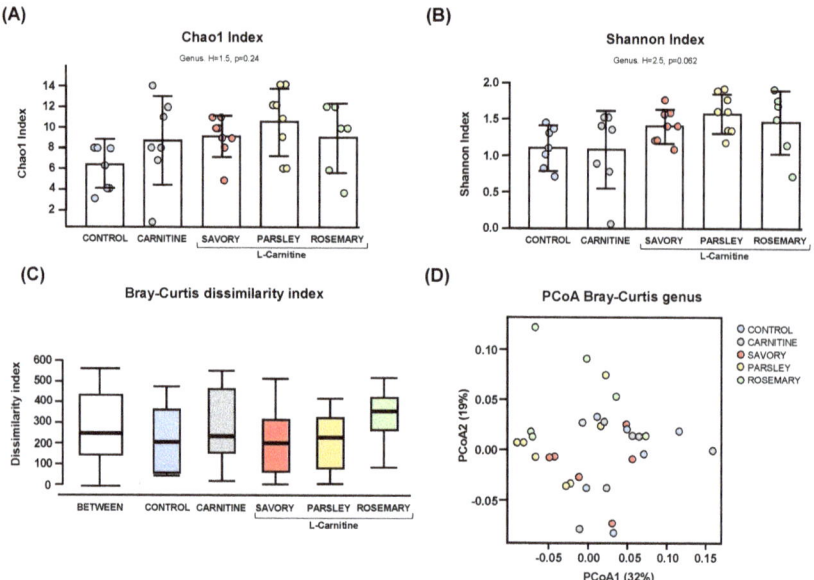

Figure 1. Alpha and beta diversity analyses of bacterial microbiota in fecal samples from the treatment groups. (**A**) Chaos1 index; (**B**) Shannon index; (**C**) Bray-Curtis dissimilarity index; and (**D**) Principal coordinates analysis of Bray-Curtis dissimilarity. Dots are individual values. Alpha diversity was assessed using the Kruskal-Wallis rank-sum test, and the Bray-Curtis dissimilarity index was assessed using the analysis of similarity (ANOSIM). Principal coordinates analysis (PCoA) based on Bray-Curtis dissimilarity index shows the distance in the bacterial communities between the treatment groups.

3.1.2. Gut Microbial Abundances at Different Taxonomic Levels

The relative abundances at the phylum level in the experimental groups showed Bacteroidetes, Firmicutes and Proteobacteria as the most predominant phyla, but there were no differences among the groups (Figure 2A). In contrast, variations in bacterial communities were observed among the different groups at the family and genus levels. Thus, while there were no differences in the relative abundance between the carnitine and control groups, the essential oil groups showed relevant differences in bacterial families and genera. At the family level, there was a higher abundance of Lactobacillaceae and a lower abundance of Bacteroidaceae in mice treated with essential oils (mainly in the parsley and rosemary groups) than in mice from the carnitine group (Figure 2B). Similarly, mice treated with essential oils had a higher abundance of *Lactobacillus* and a lower abundance of *Bacteroides* than mice from the carnitine group (Figure 3A). Furthermore, the analysis of the number of each genus revealed significant differences in *Lactobacillus* genus among the groups (p < 0.040), and mice treated with essential oils, mainly in the rosemary group, had a higher number of *Lactobacillus* than mice from the carnitine and control groups (Figure 3B). The relative abundances at the species level are shown in Figure S1.

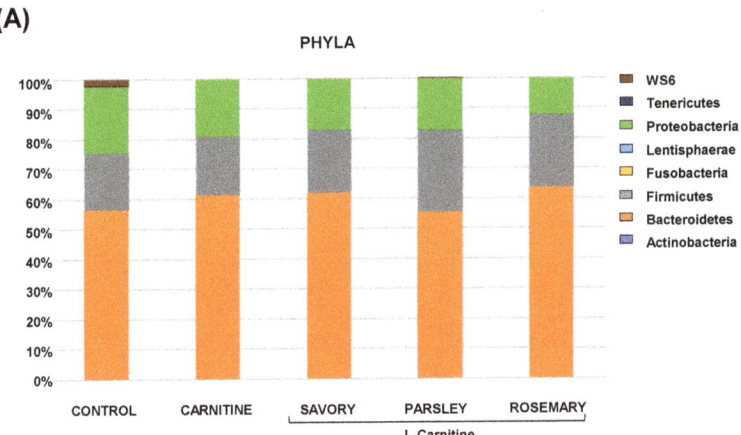

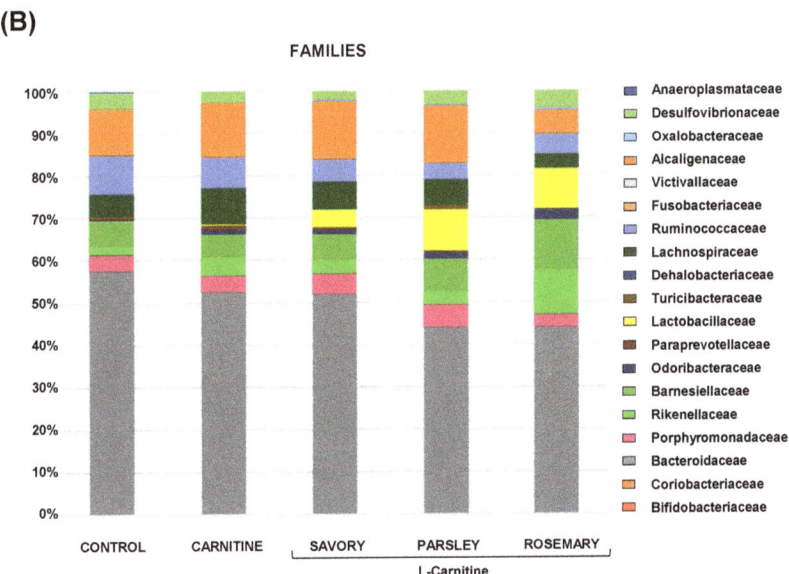

Figure 2. Bacterial profile at the phylum and family levels in fecal samples of mice from the treatment groups. (**A**) Phyla; and (**B**) Families. Bars show the relative abundances (%) for each group using 16S rRNA gene sequencing (Ion S5^{TM} System).

3.2. Treatment with Essential Oils of Parsley and Rosemary Reduced Plasma TMAO Levels

L-carnitine, TMA and TMAO levels were measured in the plasma of mice from all groups after treatment. Raw data were log10-transformed, and the estimated marginal means and SEM of the logarithmic values are represented in Figure 4.

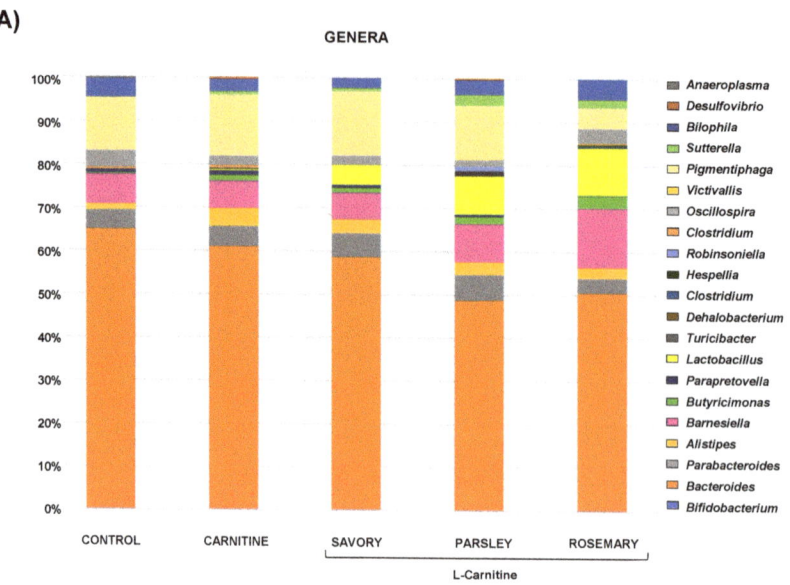

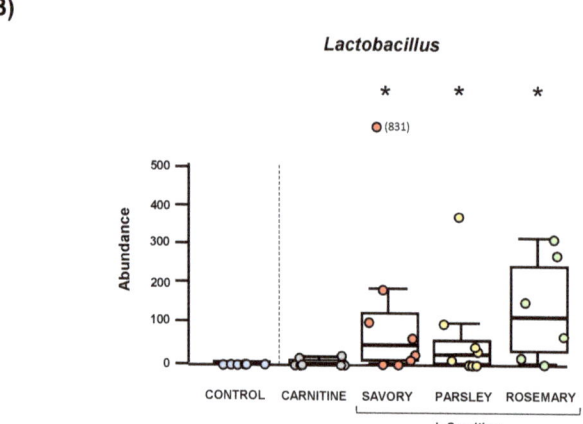

Figure 3. Bacterial profile at the genus level and abundance of Lactobacillus in fecal samples of mice from the treatment groups. (**A**) Genera; and (**B**) Lactobacillus. Bars show the relative abundance (%) for each group using 16S rRNA gene sequencing (Ion S5™ System). Dots are individual values and data from the carnitine, savory, parsley and rosemary groups were analyzed using the Kruskal-Wallis rank-sum test (*) $p < 0.05$ denotes significant differences compared with the carnitine group.

3.2.1. Plasma L-carnitine Levels

As expected, L-carnitine supplementation induced a significant increase in plasma L-carnitine levels in the carnitine group compared with the control group ($t_{7.194} = 5.269$, $p = 0.001$). However, one-way ANOVA revealed no significant differences in the L-carnitine levels in the essential oil (i.e., savory, parsley and rosemary) and carnitine groups (Figure 4A).

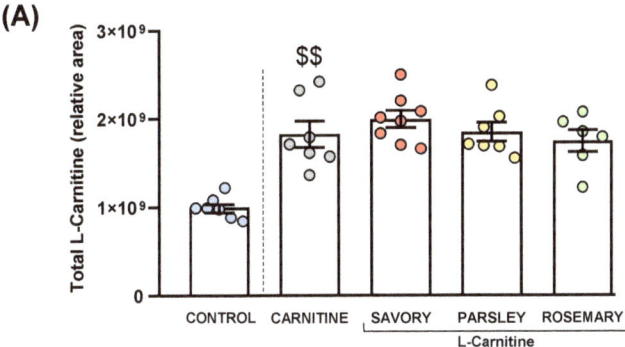
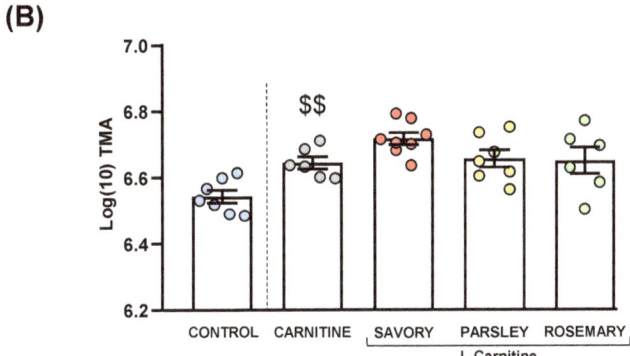
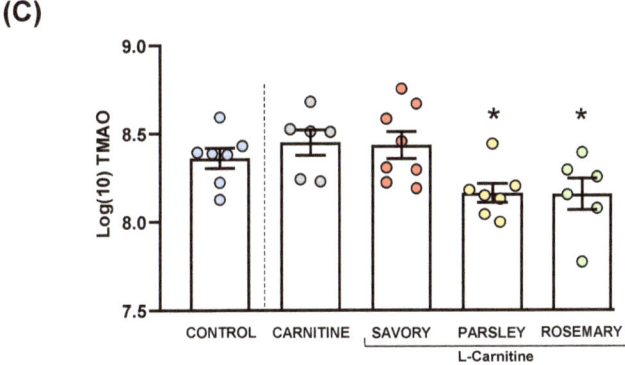

Figure 4. Plasma levels of total L-Carnitine, TMA and TMAO in mice from the treatment groups. (**A**) Total L-carnitine; (**B**) TMA; and (**C**) TMAO levels. Dots are individual values. Bars are means ± SEM of L-Carnitine concentrations (relative area) and log10-transformed concentrations of TMA and TMAO (ng mL^{-1}). Data from the control and carnitine groups were analyzed using Student's t test. Data from the carnitine, savory, parsley and rosemary groups were analyzed using one-way ANOVA. ($\$\$$) $p < 0.01$ denotes significant differences compared with the control group. (*) $p < 0.05$ denotes significant differences compared with the carnitine group.

3.2.2. Plasma Levels of TMA and TMAO

Similar to L-carnitine levels, mice from the carnitine group showed a significant increase in plasma TMA levels compared with the control group ($t_{11} = 3.706$, $p = 0.004$), but there were no significant differences in TMA levels in the essential oil and carnitine groups (Figure 4B).

Unlike L-carnitine and TMA levels, there were no significant differences in plasma TMAO levels between the carnitine and control groups. However, there were significant differences in TMAO levels among the essential oil and carnitine groups ($F_{3,23} = 4.890$, $p = 0.009$), and the post hoc test showed significant decreases in the parsley and rosemary groups compared with the carnitine group ($p < 0.05$) (Figure 4C).

3.3. Treatment with Essential Oils of Parsley and Rosemary Increased Fecal SCFAs Levels

Acetic, butyric and propionic acids were measured in the feces of mice from the experimental groups, as shown in Figure 5.

The comparisons of these SCFA species between the carnitine and control groups revealed no significant differences. In contrast, one-way ANOVA tests showed significant differences in fecal levels of acetic ($F_{3,25} = 3.624$, $p = 0.028$), butyric ($F_{3,25} = 14.07$, $p < 0.001$) and propionic ($F_{3,24} = 4.093$, $p = 0.018$) acids among mice from the essential oil and carnitine groups. Specifically, the post hoc comparison showed significant increases in acetic acid levels in the parsley and rosemary groups compared with the carnitine group ($p < 0.05$) (Figure 5A); significant increases in propionic acid levels in the parsley and rosemary groups compared with the carnitine group ($p < 0.05$ and $p < 0.001$, respectively) (Figure 5B); and a significant increase in butyric acid levels in the rosemary group compared with the carnitine group ($p < 0.05$) (Figure 5C).

3.4. Treatment with Essential Oils of Savory and Parsley Increased Plasma Thrombomodulin Levels

Plasma samples were used to measure common cardiovascular disease markers (sE-selectin, sICAM-1, Precam-1, sP-selectin, PAI-1 and thrombomodulin). Raw data were log10-transformed, and the estimated marginal means and SEM of the logarithmic values are represented in Figure 6.

The comparisons of these cardiovascular disease markers between the carnitine and control groups revealed no significant differences. The one-way ANOVA tests showed no significant differences in sE-selectin (Figure 6A), sICAM-1 (Figure 6B), Precam-1 (Figure 6C), sP-selectin (Figure 6D) and PAI-1 (Figure 6E) levels among mice from the essential oil and carnitine groups. In contrast, there were significant differences in thrombomodulin levels ($F_{3,22} = 8.523$, $p < 0.001$), and the post hoc comparisons showed significant increases in the savory and parsley groups compared with the carnitine group ($p < 0.001$ and $p < 0.01$, respectively) (Figure 6F).

3.5. Treatment with Essential Oils Altered Plasma Inflammatory Markers

Cytokines and chemokines were analyzed in the plasma of mice from the experimental groups. Because of statistical requirements, raw data were log10−transformed, and the estimated marginal means and SEM were represented and statistically analyzed. For clarity, only those cytokines and chemokines that resulted in statistical significance were shown in Figure 7.

3.5.1. Cytokines

The comparisons between mice from the carnitine and control groups only showed differences in IFNγ levels (Figure 7A), and a significant increase was found in the carnitine group compared with the control group ($t_{6.571} = 2.480$, $p = 0.044$).

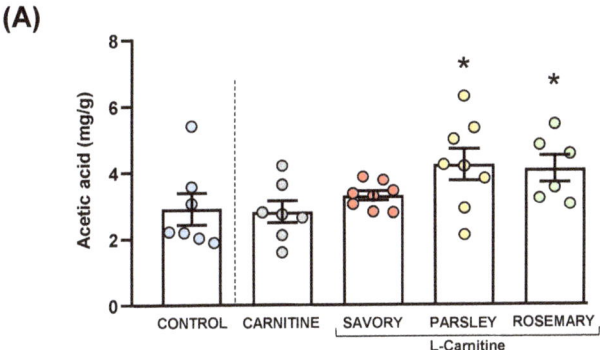
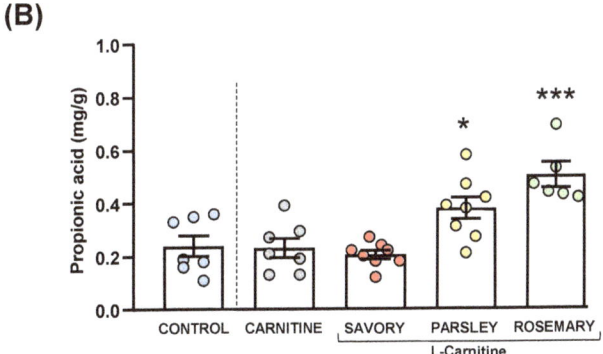
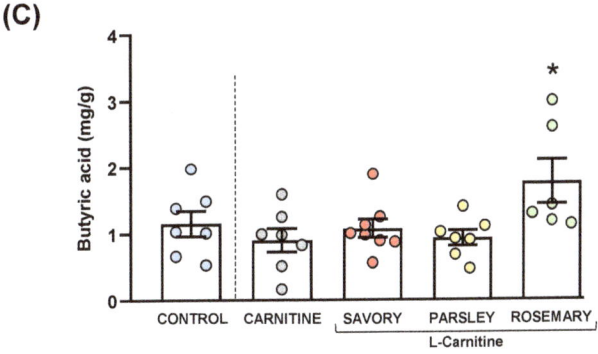

Figure 5. Fecal levels of SCFA species in mice from the treatment groups. (**A**) Acetic; (**B**) Propionic; and (**C**) Butyric acid levels. Dots are individual values. Bars are means ± SEM of SFCA concentrations (mg g^{-1}). Data from the control and carnitine groups were analyzed using Student's *t* test. Data from the carnitine, savory, parsley and rosemary groups were analyzed using one-way ANOVA. (*) $p < 0.05$ and (***) $p < 0.001$ denote significant differences compared with the carnitine group.

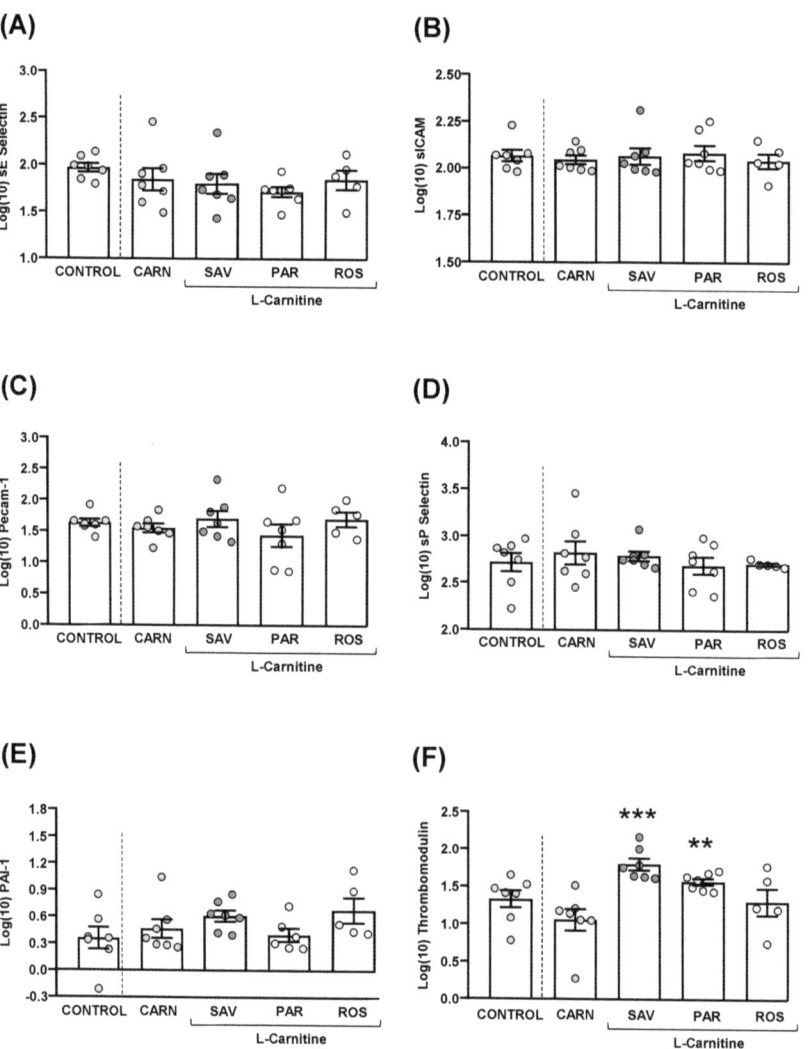

Figure 6. Plasma levels of cardiovascular markers in mice from the treatment groups. (**A**) sE-Selectin; (**B**) sICAM; (**C**) Pecam-1; (**D**) sP-Selectin; (**E**) PAI-1; and (**F**) Thrombomodulin levels. Dots are individual values. Bars are means ± SEM of log10-transformed concentrations of relevant cardiovascular markers (ng mL^{-1}). Data from the control and carnitine groups were analyzed using Student's *t* test. Data from the carnitine, savory, parsley and rosemary groups were analyzed using one-way ANOVA. (******) $p < 0.01$ and (*******) $p < 0.001$ denote significant differences compared with the carnitine group.

Regarding one-way ANOVAs and post hoc tests among the essential oil and carnitine groups, there were significant differences in the plasma levels of various cytokines: (a) IFNγ($F_{3,23}$ = 3.690, $p = 0.027$), the parsley and rosemary groups showed significant decreases compared with the carnitine group ($p < 0.05$) (Figure 8A); (b) TNFα ($F_{3,23}$ = 4.923, $p = 0.009$), the rosemary group showed a significant decrease compared with the carnitine group ($p < 0.05$) (Figure 7B); IL-4 ($F_{3,23}$ = 3.876, $p = 0.022$), the savory group showed a significant decrease compared with the carnitine group ($p < 0.05$) (Figure 7C); IL-6 ($F_{3,23}$ = 3.200, $p = 0.042$), the savory group showed a significant increase compared with the carnitine group

($p < 0.05$) (Figure 7D); IL-12p70 ($F_{3,23} = 5.090$, $p = 0.008$), the rosemary showed a significant decrease compared with the carnitine group ($p < 0.01$) (Figure 7E); IL-22 ($F_{3,23} = 5.129$, $p = 0.007$), the savory, parsley and rosemary groups showed significant decreases compared with the carnitine group ($p < 0.01$, $p < 0.05$ and $p < 0.05$, respectively) (Figure 7F); and IL-23 ($F_{3,23} = 3.302$, $p = 0.038$), the savory group showed a significant increase compared with the carnitine group ($p < 0.05$) (Figure 7G).

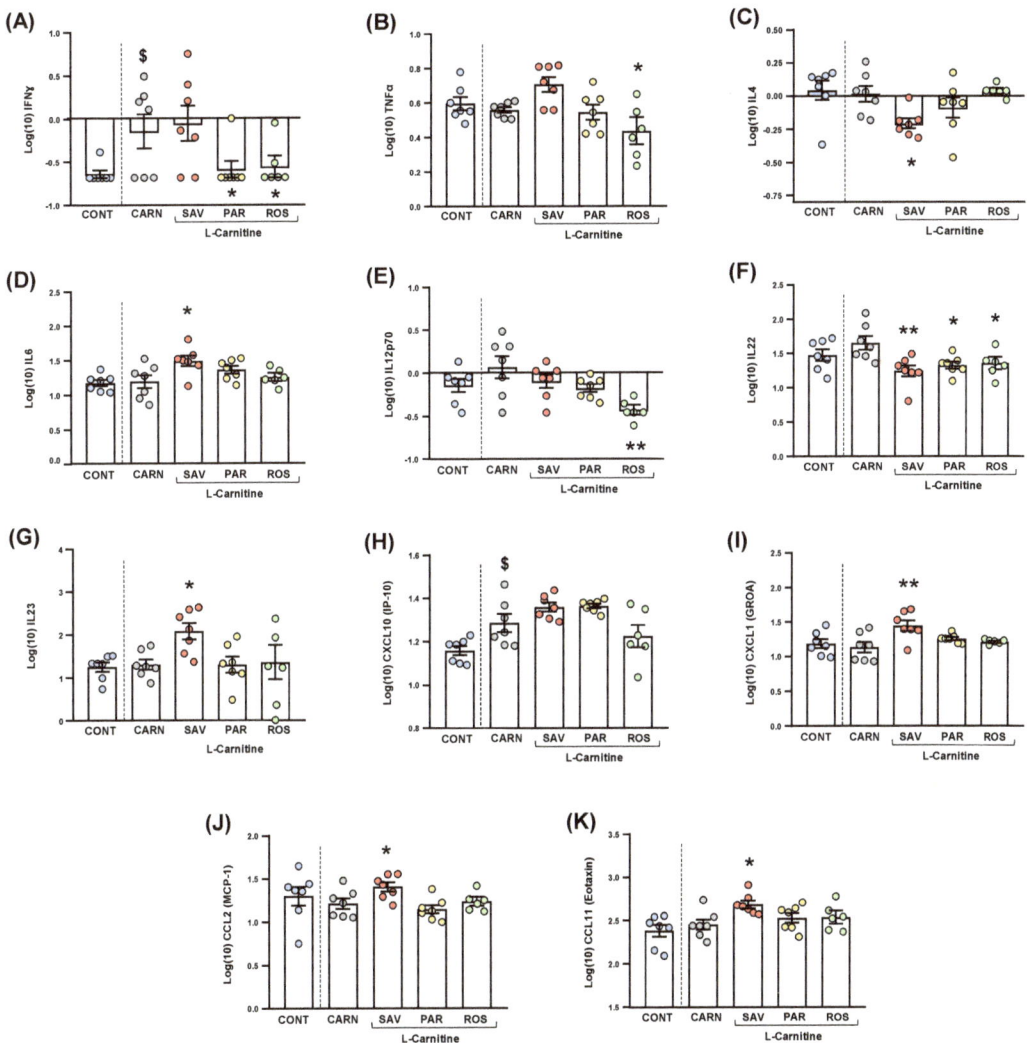

Figure 7. Plasma levels of cytokines and chemokines in mice from the treatment groups. (**A**) IFNγ; (**B**) TNFα; (**C**) IL−4; (**D**) IL−6; (**E**) IL−12p70; (**F**) IL−22; (**G**) IL−23; (**H**) CXCL10 (IP−10); (**I**) CXCL1 (GROα); (**J**) CCL2 (MCP−1); and (**K**) CCL11 (Eotaxin) levels. Dots are individual values. Bars are means ± SEM of log10-transformed concentrations of cytokines and chemokines (pg mL^{-1}). Data from the control and carnitine groups were analyzed using Student's *t* test. Data from the carnitine, savory, parsley and rosemary groups were analyzed using one-way ANOVA. ($) $p < 0.05$ denotes significant differences compared with the control group. (*) $p < 0.05$ and (**) $p < 0.01$ denote significant differences compared with the carnitine group.

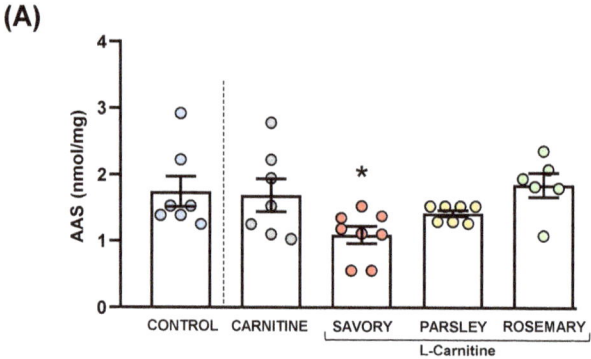
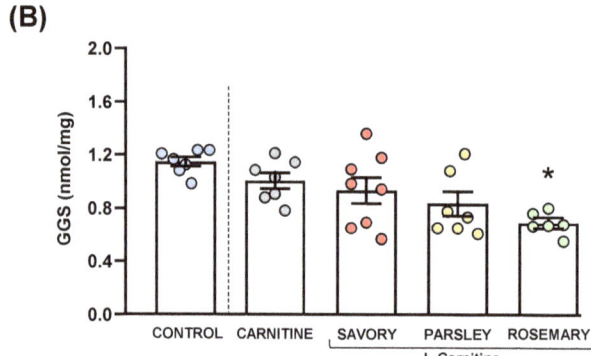
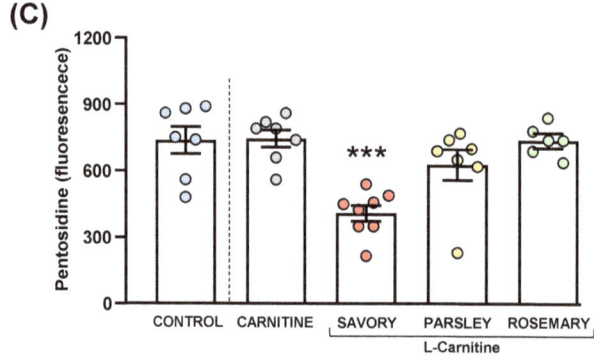

Figure 8. Plasma levels of protein carbonyls and pentosidine in mice from the treatment groups. (**A**) Aminoadipic semialdehyde (AAS); (**B**) Glutamic semialdehyde (GGS); and (**C**) Pentosidine levels. Dots are individual values. Bars are means ± SEM of AAS (nmol mg^{-1}), GGS (nmol mg^{-1}) and pentosidine (fluorescence intensity) concentrations. Data from the control and carnitine groups were analyzed using Student's *t* test. Data from the carnitine, savory, parsley and rosemary groups were analyzed using one-way ANOVA. (*) $p < 0.05$ and (***) $p < 0.001$ denotes significant differences compared with the carnitine group.

Other cytokines (i.e., GM-CSF, IL-1β, IL-2, IL-5, IL-9, IL-10, IL-13, IL-17A, IL-18 and IL-27) were not significantly altered in the experimental groups (Figure S2).

3.5.2. Chemokines

The comparisons between the carnitine and control groups only showed differences in CXCL10 levels (Figure 7H), and a significant increase was observed in the carnitine group compared with the control group ($t_{12} = 2.664$, $p = 0.037$). However, there were no significant differences in the essential oil and carnitine groups.

Unlike CXCL10, one-way ANOVA tests revealed significant differences in other chemokines as follows: (a) CXCL1 ($F_{3,23} = 5.466$, $p = 0.006$), the savory groups showed a significant increase compared with the carnitine group ($p < 0.01$) (Figure 7I); (b) CCL2 ($F_{3,23} = 4.597$, $p = 0.012$), the savory groups showed a significant increase compared with the carnitine group ($p < 0.01$) (Figure 7J); and CCL11 ($F_{3,23} = 3.109$, $p = 0.046$), the savory groups showed a significant increase compared with the carnitine group ($p < 0.05$) (Figure 7K). Therefore, only the savory group showed significant increases in chemokines.

Similar to cytokines, other chemokines (i.e., CXCL2, CCL3, CCL4, CCL5 and CCL7) were not significantly altered in the experimental groups (Figure S2).

3.6. Treatment with Essential Oils Reduced Protein Oxidative Stress

Protein carbonyls (AAS and GGS) and pentosidine were also measured in the plasma of mice from the experimental groups to examine the effects of essential oil emulsions on oxidative stress, as shown in Figure 8.

3.6.1. Protein Carbonyls

The comparisons between the carnitine and control groups revealed that supplementation with L-carnitine had no significant effects on the plasma levels of AAS and GGS. However, one-way ANOVA tests revealed significant differences in AAS ($F_{3,24} = 4.238$, $p = 0.015$) (Figure 8A) and GGS ($F_{3,24} = 3.421$, $p = 0.033$) (Figure 8B) in the essential oil and carnitine groups. Thus, the post hoc comparisons showed a significant decrease in AAS levels in the savory group and a significant decrease in GGS levels in the rosemary group compared with the carnitine group ($p < 0.05$).

3.6.2. Pentosidine

Although there were no differences between the carnitine and control groups, significant differences in pentosidine levels were found in the essential oil and carnitine groups ($F_{3,24} = 11.09$, $p < 0.001$) (Figure 8C). Similar to AAS, the savory group showed a significant decrease in pentosidine levels compared with the carnitine ($p < 0.001$).

3.7. Association between Gut Microbial Abundance and Metabolites

Because the TMAO precursor (TMA) and SCFA species are produced by gut microbiota from dietary fiber fermentation and carnitine metabolism, we investigated the association between these products and the microbial abundance at different taxonomic ranks. Additionally, we explored the association between inflammatory and oxidative markers and the microbial abundance.

3.7.1. L-carnitine, TMA and TMAO

As shown in Table 1, we analyzed the association between the abundance of gut microbiota and plasma levels of L-carnitine, TMA and TMAO. The analysis of these metabolites revealed significant and positive correlations between L-carnitine and TMA levels ($r = +0.77$, $p < 0.001$) and between TMA and TMAO levels ($r = +0.49$, $p < 0.01$). Regarding the microbial abundance, significant associations with L-carnitine and TMA levels were found at different taxonomic ranks. At the phylum level, L-carnitine levels were inversely correlated with Tenericutes (rho = −0.36, $p < 0.05$) and TMA levels were positively correlated with Lentisphaerae (rho = +0.34, $p < 0.05$), but inversely correlated with Tenericutes (rho = −0.37, $p < 0.05$). At the family level, L-carnitine levels were inversely correlated with Anaeroplasmataceae (rho = −0.36, $p < 0.05$) and TMA levels were positively correlated with Lactobacillaceae (rho = +0.35, $p < 0.05$), Alcaligenaceae (rho = +0.34, $p < 0.05$)

and Victivallaceae (rho = +0.34, $p < 0.05$), but inversely correlated with Anaeroplasmataceae (rho = −0.37, $p < 0.05$). At the genus level, L-carnitine levels were inversely correlated with *Anaeroplasma* (rho = −0.36, $p < 0.05$) and TMA levels were positively correlated with *Lactobacillus* (rho = +0.35, $p < 0.05$), *Pigmentiphaga* (rho = +0.39, $p < 0.05$) and *Victivallis* (rho = +0.34, $p < 0.05$), but inversely correlated with *Anaeroplasma* (rho = −0.37, $p < 0.05$). In contrast, TMAO levels were not significantly associated with the abundance of gut microbiota.

Table 1. Correlation analysis among plasma levels of L-carnitine, TMA and TMAO, as well as between gut microbial abundance and plasma levels of L-carnitine, TMA and TMAO.

	L-carnitine (Area)		TMA (ng mL^{-1})		TMAO (ng mL^{-1})	
	r	p-Value	r	p-Value	r	p-Value
TMAO (ng mL^{-1})	+0.152	0.383	+0.492	0.003	1	—
TMA (ng mL^{-1})	+0.767	<0.001	1	—	+0.492	0.003
L-carnitine (area)	1	—	+0.767	<0.001	+0.152	0.383
Phylum	rho	p-value	rho	p-value	rho	p-value
Lentisphaerae	+0.329	0.058	+0.342	0.047	+0.007	0.970
Tenericutes	−0.362	0.035	−0.369	0.032	+0.003	0.988
Family	rho	p-value	rho	p-value	rho	p-value
Lactobacillaceae	+0.337	0.051	+0.353	0.041	−0.210	0.234
Alcaligenaceae	+0.271	0.122	+0.342	0.048	+0.203	0.250
Victivallaceae	+0.329	0.058	+0.342	0.047	+0.007	0.970
Anaeroplasmataceae	−0.362	0.035	−0.369	0.032	+0.003	0.988
Genus	rho	p-value	rho	p-value	rho	p-value
Lactobacillus	+0.337	0.051	+0.353	0.041	−0.210	0.234
Pigmentiphaga	+0.248	0.157	+0.390	0.023	+0.259	0.139
Victivallis	+0.329	0.058	+0.342	0.047	+0.007	0.970
Anaeroplasma	−0.362	0.035	−0.369	0.032	+0.003	0.988

Abbreviations: r, Pearson correlation coefficient; rho, Spearman correlation coefficient; TMA, trimethylamine; TMAO, trimethylamine N−oxide.

3.7.2. SCFA Species

The association between the abundance of gut microbiota and fecal levels of acetic, propionic and butyric acids was also analyzed (Table 2). A first correlation analysis between SCFA levels showed significant and positive correlations (acetic acid vs. propionic acid, r = +0.77, $p < 0.001$; acetic acid vs. butyric acid, r = +0.69, $p < 0.001$; and propionic acid vs. butyric acid, r = +0.66, $p < 0.001$). At the family level, acetic acid levels were positively correlated with Lactobacillaceae (rho = +0.39, $p < 0.05$) and propionic acid levels were positively correlated with Barnesiellaceae (rho = +0.40, $p < 0.05$), Odoribacteraceae (rho = +0.38, $p < 0.05$) and Lactobacillaceae (rho = +0.36, $p < 0.05$). At the genus level, we confirm these significant associations with acetic (*Lactobacillus*) and propionic (*Barnesiella*, *Butyricimonas* and *Lactobacillus*) acids. Unlike acetic and propionic acids, there were no significant correlations between the gut microbial abundance and butyric acid levels.

Table 2. Correlation analysis among fecal levels of SCFA species, as well as between gut microbial abundance and fecal levels of SCFA species.

	Acetic Acid (mg g^{-1})		Propionic Acid (mg g^{-1})		Butyric Acid (mg g^{-1})	
	r	p-Value	r	p-Value	r	p-Value
Acetic acid (mg g^{-1})	1	—	+0.770	<0.001	+0.692	<0.001
Propionic acid (mg g^{-1})	+0.770	<0.001	1	—	+0.655	<0.001
Butyric acid (mg g^{-1})	+0.692	<0.001	+0.655	<0.001	1	—
Family	rho	p-value	rho	p-value	rho	p-value
Barnesiellaceae	+0.233	0.177	+0.403	0.016	+0.162	0.352
Odoribacteraceae	+0.272	0.114	+0.375	0.027	+0.095	0.589
Lactobacillaceae	+0.387	0.022	+0.362	0.033	+0.054	0.758
Genus	rho	p-value	rho	p-value	rho	p-value
Barnesiella	+0.236	0.172	+0.411	0.014	+0.165	0.345
Butyricimonas	+0.272	0.114	+0.375	0.027	+0.095	0.589
Lactobacillus	+0.387	0.022	+0.362	0.033	+0.054	0.758

Abbreviations: r, Pearson correlation coefficient; rho, Spearman correlation coefficient; SCFA, short-chain fatty acid.

3.7.3. Cytokines and Chemokines

Additionally, we also performed a correlation analysis to explore the association between gut microbiota and inflammatory markers (Table S2). After adjustment for multiple correlations, we found significant associations with some inflammatory markers at family and genus levels. At the family level, there were inverse correlations between IL−1ß levels and Oxalobacteraceae (rho = −0.46, adjusted $p < 0.05$), GM-CSF levels and Lactobacillaceae (rho = −0.53, adjusted $p < 0.05$), and CXCL12 levels and Ruminococcaceae (rho = −0.46, adjusted $p < 0.05$). At the genus level, there were inverse correlations between GM-CSF levels and *Lactobacillus* (rho = −0.53, adjusted $p < 0.05$), CXCL12 levels and *Ocillospira* (rho = −0.46, adjusted $p < 0.05$), CXCL12 levels and *Bilophila* (rho = −0.46, adjusted $p < 0.05$), and CCL7 levels and *Ocillospira* (rho = −0.49, adjusted $p < 0.05$); but there was a positive correlation between IL−22 levels and *Clostridium* (rho = +0.47, adjusted $p < 0.05$).

3.7.4. AAS, GGS and Pentosidine

Overall, there was a negative association between the gut microbial abundance and plasma levels of carbonyl products and pentosidine (Table S3). After adjustment for multiple correlations, we found significant correlations with AAS and GGS levels at family and genus levels. Namely, AAS levels were inversely correlated with Paraprevotellaceae and *Paraprevotella* (rho = −0–47, adjusted $p < 0.05$), GGS levels were inversely correlated with Barnesiellaceae and *Barnesiella* (rho = −0.56, adjusted $p < 0.05$) and Lactobacillaceae and *Lactobacillus* (rho = −0.50, adjusted $p < 0.05$). Unlike AAS and GGS, pentosidine levels were not significantly associated with the gut microbial abundance.

4. Discussion

Evidence supports that adherence to the Mediterranean diet is strongly associated with a reduction in the risk of cardiovascular disease [45–47]. In fact, the Mediterranean diet is recommended to patients, as it was shown to be effective for prevention of cardiovascular events [48,49]. Some components of the Mediterranean diet such as olive oil provide cardiovascular benefits, antithrombotic properties [50,51] and improves postprandial lipemia concentration, which is typically elevated in patients with T2DM [52]. In recent years, interest in functional components from herbal medicines has increased, supported by the confirmed medicinal potential of essential oils [53]. In this study, we aimed to assess the effects of essential oils from savory, parsley and rosemary, which are commonly used condiments in the Mediterranean diet, using a higher dose than within a regular diet. We used the essential oils as potential nutraceuticals and assessed their effects on microbial populations, their metabolites (TMA and TMAO in plasma and SCFAs in feces) and plasma markers (cardiovascular disease, inflammation and oxidative stress), using a humanized mouse model harboring colonic microbiota derived from that of patients with IHD and T2DM. The main results of this study are as follows: (a) Treatments with essential oil emulsions of savory, parsley and rosemary had prebiotic effects on gut microbiota by inducing an increase in *Lactobacillus* genus, which are considered beneficial bacteria; (b) Plasma TMAO levels, a pro-atherogenic substance related to the pathogenicity of IHD and the production of pro-inflammatory cytokines [54], were significantly reduced after treatment with essential oils, more specifically with parsley and rosemary; (c) Fecal levels of SCFA species were increased after treatment with parsley and rosemary essential oils, which suggests a beneficial effect of these essential oils on the gastrointestinal health; (d) Plasma thrombomodulin levels were increased after treatments with essential oils of savory and parsley; (e) Overall, essential oils had anti-inflammatory effects through alterations in the plasma levels of cytokines and chemokines; and (f) Finally, there was a reduction in the expression of protein carbonyls and pentosidine.

High-level adherence to the Mediterranean diet has been positively associated with changes in gut microbiota composition and their metabolites [55]. Gut microbiota uses L-carnitine as a precursor to generate TMA, which is rapidly absorbed into the portal circulation by passive diffusion across the enterocyte membranes and then oxidized to TMAO by the action of hepatic flavin-containing monooxygenases (mainly FMO3) [56]. As expected, our results showed that TMA was only increased after administration of L-carnitine, but we did not observe changes in TMA levels after treatments with different essential oil emulsions. In contrast, we observed a significant reduction of plasma TMAO levels in the parsley and rosemary groups that cannot be explained by changes in the TMA levels. Therefore, the treatments with parsley and rosemary essential oils likely affect the metabolism of TMAO by decreasing the oxidative activity of FMO3 and/or increasing the mobilization of TMAO (i.e., absorption by tissues or excretion in urine) [57]. However, the exact mechanism has to be elucidated, and further research is needed.

Among others, the microorganisms linked to high concentrations of pro-atherogenic substances, mainly TMAO, include species from Firmicutes, Pseudomonas, Bacillota and Proteobacteria phyla, such as *Anaerococcus hydrogenalis*, *Clostridium asparagiforme*, *Clostridium hathewayi*, *Clostridium sporogenes*, *Escherichia fergusonii*, *Proteus penneri* or *Providencia rettgeri* [58]. In fact, these microorganisms were found to a lesser extent in the colonic microbiota of patients presenting low levels of TMAO in plasma [59]. However, after correlation analysis, we found that TMAO levels were not significantly associated with the abundance of different groups of gut microbiota. This fact would support the idea that the TMAO inhibition provoked by these essential oils would be based on the TMAO oxidation hampering, instead of the bacterial role.

Specific dietary components could also alter gut microbiota composition and activity [60]. Colonic microbiota populations play a key role in the generation of SCFAs, with a positive impact on the metabolism of the host [16]. Within the SCFA, acetate is present in highest proportions in subjects with adherence to the Mediterranean diet [60]. In our results, we observed that Mediterranean plant-derived essential oils alter the fecal composition of SCFA species, as previously reported [61]. More specifically, essential oil emulsions of parsley and rosemary induced an increase in the acetic acid levels, the most abundant SCFA. These results are consistent with the increase in *Lactobacillus* genus population observed in our results, which is one of the highest contributors to the production of acetic acid [62]. In addition, we also observed an increase in the fecal levels of propionic and butyric acids in the rosemary group. In this regard, the higher content of SCFAs seems to be also linked to the increased percentage of *Barnesiella* genus in the gut microbiota by the effect of rosemary essential oil. Consistently, the positive correlation of this genus with the SCFA levels [63] has been previously reported.

Previous studies demonstrated that SCFAs have a beneficial effect on regulating regulatory T cells [64], revealing the important role of both microbiota and microbiota-derived SCFAs on immune system modulation [65,66]. Our data showed a marked differential effect on plasma inflammatory markers depending on the essential oil administered. Thus, our results suggest a role of savory essential oil in a pro-inflammatory response, while both parsley and rosemary essential oils induce an anti-inflammatory profile, likely linked to a high production of SFCAs. It is worth emphasizing that not all SFCAs play the same role in relation to gut health, lipid metabolism and health status. Acetic and butyric acids are used by rat colonic epithelial cells as an energy source and strengthen the epithelial homeostasis preventing inflammation [67,68]. Considering the observed prebiotic effect, boosting *Lactobacillus* genus among others, in parallel to the higher levels found for the three main SFCAs and the anti-inflammatory response, rosemary essential oil seems to exert the most beneficial effect.

In previous studies, the Mediterranean diet has been associated with reduced inflammation [69] due to the effect of some of its components. In our study, the analysis of plasma inflammatory markers, cytokines and chemokines, showed different profiles depending on the type of essential oil used in the treatment. Thus, savory essential oil induced an increase in the levels of chemokines CXCL1, CCL2 and CCL11 and pro-inflammatory cytokines IL−6 and IL−23. Moreover, savory essential oil induced a decrease in IL−4 levels, which is a typical anti-inflammatory cytokine. On the contrary, parsley essential oil induced a more anti-inflammatory pattern showing low levels of IFNγ and IL−22 cytokines. Finally, treatment with rosemary essential oil emulsion clearly showed an anti-inflammatory profile, reducing the levels of IFNγ, TNFα, IL−12p and IL−22. In addition, we found increased levels of CXCL10 in all groups supplemented with L-carnitine when compared with the control group. CXCL10 is a pro-inflammatory chemokine that can be secreted by numerous cell types in response to an inflammatory process, regulating cell recruitment [70]. Its function can be regulated by cytokines, such as IFNγ and TNFα [71–73], and it has been proposed, together with CXCL9 and CXCL11, as a biomarker for heart failure and left ventricular dysfunction [74,75]. It has been previously reported that essential oils can modulate the secretion of important cytokines, having an effect in inflammatory pathways such as nuclear factor kappa-light-chain-enhancer of activated B cells (NF-kB) [76]. Our results suggest that treatment with parsley and rosemary essential oils may partially compensate for the elevation of the pro-inflammatory chemokine CXCL10 by inducing an anti-inflammatory profile.

These pro- and anti-inflammatory profiles may be also related to the production of thrombomodulin, an anti-coagulant cofactor. Interestingly, recent studies have shown that thrombomodulin exhibits anti-inflammatory effects by inhibiting leukocyte recruitment [77]. In addition, the prototypical pro-inflammatory NF-kB signaling pathway has been shown to down-regulate thrombomodulin expression [78]; however, the elevated thrombomodulin expression in the savory and parsley groups was only associated with the decrease in the expression of the pro-inflammatory cytokine IL−22, because the expression of other pro-inflammatory cytokines was inconsistent in both groups.

The antioxidant effect of some plant-derived compounds has been previously applied against a series of chronic diseases, such as IHD and T2DM [30]. Recently, essential oils of some plants have shown to exhibit important antioxidant activity [79]. To evaluate the antioxidant potential of savory, parsley and rosemary essential oils, we assessed the plasma levels of protein carbonyls and pentosidine after treatment. Protein carbonyls are the result of oxidation of lysine, arginine and proline residues in proteins, mostly to AAS and GGS. A pentosidine is a glycosylation end-product formed by the cross-link of a pentose between arginine and lysine residues of proteins. Production of both carbonyls and pentosidine are induced by oxidative reactions and, therefore, their levels are considered as biomarkers of oxidative stress [80]. Protein oxidation and the accretion of protein carbonyls is a pathological hallmark of multiple chronic diseases, such as T2DM, inflammatory bowel diseases and neurodegenerative disorders, among others [81]. Scientific evidence reports the onset of carbonyl stress in hyperglycemic conditions leading to pancreatic failure, insulin resistance and onset of T2DM [31,82]. In addition, pentosidine is commonly used as an indicator of T2DM complications, such as hypertension and heart failure [83]. We did not observe changes induced by L-carnitine supplementation, despite being an antioxidant compound. However, we found a general reduction in the plasma levels of AAS, GGS and pentosidine levels after treatments with essential oil emulsions. Specifically, AAS and pentosidine levels were reduced in mice treated with savory essential oil, while GGS levels were reduced with rosemary essential oil treatment. Consistently, gut microbiota populations were found negatively correlated with AAS and GGS levels in the plasma. Reduction in inflammation in the parsley and rosemary groups may alleviate the oxidative stress, leading to lower levels of protein carbonyls and pentosidine. The savory group also showed reduced oxidative stress, pointing out that the essential oil may contain compounds with intrinsic antioxidant properties. Our results suggest an antioxidant profile of plant-derived compounds widely used in the Mediterranean diet, such as savory, parsley and rosemary essential oils, when used as nutraceuticals.

We are aware that there are some limitations to the findings reported in this study. First, sample size was low, and a higher sample size would allow us to consolidate our results. Second, we used a preclinical humanized model, which entails a number of limitations when transferring the findings directly to patients. Third, randomly cycling female mice were used because the variability in 30 categories of behavioral, morphological, physiological, and molecular traits is not higher than in male mice [84], and because female mice housed in groups do not fight [85]; however, we are aware that future studies need to incorporate females and males in equal numbers with explicit comparison of the two sexes and that the inclusion of the estrous cycle stage of female mice contributes to a better characterization in several of these biochemical variables. Finally, we only assessed a single high dose of essential oil emulsions of savory, parsley and rosemary to evaluate their potential to protect against cardiovascular diseases. Furthermore, the combination of these essential oils could give rise to a synergistic beneficial effect higher than the one observed by each essential oil separately. Thus, our results pave the way for future translational studies assessing the minimal dose with the maximum effect and the potential toxic effect.

5. Conclusions

In summary, this study demonstrates that dietary supplementation of essential oils from parsley, savory and rosemary exert prebiotic effects by promoting or restoring beneficial bacteria populations in the gut of humanized mice with fecal transplantation from patients with IHD and T2DM. These effects on gut microbiota caused a decrease in plasma TMAO levels and an increase in fecal SCFA levels. Interestingly, treatments with essential oil emulsions were associated with an anti-inflammatory and antioxidant profile. It is worth mentioning that rosemary essential oil was the most promising nutraceutical for the treatment and/or prevention of cardiovascular events. Moreover, this work displays novel evidence by which plant-derived essential oils, commonly used in the Mediterranean diet, promote health and protect against inflammation and oxidative stress typically observed in IHD and/or T2DM. Further studies are warranted to validate our results in humans with the aim to modulate the gut microbiota and enhance biochemical biomarkers in patients with IHD and T2DM.

Supplementary Materials: The following supporting information can be downloaded at: https://www.mdpi.com/article/10.3390/nu14214650/s1, Figure S1: Relative gut microbial abundances at the species level. Figure S2: Plasma levels of additional cytokines and chemokines in mice from the treatment groups; Table S1: Experimental diet used in animals. Table S2: Correlation analysis between gut microbial abundance and plasma levels of cytokines and chemokines. Table S3: Correlation analysis between gut microbial abundance and plasma levels of AAS, GGS and pentosidine.

Author Contributions: Conceptualization, M.J.S.-Q., J.D., V.M.B.-M., M.F.J.-N. and F.J.P.-M.; methodology, M.J.S.-Q., J.D., D.M.-V., M.I.Q.-O. and I.P.-A.; software, M.I.Q.-O. and F.J.P.-M.; resources, V.M.B.-M., M.I.Q.-O., M.E., J.R.-C., P.L.S., M.G.C.-L. and F.J.P.-M.; data curation, M.J.S.-Q., J.D., D.M.-V., M.I.Q.-O., M.E. and F.J.P.-M.; writing—review and editing, M.J.S.-Q., J.D. and F.J.P.-M.; project administration, J.D.; funding acquisition, J.D., V.M.B.-M. and M.F.J.-N. All authors have read and agreed to the published version of the manuscript.

Funding: This work was supported by the following projects and programs: Research project (PI-0170-2018) funded by Consejería de Salud y Familias-Junta de Andalucía and the European Regional Development Funds/European Social Fund (ERDF/ESF); Projects funded by the Sociedad Española de Cardiología and Fundación Andaluza de Cardiología; Plataforma ISCIII de Biobancos y Biomodelos de IBIMA (PT20/00101) funded by Instituto de Salud Carlos III, Ministerio de Ciencia e Innovación-Gobierno de España; CIBERCV (CB16/11/00360) funded by Instituto de Salud Carlos III, Ministerio de Ciencia e Innovación-Gobierno de España and ERDF/ESF. M.J.S.Q. holds a Senior Postdoc Researcher contract (RH-0078-2021) funded by Consejería de Salud y Familias-Junta de Andalucía and ERDF/ESF; F.J.P.M. holds a Miguel Servet II research contract (CPII19/00022) and D.M.-V. holds a PFIS contract (FI20/00227) funded by Instituto de Salud Carlos III and ERDF/ESF. J.D. was recipient of mobility grants (MOV19-003) funded by IBIMA and CIBERCV. This study has received support from the Cátedra de Terapias Avanzadas en Patología Cardiovascular (CIF Q-2918001-E), Universidad de Málaga.

Institutional Review Board Statement: The study was conducted in accordance with the Declaration of Helsinki and approved by the "*Animal Experimentation Ethics Committee of BIONAND*", Málaga, Spain (23/10/2018/151).

Informed Consent Statement: Not applicable.

Data Availability Statement: Data is presented as individual data points in this study. Raw data is contained within the Supplementary Material. Additional information is available on request from the corresponding author.

Conflicts of Interest: The authors declare no conflict of interest.

References

1. Timmis, A.; Townsend, N.; Gale, C.P.; Torbica, A.; Lettino, M.; Petersen, S.E.; Mossialos, E.A.; Maggioni, A.P.; Kazakiewicz, D.; May, H.T.; et al. European Society of Cardiology: Cardiovascular Disease Statistics 2019. *Eur. Heart J.* **2020**, *41*, 12–85. [CrossRef]
2. Timmis, A.; Vardas, P.; Townsend, N.; Torbica, A.; Katus, H.; De Smedt, D.; Gale, C.P.; Maggioni, A.P.; Petersen, S.E.; Huculeci, R.; et al. European Society of Cardiology: Cardiovascular Disease Statistics 2021: Executive Summary. *Eur. Hear. J.—Qual. Care Clin. Outcomes* **2022**, *8*, 377–382. [CrossRef]
3. Lau, D.C.W. Metabolic Syndrome: Perception or Reality? *Curr. Atheroscler. Rep.* **2009**, *11*, 264–271. [CrossRef]
4. Sanchez-Alcoholado, L.; Castellano-Castillo, D.; Jordán-Martínez, L.; Moreno-Indias, I.; Cardila-Cruz, P.; Elena, D.; Muñoz-Garcia, A.J.; Queipo-Ortuño, M.I.; Jimenez-Navarro, M. Role of Gut Microbiota on Cardio-Metabolic Parameters and Immunity in Coronary Artery Disease Patients with and without Type-2 Diabetes Mellitus. *Front. Microbiol.* **2017**, *8*, 1936. [CrossRef]
5. Morelli, M.B.; Wang, X.; Santulli, G. Functional Role of Gut Microbiota and PCSK9 in the Pathogenesis of Diabetes Mellitus and Cardiovascular Disease. *Atherosclerosis* **2019**, *289*, 176–178. [CrossRef]
6. Stock, J. Gut Microbiota: An Environmental Risk Factor for Cardiovascular Disease. *Atherosclerosis* **2013**, *229*, 440–442. [CrossRef]
7. Beam, A.; Clinger, E.; Hao, L. Effect of Diet and Dietary Components on the Composition of the Gut Microbiota. *Nutrients* **2021**, *13*, 2795. [CrossRef]
8. Bentham Science Publisher, B.S.P. The Gut Microbiota and Lipid Metabolism: Implications for Human Health and Coronary Heart Disease. *Curr. Med. Chem.* **2006**, *13*, 3005–3021. [CrossRef]
9. Li, S.Y.; Ru, Y.J.; Liu, M.; Xu, B.; Péron, A.; Shi, X.G. The Effect of Essential Oils on Performance, Immunity and Gut Microbial Population in Weaner Pigs. *Livest. Sci.* **2012**, *145*, 119–123. [CrossRef]
10. Koeth, R.A.; Wang, Z.; Levison, B.S.; Buffa, J.A.; Org, E.; Sheehy, B.T.; Britt, E.B.; Fu, X.; Wu, Y.; Li, L.; et al. Intestinal Microbiota Metabolism of L-Carnitine, a Nutrient in Red Meat, Promotes Atherosclerosis. *Nat. Med.* **2013**, *19*, 576–585. [CrossRef]
11. Tang, W.H.W.; Wang, Z.; Levison, B.S.; Koeth, R.A.; Britt, E.B.; Fu, X.; Wu, Y.; Hazen, S.L. Intestinal Microbial Metabolism of Phosphatidylcholine and Cardiovascular Risk. *N. Engl. J. Med.* **2013**, *368*, 1575–1584. [CrossRef] [PubMed]
12. Wang, Z.; Tang, W.H.W.; Buffa, J.A.; Fu, X.; Britt, E.B.; Koeth, R.A.; Levison, B.S.; Fan, Y.; Wu, Y.; Hazen, S.L. Prognostic Value of Choline and Betaine Depends on Intestinal Microbiota-Generated Metabolite Trimethylamine-N-Oxide. *Eur. Heart J.* **2014**, *35*, 904–910. [CrossRef]

13. Trøseid, M.; Ueland, T.; Hov, J.R.; Svardal, A.; Gregersen, I.; Dahl, C.P.; Aakhus, S.; Gude, E.; Bjørndal, B.; Halvorsen, B.; et al. Microbiota-Dependent Metabolite Trimethylamine-N-Oxide Is Associated with Disease Severity and Survival of Patients with Chronic Heart Failure. *J. Intern. Med.* **2015**, *277*, 717–726. [CrossRef]
14. Trøseid, M. Gutmicrobiota and Acute Coronary Syndromes: Ready for Use in the Emergency Room? *Eur. Heart J.* **2017**, *38*, 825–827. [CrossRef]
15. Wu, W.K.; Panyod, S.; Ho, C.T.; Kuo, C.H.; Wu, M.S.; Sheen, L.Y. Dietary Allicin Reduces Transformation of L-Carnitine to TMAO through Impact on Gut Microbiota. *J. Funct. Foods* **2015**, *15*, 408–417. [CrossRef]
16. Miller, T.L.; Wolin, M.J. Pathways of Acetate, Propionate, and Butyrate Formation by the Human Fecal Microbial Flora. *Appl. Environ. Microbiol.* **1996**, *62*, 1589–1592. [CrossRef]
17. Louis, P.; Flint, H.J. Diversity, Metabolism and Microbial Ecology of Butyrate-Producing Bacteria from the Human Large Intestine. *FEMS Microbiol. Lett.* **2009**, *294*, 1–8. [CrossRef]
18. Holscher, H.D. Dietary Fiber and Prebiotics and the Gastrointestinal Microbiota. *Gut Microbes* **2017**, *8*, 172–184. [CrossRef]
19. Venegas, D.P.; De La Fuente, M.K.; Landskron, G.; González, M.J.; Quera, R.; Dijkstra, G.; Harmsen, H.J.M.; Faber, K.N.; Hermoso, M.A. Short Chain Fatty Acids (SCFAs)Mediated Gut Epithelial and Immune Regulation and Its Relevance for Inflammatory Bowel Diseases. *Front. Immunol.* **2019**, *10*, 277. [CrossRef]
20. Fernandes, J.; Su, W.; Rahat-Rozenbloom, S.; Wolever, T.M.S.; Comelli, E.M. Adiposity, Gut Microbiota and Faecal Short Chain Fatty Acids Are Linked in Adult Humans. *Nutr. Diabetes* **2014**, *4*, e121. [CrossRef]
21. Luu, M.; Pautz, S.; Kohl, V.; Singh, R.; Romero, R.; Lucas, S.; Hofmann, J.; Raifer, H.; Vachharajani, N.; Carrascosa, L.C.; et al. The Short-Chain Fatty Acid Pentanoate Suppresses Autoimmunity by Modulating the Metabolic-Epigenetic Crosstalk in Lymphocytes. *Nat. Commun.* **2019**, *10*, 760. [CrossRef]
22. Cummings, J.H.; Pomare, E.W.; Branch, H.W.J.; Naylor, C.P.E.; MacFarlane, G.T. Short Chain Fatty Acids in Human Large Intestine, Portal, Hepatic and Venous Blood. *Gut* **1987**, *28*, 1221–1227. [CrossRef]
23. Bergman, E.N. Energy Contributions of Volatile Fatty Acids from the Gastrointestinal Tract in Various Species. *Physiol. Rev.* **1990**, *70*, 567–590. [CrossRef] [PubMed]
24. Macfarlane, S.; Macfarlane, G.T. Regulation of Short-Chain Fatty Acid Production. *Proc. Nutr. Soc.* **2003**, *62*, 67–72. [CrossRef] [PubMed]
25. Pituch, A.; Walkowiak, J.; Banaszkiewicz, A. Butyric Acid in Functional Constipation. *Prz. Gastroenterol.* **2013**, *8*, 295–298. [CrossRef] [PubMed]
26. Hernández, M.A.G.; Canfora, E.E.; Jocken, J.W.E.; Blaak, E.E. The Short-Chain Fatty Acid Acetate in Body Weight Control and Insulin Sensitivity. *Nutrients* **2019**, *11*, 943. [CrossRef]
27. Hashemipour, H.; Kermanshahi, H.; Golian, A.; Veldkamp, T. Metabolism and Nutrition: Effect of Thymol and Carvacrol Feed Supplementation on Performance, Antioxidant Enzyme Activities, Fatty Acid Composition, Digestive Enzyme Activities, and Immune Response in Broiler Chickens. *Poult. Sci.* **2013**, *92*, 2059–2069. [CrossRef]
28. Alagawany, M. Biological Effects and Modes of Action of Carvacrol in Animal and Poultry Production and Health—A Review. *Adv. Anim. Vet. Sci.* **2015**, *3*, 73–84. [CrossRef]
29. Lontchi-Yimagou, E.; Sobngwi, E.; Matsha, T.E.; Kengne, A.P. Diabetes Mellitus and Inflammation. *Curr. Diab. Rep.* **2013**, *13*, 435–444. [CrossRef]
30. Bucciantini, M.; Leri, M.; Nardiello, P.; Casamenti, F.; Stefani, M. Olive Polyphenols: Antioxidant and Anti-Inflammatory Properties. *Antioxidants* **2021**, *10*, 1044. [CrossRef]
31. Luna, C.; Arjona, A.; Dueñas, C.; Estevez, M. Allysine and α-Aminoadipic Acid as Markers of the Glyco-Oxidative Damage to Human Serum Albumin under Pathological Glucose Concentrations. *Antioxidants* **2021**, *10*, 474. [CrossRef] [PubMed]
32. Kalousová, M.; Sulková, S.; Fialová, L.; Soukupová, J.; Malbohan, I.M.; Špaček, P.; Braun, M.; Mikulíková, L.; Fořtová, M.; Hořejší, M.; et al. Glycoxidation and Inflammation in Chronic Haemodialysis Patients. *Nephrol. Dial. Transplant.* **2003**, *18*, 2577–2581. [CrossRef] [PubMed]
33. Requena, J.R.; Chao, C.C.; Levine, R.L.; Stadtman, E.R. Glutamic and Aminoadipic Semialdehydes Are the Main Carbonyl Products of Metal-Catalyzed Oxidation of Proteins. *Proc. Natl. Acad. Sci. USA* **2001**, *98*, 69–74. [CrossRef] [PubMed]
34. Arcanjo, N.M.O.; Luna, C.; Madruga, M.S.; Estévez, M. Antioxidant and Pro-Oxidant Actions of Resveratrol on Human Serum Albumin in the Presence of Toxic Diabetes Metabolites: Glyoxal and Methyl-Glyoxal. *Biochim. Biophys. Acta—Gen. Subj.* **2018**, *1862*, 1938–1947. [CrossRef]
35. Sell, D.R.; Strauch, C.M.; Shen, W.; Monnier, V.M. 2-Aminoadipic Acid Is a Marker of Protein Carbonyl Oxidation in the Aging Human Skin: Effects of Diabetes, Renal Failure and Sepsis. *Biochem. J.* **2007**, *404*, 269–277. [CrossRef]
36. Kennedy, E.A.; King, K.Y.; Baldridge, M.T. Mouse Microbiota Models: Comparing Germ-Free Mice and Antibiotics Treatment as Tools for Modifying Gut Bacteria. *Front. Physiol.* **2018**, *9*, 1534. [CrossRef]
37. Reikvam, D.H.; Erofeev, A.; Sandvik, A.; Grcic, V.; Jahnsen, F.L.; Gaustad, P.; McCoy, K.D.; Macpherson, A.J.; Meza-Zepeda, L.A.; Johansen, F.E. Depletion of Murine Intestinal Microbiota: Effects on Gut Mucosa and Epithelial Gene Expression. *PLoS ONE* **2011**, *6*, e0017996. [CrossRef]
38. Le Bastard, Q.; Ward, T.; Sidiropoulos, D.; Hillmann, B.M.; Chun, C.L.; Sadowsky, M.J.; Knights, D.; Montassier, E. Fecal Microbiota Transplantation Reverses Antibiotic and Chemotherapy-Induced Gut Dysbiosis in Mice. *Sci. Rep.* **2018**, *8*, 6219. [CrossRef]

39. Zhang, Y.; Huang, R.; Cheng, M.; Wang, L.; Chao, J.; Li, J.; Zheng, P.; Xie, P.; Zhang, Z.; Yao, H. Gut Microbiota from NLRP3-Deficient Mice Ameliorates Depressive-like Behaviors by Regulating Astrocyte Dysfunction via CircHIPK2. *Microbiome* **2019**, *7*, 116. [CrossRef]
40. Ubeda, C.; Bucci, V.; Caballero, S.; Djukovic, A.; Toussaint, N.C.; Equinda, M.; Lipuma, L.; Ling, L.; Gobourne, A.; No, D.; et al. Intestinal Microbiota Containing Barnesiella Species Cures Vancomycin-Resistant Enterococcus Faecium Colonization. *Infect. Immun.* **2013**, *81*, 965–973. [CrossRef]
41. Wilson Tang, W.H.; Wang, Z.; Kennedy, D.J.; Wu, Y.; Buffa, J.A.; Agatisa-Boyle, B.; Li, X.S.; Levison, B.S.; Hazen, S.K. Gut Microbiota-Dependent Trimethylamine N-Oxide (TMAO) Pathway Contributes to Both Development of Renal Insufficiency and Mortality Risk in Chronic Kidney Disease. *Circ. Res.* **2015**, *116*, 448–455. [CrossRef] [PubMed]
42. Utrera, M.; Morcuende, D.; Rodríguez-Carpena, J.G.; Estévez, M. Fluorescent HPLC for the Detection of Specific Protein Oxidation Carbonyls—α-Aminoadipic and γ-Glutamic Semialdehydes—In Meat Systems. *Meat Sci.* **2011**, *89*, 500–506. [CrossRef] [PubMed]
43. Bolyen, E.; Rideout, J.R.; Dillon, M.R.; Bokulich, N.A.; Abnet, C.C.; Al-Ghalith, G.A.; Alexander, H.; Alm, E.J.; Arumugam, M.; Asnicar, F.; et al. Reproducible, Interactive, Scalable and Extensible Microbiome Data Science Using QIIME 2. *Nat. Biotechnol.* **2019**, *37*, 852–857. [CrossRef]
44. Sánchez-Alcoholado, L.; Ordóñez, R.; Otero, A.; Plaza-Andrade, I.; Laborda-Illanes, A.; Medina, J.A.; Ramos-Molina, B.; Gómez-Millán, J.; Queipo-Ortuño, M.I. Gut Microbiota-Mediated Inflammation and Gut Permeability in Patients with Obesity and Colorectal Cancer. *Int. J. Mol. Sci.* **2020**, *21*, 6782. [CrossRef]
45. Razquin, C.; Martinez-Gonzalez, M.A. A Traditional Mediterranean Diet Effectively Reduces Inflammation and Improves Cardiovascular Health. *Nutrients* **2019**, *11*, 1842. [CrossRef] [PubMed]
46. Estruch, R.; Ros, E.; Salvadó, J.S.; Covas, M.; Corella, D.; Arós, F.; Gracia, E.G.; Gutiérrez, V.R.; Fiol, M.; Lapetra, J.; et al. Primary Prevention of Cardiovascular Disease with a Mediterranean Diet Supplemented with Extra-Virgin Olive Oil or Nuts. *N. Engl. J. Med.* **2018**, *379*, 1387. [CrossRef]
47. Liang, K.W.; Lee, C.L.; Liu, W.J. Lower All-Cause Mortality for Coronary Heart or Stroke Patients Who Adhere Better to Mediterranean Diet-An. *Nutrients* **2022**, *14*, 3203. [CrossRef]
48. Novaković, M.; Rajkovič, U.; Košuta, D.; Tršan, J.; Fras, Z.; Jug, B. Effects of Cardiac Rehabilitation and Diet Counselling on Adherence to the Mediterranean Lifestyle in Patients after Myocardial Infarction. *Nutrients* **2022**, *14*, 4048. [CrossRef]
49. Delgado-Lista, J.; Alcala-Diaz, J.F.; Torres-Peña, J.D.; Quintana-Navarro, G.M.; Fuentes, F.; Garcia-Rios, A.; Ortiz-Morales, A.M.; Gonzalez-Requero, A.I.; Perez-Caballero, A.I.; Yubero-Serrano, E.M.; et al. Long-Term Secondary Prevention of Cardiovascular Disease with a Mediterranean Diet and a Low-Fat Diet (CORDIOPREV): A Randomised Controlled Trial. *Lancet* **2022**, *399*, 1876–1885. [CrossRef]
50. Jiménez-Sánchez, A.; Martínez-Ortega, A.J.; Remón-Ruiz, P.J.; Piñar-Gutiérrez, A.; Pereira-Cunill, J.L.; García-Luna, P.P. Therapeutic Properties and Use of Extra Virgin Olive Oil in Clinical Nutrition: A Narrative Review and Literature Update. *Nutrients* **2022**, *14*, 1440. [CrossRef]
51. Claro-cala, C.M.; Jim, F.; Rodriguez-Rodriguez, R. Molecular Mechanisms Underlying the Effects of Olive Oil Triterpenic Acids in Obesity and Related Diseases. *Nutrients* **2022**, *14*, 1606. [CrossRef] [PubMed]
52. Gomez-Marin, B.; Gomez-Delgado, F.; Lopez-Moreno, J.; Alcala-Diaz, J.F.; Jimenez-Lucena, R.; Torres-Peña, J.D.; Garcia-Rios, A.; Ortiz-Morales, A.M.; Yubero-Serrano, E.M.; Malagon, M.D.M.; et al. Long-Term Consumption of a Mediterranean Diet Improves Postprandial Lipemia in Patients with Type 2 Diabetes: The Cordioprev Randomized Trial. *Am. J. Clin. Nutr.* **2018**, *108*, 963–970. [CrossRef] [PubMed]
53. Long, Y.; Li, D.; Yu, S.; Zhang, Y.-L.; Liu, S.-Y.; Wan, J.-Y.; Shi, A.; Deng, J.; Wen, J.; Li, X.-Q.; et al. Natural essential oils: A promising strategy for treating cardio-cerebrovascular diseases. *J. Ethnopharmacol.* **2022**, *297*, 115421. [CrossRef]
54. Verhaar, B.J.; Prodan, A.; Nieuwdorp, M.; Muller, M. Gut Microbiota in Hypertension and Atherosclerosis: A Review. *Nutrients* **2020**, *12*, 2982. [CrossRef] [PubMed]
55. Garcia-mantrana, I.; Selma-royo, M.; Alcantara, C.; Collado, M.C. Shifts on Gut Microbiota Associated to Mediterranean Diet Adherence and Specific Dietary Intakes on General Adult Population. *Front. Microbiol.* **2018**, *9*, 890. [CrossRef]
56. Bennett, B.J.; de Aguiar Vallim, T.Q.; Wang, Z.; Shih, D.M.; Meng, Y.; Gregory, J.; Allayee, H.; Lee, B.; Graham, M.; Crooke, R.; et al. Trimethylamine-N-oxide, a metabolite associated with atherosclerosis, exhibits complex genetic and dietary regulation. *Cell Metab.* **2014**, *17*, 49–60. [CrossRef]
57. Cho, C.E.; Caudill, M.A. Trimethylamine-N-Oxide: Friend, Foe, or Simply Caught in the Cross-Fire? *Trends Endocrinol. Metab.* **2017**, *28*, 121–130. [CrossRef]
58. Zysset-burri, D.C.; Keller, I.; Berger, L.E.; Neyer, P.J.; Steuer, C.; Wolf, S.; Zinkernagel, M.S. Retinal Artery Occlusion Is Associated with Compositional and Functional Shifts in the Gut Microbiome and Altered Trimethylamine-N-Oxide Levels. *Sci. Rep.* **2019**, *9*, 15303. [CrossRef]
59. Romano, K.A.; Vivas, E.I.; Amador-noguez, D.; Rey, F.E. From Diet and Accumulation of the Proatherogenic Metabolite. *Intest. Microbiota Choline Metab.* **2015**, *6*, 1–8. [CrossRef]
60. Muralidharan, J.; Galiè, S.; Hernández-alonso, P. Plant-Based Fat, Dietary Patterns Rich in Vegetable Fat and Gut Microbiota Modulation. *Front. Nutr.* **2019**, *6*, 157. [CrossRef]
61. Yan, J.; Wang, L.; Gu, Y.; Hou, H.; Liu, T.; Ding, Y.; Cao, H. Dietary Patterns and Gut Microbiota Changes in Inflammatory Bowel Disease: Current Insights and Future Challenges. *Nutrients* **2022**, *14*, 4003. [CrossRef] [PubMed]

62. Feng, W.; Ao, H.; Peng, C. Gut Microbiota, Short-Chain Fatty Acids, and Herbal Medicines. *Front. Pharmacol.* **2018**, *9*, 1354. [CrossRef] [PubMed]
63. Zhao, Y.; Wu, J.; Li, J.V.; Zhou, N.Y.; Tang, H.; Wang, Y. Gut Microbiota Composition Modifies Fecal Metabolic Profiles in Mice. *J. Proteome Res.* **2013**, *12*, 2987–2999. [CrossRef]
64. Dąbek-Drobny, A.; Kaczmarczyk, O.; Piątek-Guziewicz, A.; Woźniakiewicz, M.; Paśko, P.; Dobrowolska-Iwanek, J.; Woźniakiewicz, A.; Targosz, A.; Ptak-Belowska, A.; Zagrodzki, P.; et al. Application of the Clustering Technique to Multiple Nutritional Factors Related to Inflammation and Disease Progression in Patients with Inflammatory Bowel Disease. *Nutrients* **2022**, *14*, 3960. [CrossRef]
65. Tang, T.W.H.; Chen, H.C.; Chen, C.Y.; Yen, C.Y.T.; Lin, C.J.; Prajnamitra, R.P.; Chen, L.L.; Ruan, S.C.; Lin, J.H.; Lin, P.J.; et al. Loss of Gut Microbiota Alters Immune System Composition and Cripples Postinfarction Cardiac Repair. *Circulation* **2019**, *139*, 647–659. [CrossRef] [PubMed]
66. Sadler, R.; Cramer, J.V.; Heindl, S.; Kostidis, S.; Betz, D.; Zuurbier, K.R.; Northoff, B.H.; Heijink, M.; Goldberg, M.P.; Plautz, E.J.; et al. Short-Chain Fatty Acids Improve Poststroke Recovery via Immunological Mechanisms. *J. Neurosci.* **2020**, *40*, 1162–1173. [CrossRef]
67. Den Besten, G.; Van Eunen, K.; Groen, A.K.; Venema, K.; Reijngoud, D.J.; Bakker, B.M. The Role of Short-Chain Fatty Acids in the Interplay between Diet, Gut Microbiota, and Host Energy Metabolism. *J. Lipid Res.* **2013**, *54*, 2325–2340. [CrossRef]
68. He, J.; Zhang, P.; Shen, L.; Niu, L.; Tan, Y.; Chen, L.; Zhao, Y.; Bai, L.; Hao, X.; Li, X.; et al. Short-Chain Fatty Acids and Their Association with Signalling Pathways in Inflammation, Glucose and Lipid Metabolism. *Int. J. Mol. Sci.* **2020**, *21*, 6356. [CrossRef]
69. Finicelli, M.; Di Salle, A.; Galderisi, U. The Mediterranean Diet: An Update of the Clinical Trials. *Nutrients* **2022**, *14*, 2956. [CrossRef]
70. Nie, M.; Li, H.; Liu, P.; Dang, P. HMBOX1 Attenuates LPS-induced Periodontal Ligament Stem Cell Injury by Inhibiting CXCL10 Expression through the NF-κB Signaling Pathway. *Exp. Ther. Med.* **2022**, *23*, 224. [CrossRef]
71. Zhang, F.; Mears, J.R.; Shakib, L.; Beynor, J.I.; Shanaj, S. Expanded in Severe COVID-19 and Other Diseases with Tissue Inflammation. *bioRxiv* **2020**. [CrossRef]
72. Luster, A.; Unkeless, J.; Ravetch, J. γ-Interferon Transcriptionally Regulates an Early-Response Gene Containing Homology to Platelet Proteins. *Nature* **1985**, *315*, 672–676. [CrossRef] [PubMed]
73. Gao, J.; Wu, L.; Wang, S.; Chen, X. Role of Chemokine (C-X-C Motif) Ligand 10 (CXCL10) in Renal Diseases. *Mediat. Inflamm.* **2020**, *2020*, 6194864. [CrossRef]
74. Altara, R.; Gu, Y.M.; Struijker-Boudier, H.A.J.; Thijs, L.; Staessen, J.A.; Blankesteijn, W.M. Left Ventricular Dysfunction and CXCR3 Ligands in Hypertension: From Animal Experiments to a Population-Based Pilot Study. *PLoS ONE* **2015**, *10*, e0141394. [CrossRef]
75. Altara, R.; Manca, M.; Hessel, M.H.; Gu, Y.; van Vark, L.C.; Akkerhuis, K.M.; Staessen, J.A.; Struijker-Boudier, H.A.J.; Booz, G.W.; Blankesteijn, W.M. CXCL10 Is a Circulating Inflammatory Marker in Patients with Advanced Heart Failure: A Pilot Study. *J. Cardiovasc. Transl. Res.* **2016**, *9*, 302–314. [CrossRef]
76. Valdivieso-Ugarte, M.; Gomez-llorente, C.; Plaza-Díaz, J.; Gil, Á. Antimicrobial, Antioxidant, and Immunomodulatory Properties of Essential Oils: A Systematic Review. *Nutrients* **2019**, *11*, 2786. [CrossRef] [PubMed]
77. Nishizawa, S.; Kikuta, J.; Seno, S.; Kajiki, M.; Tsujita, R.; Mizuno, H.; Sudo, T.; Ao, T.; Matsuda, H.; Ishii, M. Thrombomodulin Induces Anti-Inflammatory Effects by Inhibiting the Rolling Adhesion of Leukocytes in Vivo. *J. Pharmacol. Sci.* **2020**, *143*, 17–22. [CrossRef]
78. Lentz, S.R.; Tsiang, M.; Sadler, J.E. Regulation of Thrombomodulin by Tumor Necrosis Factor-α: Comparison of Transcriptional and Posttranscriptional Mechanisms. *Blood* **1991**, *77*, 542–550. [CrossRef]
79. Mutlu-Ingok, A.; Devecioglu, D.; Dikmetas, D.N.; Karbancioglu-Guler, F.; Capanoglu, E. Antibacterial, Antifungal, Antimycotoxigenic, and Antioxidant Activities of Essential Oils: An Updated Review. *Nutrients* **2020**, *25*, 4711. [CrossRef]
80. Colombo, G.; Reggiani, F.; Angelini, C.; Finazzi, S.; Astori, E.; Garavaglia, M.L.; Landoni, L.; Portinaro, N.M.; Giustarini, D.; Rossi, R.; et al. Plasma Protein Carbonyls as Biomarkers of Oxidative Stress in Chronic Kidney Disease, Dialysis, and Transplantation. *Oxid. Med. Cell Longev.* **2020**, *2020*, 2975256. [CrossRef] [PubMed]
81. Dalle-Donne, I.; Giustarini, D.; Colombo, R.; Rossi, R.; Milzani, A. Protein Carbonylation in Human Diseases. *Trends Mol. Med.* **2003**, *9*, 169–176. [CrossRef]
82. Hecker, M.; Wagner, A.H. Role of Protein Carbonylation in Diabetes. *J. Inherit. Metab. Dis.* **2018**, *41*, 29–38. [CrossRef]
83. Sugiyama, S.; Miyata, T.; Ueda, Y.; Tanaka, H.; Maeda, K.; Kawashima, S.; Van Ypersele De Strihou, C.; Kurokawa, K. Plasma Levels of Pentosidine in Diabetic Patients: An Advanced Glycation End Product. *J. Am. Soc. Nephrol.* **1998**, *9*, 1681–1688. [CrossRef] [PubMed]
84. Prendergast, B.J.; Onishi, K.G.; Zucker, I. Female mice liberated for inclusion in neuroscience and biomedical research. *Neurosci. Biobehav. Rev.* **2014**, *40*, 1–5. [CrossRef] [PubMed]
85. Meakin, L.B.; Sugiyama, T.; Galea, G.L.; Browne, W.J.; Lanyon, L.E.; Price, J.S. Male Mice Housed in Groups Engage in Frequent Fighting and Show a Lower Response to Additional Bone Loading than Females or Individually Housed Males That Do Not Fight. *Bone* **2013**, *54*, 113–117. [CrossRef]

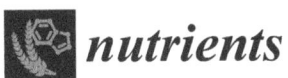

Article

The Role of 20-HETE, COX, Thromboxane Receptors, and Blood Plasma Antioxidant Status in Vascular Relaxation of Copper-Nanoparticle-Fed WKY Rats

Michał Majewski [1,*], Jerzy Juśkiewicz [2], Magdalena Krajewska-Włodarczyk [3], Leszek Gromadziński [4], Katarzyna Socha [5], Ewelina Cholewińska [6] and Katarzyna Ognik [6]

1. Department of Pharmacology and Toxicology, UWM, 10-082 Olsztyn, Poland
2. Division of Food Science, Institute of Animal Reproduction and Food Research, Polish Academy of Sciences, 10-748 Olsztyn, Poland; j.juskiewicz@pan.olsztyn.pl
3. Department of Mental and Psychosomatic Diseases, Faculty of Medicine, UWM, 10-228 Olsztyn, Poland; magdalenakw@op.pl
4. Department of Cardiology and Internal Medicine, Faculty of Medicine, UWM, 10-082 Olsztyn, Poland; leszek.gromadzinski@uwm.edu.pl
5. Department of Bromatology, Medical University of Białystok, 15-222 Białystok, Poland; katarzyna.socha@umb.edu.pl
6. Department of Biochemistry and Toxicology, Faculty of Biology, Animal Sciences and Bioeconomy, University of Life Sciences, 20-950 Lublin, Poland; ewelina.cholewinska@up.lublin.pl (E.C.); kasiaognik@poczta.fm (K.O.)
* Correspondence: michal.majewski@uwm.edu.pl; Tel.: +48-89-524-56-68

Citation: Majewski, M.; Juśkiewicz, J.; Krajewska-Włodarczyk, M.; Gromadziński, L.; Socha, K.; Cholewińska, E.; Ognik, K. The Role of 20-HETE, COX, Thromboxane Receptors, and Blood Plasma Antioxidant Status in Vascular Relaxation of Copper-Nanoparticle-Fed WKY Rats. *Nutrients* **2021**, *13*, 3793. https://doi.org/10.3390/nu13113793

Academic Editors: Gaetano Santulli and Bruno Trimarco

Received: 25 September 2021
Accepted: 24 October 2021
Published: 26 October 2021

Publisher's Note: MDPI stays neutral with regard to jurisdictional claims in published maps and institutional affiliations.

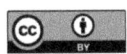

Copyright: © 2021 by the authors. Licensee MDPI, Basel, Switzerland. This article is an open access article distributed under the terms and conditions of the Creative Commons Attribution (CC BY) license (https://creativecommons.org/licenses/by/4.0/).

Abstract: Recently, the addition of copper nanoparticles (NPs) in a daily diet (6.5 mg/kg) was studied in different animal models as a possible alternative to ionic forms. Male Wistar–Kyoto rats (24-week-old, $n = 11$) were fed with copper, either in the form of carbonate salt ($Cu_{6.5}$) or metal-based copper NPs ($NP_{6.5}$), for 8 weeks. The third group was fed with a half dose of each ($NP_{3.25} + Cu_{3.25}$). The thoracic aorta and blood plasma was studied. Supplementation with $NP_{6.5}$ decreased the Cu ($\times 0.7$), Cu/Zn-ratio ($\times 0.6$) and catalase (CAT, $\times 0.7$), and increased Zn ($\times 1.2$) and superoxide dismutase (SOD, $\times 1.4$). Meanwhile, $NP_{3.25} + Cu_{3.25}$ decreased the Cu/Zn-ratio ($\times 0.7$), and CAT ($\times 0.7$), and increased the daily feed intake ($\times 1.06$). Preincubation with either the selective cyclooxygenase (COX)-2 inhibitor, or the non-selective COX-1/2 inhibitor attenuated vasodilation of rat thoracic aorta in the $NP_{6.5}$ group exclusively. However, an increased vasodilator response was observed in the $NP_{6.5}$ and $NP_{3.25} + Cu_{3.25}$ group of rats after preincubation with an inhibitor of 20-hydroxyeicosatetraenoic acid (20-HETE) formation, and the thromboxane receptor (TP) antagonist. Significant differences were observed between the $NP_{6.5}$ and $NP_{3.25} + Cu_{3.25}$ groups of rats in: dietary intake, acetylcholine-induced vasodilation, and response to COX-inhibitors. Copper NPs in a standard daily dose had more significant effects on the mechanism(s) responsible for the utilization of reactive oxygen species in the blood plasma with the participation of prostanoids derived from COX-2 in the vascular relaxation. Dietary copper NPs in both doses modified vasodilation through the vasoconstrictor 20-HETE and the TP receptors.

Keywords: aging; 20-HETE; furegrelate; HET0016; indomethacin; NS-398; SQ-29,548; thromboxane-A_2

1. Introduction

Copper fluctuations in a diet may have either pro- or antioxidant effects on animal or human health, dependent on the daily dose [1–4]. A high intake of copper (including the recommended daily dose) may induce oxidation of lipids and proteins in cells that are potentiated in situations of a high-risk susceptibility to toxic compounds, such as in diabetes mellitus or hypertension [5,6]. Many of the major enzymes of biological processes are influenced by copper intake, including Cu–Zn superoxide dismutase (SOD), cytochrome c oxidase, lysyl oxidase, L-ascorbate oxidase, monoamine oxidase, tyrosinase, and the enzymes of tryptophan degradation [7]. This may bring oxidative damage to lipids, proteins, and DNA, and result in neurodegenerative changes when dysregulated by either copper deficiency or its surplus [8,9].

Moreover, administration of copper nanoparticles (NPs) to animal feed, in a standard daily dose, may be of toxicological relevance due to its negative impact on animal health and the excretion of a large amount of this element into the environment and thus contamination [10]. Copper NPs induce a toxic effect by the increased production of free radicals, including hydroxyl radicals, hydrogen peroxides, and superoxide anions. The properties of metal NPs, including small size and high reactivity, increase their biological action, which may interfere with the physiological processes and the bioavailability of other macro- and microelements; therefore, the standard daily dose (6.5 mg/kg of diet) should probably be reduced to prevent increased toxicity [11].

As there are just a few studies regarding the safety of copper NPs in rats, and some of these results are controversial, we aimed to examine the influence of a standard 6.5 mg/kg dose of copper as NPs. In another group, the daily dose of NPs was reduced by half, to 3.25 mg/kg, and 3.25 mg/kg of copper carbonate was added instead. The third group was fed with 6.5 mg/kg of copper carbonate. The blood plasma antioxidant status was studied together with the participation of arachidonic acid metabolites in the vasodilator response of rat thoracic aorta to acetylcholine.

2. Materials and Methods

2.1. Drugs and Chemicals

Acetylcholine (chloride), indomethacin, noradrenaline (hydrochloride), and NS-398 were obtained from Sigma-Aldrich (St. Louise, MO, USA); copper as carbonate (purity $\geq 99\%$) from Poch (Gliwice, Poland); SQ-29,548, furegrelate, and HET0016 from Cayman Chemical (Ann Arbor, MI, USA). Stock solutions (10 mM) of these drugs were prepared in distilled water, except for noradrenaline, which was dissolved in NaCl (0.9%) + ascorbic acid (0.01% w/v) solution; HET0016, SQ-29,548, and indomethacin were dissolved in ethanol; 1400 W in methanol; and NS-398 in DMSO. The solvent concentration was less than 0.01% (v/v).

These solutions were stored at $-20\,^\circ$C, and appropriate dilutions were made in Krebs–Henseleit solution (KH in mM: NaCl 115; $CaCl_2$ 2.5; KCl 4.6; KH_2PO_4 1.2; $MgSO_4$ 1.2; $NaHCO_3$ 25; glucose 11.1) on the day of the experiment.

Metal-Based Copper Nanoparticles

Copper NPs (99.9% purity powder, 40–60 nm size, 12 m^2/g SSA, spherical morphology, 0.19 g/cm^3 bulk density, 8.9 g/cm^3 true density) were purchased from Sky Spring Nanomaterials (Inc., Houston, TX, USA). Stock solution (5 g/L) was prepared in a rapeseed oil, and about 9% of NPs dissolved as Cu (II) ions; thus, the final suspension contained both NPs and released copper species. The zeta potential of the copper NP suspension was determined to be -30.3 mV (in PBS) and -38.3 mV (pH 5), and the size was 104 nm (in rapeseed oil) determined by dynamic light scattering with a Zetasizer Nano ZS (Malvern Instruments, Malvern, UK) [12].

2.2. Experimental Protocol

24-week-old normotensive Wistar–Kyoto (WKYs/NCrl) rats from Charles River (Sulzfeld, Germany) were allocated randomly to 3 groups ($n = 11$) and were fed individually for 8 weeks with experimental diets under standard laboratory conditions [1]. Exclusively male rats were studied, to enable comparison with the previous experimentations. The rats were fed with copper in a standard daily dose of 6.5 mg/kg, either as carbonate salt ($Cu_{6.5}$) or metal NPs ($NP_{6.5}$). Moreover, the third group ($NP_{3.25} + Cu_{3.25}$) was fed with 3.25 mg of copper NPs plus 3.25 mg of copper carbonate. Animal pellets were prepared according to the American Institute of Nutrition, and the copper NPs were dissolved in pure rapeseed oil (5 g/L) and mixed with the diet weekly [1].

2.3. Experimental Procedures

Intraperitoneal injections of ketamine (100 mg/kg BW) and xylazine (10 mg/kg BW) were used for anesthesia, followed by exsanguination [13]. Blood was centrifuged at $3000 \times g$ for 10 min to separate the plasma, which was further stored at -80 °C until analysis. The thoracic aorta was dissected and kept in an ice-cold Krebs–Henseleit buffer.

2.4. Blood Analysis

Copper and zinc were measured by the ICP–OES method. Bovine liver was used as a certified reference material (NIST1577C) for quality control. The units are expressed as µM. Superoxide dismutase activity was measured with Ransod and Ransel diagnostic kits (Randox); meanwhile, catalase (CAT) was determined by the enzymatic decomposition of hydrogen peroxide into water and oxygen. Data are expressed in U/mL. The sums of reduced glutathione (GSH) and oxidized glutathione (GSSG) were determined using an enzymatic method (Cell Biolabs) [14]. The units are expressed as µM. The total antioxidant potency FRAP (Ferric Reducing Antioxidant Power) was measured colorimetrically at 594 nm through the reduction of Fe(III) to Fe(II) by antioxidants present in the sample. Data are expressed as µM. The malondialdehyde (MDA) generates the MDA–TBA adduct, which was quantified with a fluorometric assay kit (ab118970) at Ex/Em = 532/553 nm. Data are expressed as mM.

2.5. Vascular Reactivity Studies

Briefly, aortic rings of 4 mm length were mounted in a stagnant 5 mL Graz Tissue Bath System (Barcelona, Spain) under the pre-load tension of 1 cN and aerated with carbogen gas for 60 min (TAM-A Hugo Sachs Elektronik, March, Germany) [15,16]. The functional integrity of aortic rings was checked with high K^+ (75 mM KCl) and ACh (10 µM). Next, aortic rings were incubated for 30 min with either the inducible nitric oxide synthase (iNOS) inhibitor (1 µM, 1400 W), the selective cyclooxygenase-2 (COX-2) inhibitor (10 µM, NS-398), the non-selective COX-1/2 inhibitor (10 µM, indomethacin), the inhibitor of 20-hydroxyeicosatetraenoic acid (20-HETE) formation (0.1 µM, HET0016), the thromboxane-A_2 synthase inhibitor (1 µM, furegrelate), or the thromboxane-A_2 receptor (TP) antagonist (1 µM, SQ-29,548), and contracted with noradrenaline (0.1 µM). Then, the cumulative doses of ACh (0.1 nM–10 µM) were added into the incubation chambers. Only one cumulative concentration–response curve (CCRC) was performed on each aortic ring.

2.6. Data Analysis and Statistics

Vascular relaxation was expressed as a percentage of the contractile response to noradrenaline NA (0.1 µM). The CCRCs were analyzed by a nonlinear regression model (log agonist vs. response), which determined the area under the curve (dAUC), the maximal response (E_{max}, %), and the potency ($pEC_{50} = -logEC_{50}$). The Gaussian distribution of residuals and homoscedasticity of variance were tested for all data with $n = 11$; "n" refers to independent values, not replicates. The group comparison was performed by either a parametric (t-test or ANOVA) or non-parametric test (Mann–Whitney U-test or Kruskal–Wallis test). Results are expressed as the means ± SEM (for CCRCs) and means ± SD. Due to the small group sizes ($n < 12$), outliers detected by Grubbs' test were included in a data set [13]. The level of significance was when * $p < 0.05$.

3. Results

3.1. The General Characterization of WKY Rats

These results are presented in Figure 1A–D. Experimental supplementation with $NP_{6.5}$ neither changed the body weight (BW) gain ($\times 1.0$, Figure 1C), nor the dietary intake ($\times 1.02$, Figure 1D). In the $NP_{3.25} + Cu_{3.25}$ group of rats, BW gain was not changed in a significant way ($\times 1.4$, Figure 1C), contrary to the significant increase in daily feed intake ($\times 1.06$, $p = 0.0008$, Figure 1D). No significant difference was observed in the BW gain between

NP$_{3.25}$ + Cu$_{3.25}$ and NP$_{6.5}$ supplemented rats (×1.4, Figure 1C), as opposed to the increased daily feed intake (×1.04, p = 0.0462, Figure 1D).

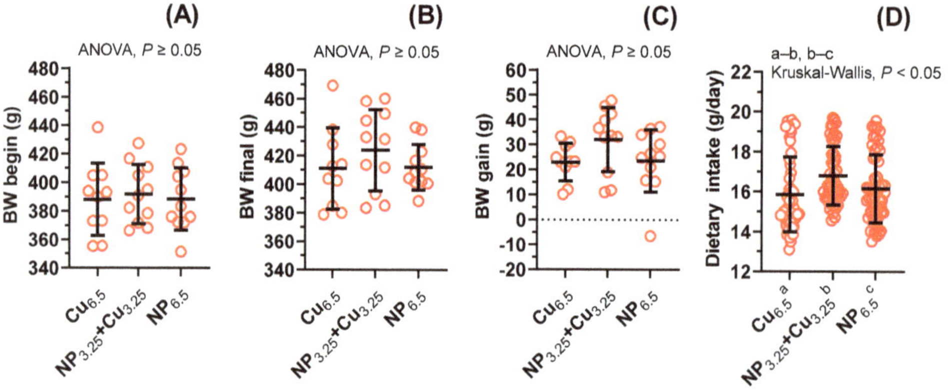

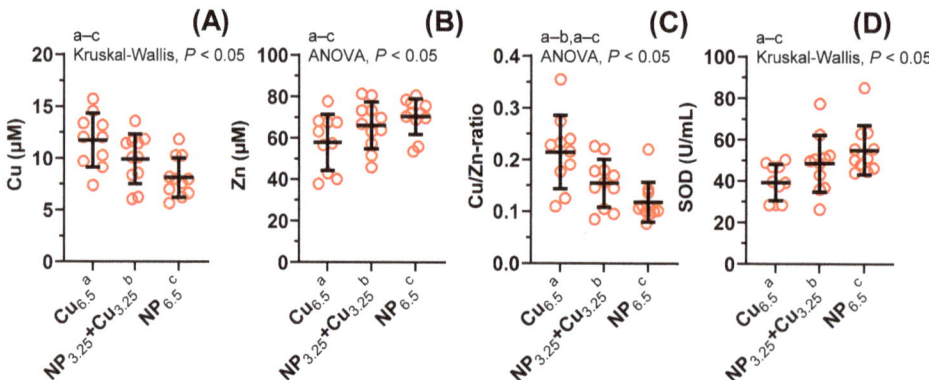

Figure 1. The influence of experimental diets on rat body weight (**A–C**), and daily feed intake (**D**). Values are expressed as means ± SD of n = 11 rats (**A–C**), and of m = 56 days of supplementation (**D**). NP$_{3.25}$ + Cu$_{3.25}$ increased by 1.06-fold the daily feed intake.

3.2. Biomarkers of Oxidative Stress in the Blood Plasma

Supplementation with NP$_{6.5}$ modified the Cu/Zn-ratio (×0.6, p = 0.007), Cu (×0.7, p = 0.0083), CAT (×0.7, p = 0.0134), Zn (×1.2, p = 0.0429), and SOD (×1.4, p = 0.0137); meanwhile, NP$_{3.25}$ + Cu$_{3.25}$ decreased the Cu/Zn-ratio (×0.7, p = 0.0397), and CAT (×0.7, p = 0.0134). NP$_{6.5}$ did not change FRAP (×1.0), GSH + GSSG (×1.1) and MDA (×1.4); and NP$_{3.25}$ + Cu$_{3.25}$ did not change Cu (×0.8), MDA (×1.0), GSH + GSSG (×1.0), Zn (×1.1), FRAP (×1.1), and SOD (×1.2). There was no significant difference between NP$_{3.25}$ + Cu$_{3.25}$ and NP$_{6.5}$ in the level of MDA (×0.7), GSH + GSSG (×0.9), SOD (×0.9), Zn (×0.9), CAT (×1.0), FRAP (×1.1), Cu (×1.2), and Cu/Zn-ratio (×1.3). Data are presented in Figure 2A–H.

Figure 2. *Cont.*

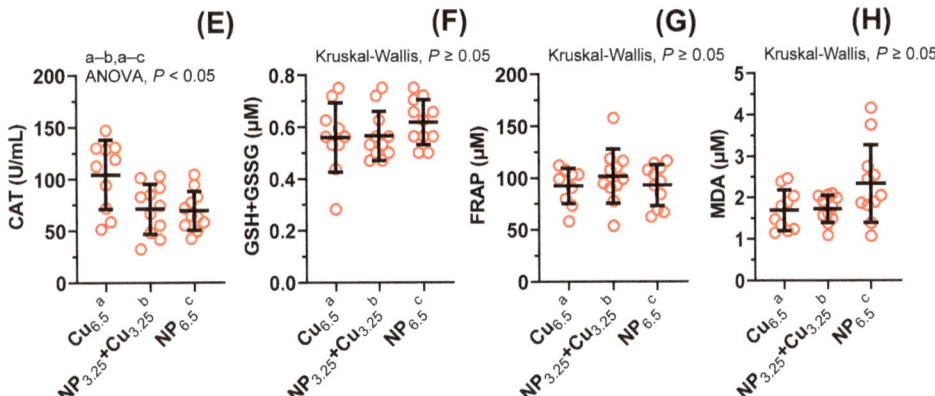

Figure 2. The influence of experimental diets on Cu, Zn content (**A–C**), and antioxidant mechanism (**D–H**) in blood plasma. Values are expressed as means ± SD of $n = 11$ rats. Supplementation with $NP_{6.5}$ decreased the Cu ($\times 0.7$), Cu/Zn-ratio ($\times 0.6$), catalase (CAT, $\times 0.7$), and increased Zn ($\times 1.2$), and superoxide dismutase (SOD, $\times 1.4$). $NP_{3.25} + Cu_{3.25}$ decreased the Cu/Zn-ratio ($\times 0.7$), and CAT ($\times 0.7$).

3.3. Vascular Reactivity Studies

Neither $NP_{3.25} + Cu_{3.25}$ (AUC: $\times 0.85$) nor $NP_{6.5}$ (AUC: $\times 1.18$) changed the vasodilation compared to the control $Cu_{6.5}$. However, there was a tendency to increased vasodilation at 10 nM of ACh in $NP_{6.5}$ (see Figure 3). Moreover, significant change was observed in $NP_{3.25} + Cu_{3.25}$ compared to $NP_{6.5}$ (AUC: $\times 0.72$). Preincubation with NS-398 diminished that response (between $NP_{3.25} + Cu_{3.25}$ and $NP_{6.5}$), which was completely abolished with indomethacin (see Table 1).

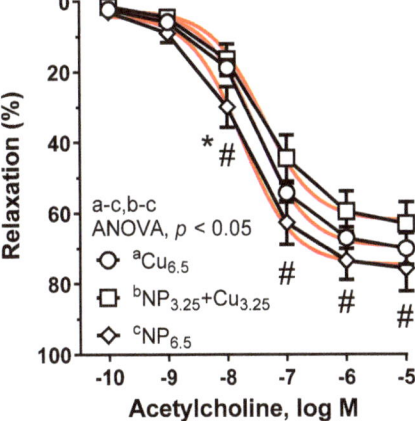

Figure 3. The relaxant response to acetylcholine in the isolated thoracic rings from rats supplemented with $Cu_{6.5}$, $NP_{3.25} + Cu_{3.25}$, and $NP_{6.5}$. Results are means ± SEM, * compared to $Cu_{6.5}$, # compared to $NP_{3.25} + Cu_{3.25}$, $p < 0.05$ of $n = 11$ rats; ANOVA/Tukey's. The red curve is the nonlinear regression model (log agonist vs. response). A significant change in the relaxant response was observed between the $NP_{3.25} + Cu_{3.25}$ and $NP_{6.5}$ groups of rats.

Table 1. The influence of iNOS inhibitor (1400 W, 1.0 µM), the selective COX-2 inhibitor (NS-398, 10 µM), the non-selective COX-1/2 inhibitor (indomethacin, 10 µM), the inhibitor of 20-HETE formation (HET0016, 0.1 µM), the thromboxane-A_2 synthase inhibitor (furegrelate, 1.0 µM), and the thromboxane receptor antagonist (SQ-29,548, 1.0 µM) on the vasorelaxant effects to acetylcholine of thoracic arteries from Wistar–Kyoto rats supplemented with $Cu_{6.5}$, $NP_{3.25} + Cu_{3.25}$ and $NP_{6.5}$.

Group		$Cu_{6.5}$				$NP_{3.25} + Cu_{3.25}$				$NP_{6.5}$		
	n	Emax (%)	pEC_{50}	AUC	n	Emax (%)	pEC_{50}	AUC	n	Emax (%)	pEC_{50}	AUC
Control conditions	11	69.76	7.509	182.0	11	62.19	7.413	157.0	11	76.80 $^\$$	7.748	214.3 $^\$$
±SEM		1.899	0.087	12.73		3.460	0.172	25.01		3.294	0.147	25.10
+1400 W	5	74.95	7.581	205.9	5	66.40	7.454	173.2	5	80.15 $^\$$	7.839	232.1 $^\$$
±SEM		4.092	0.183	21.09		4.326	0.209	25.66		3.212	0.131	18.19
+HET0016	5	60.64	7.795	175.1	6	76.50 *#	7.386	190.3 *	7	88.44 *#$^\$$	7.874 $^\$$	252.9 *#$^\$$
±SEM		4.180	0.227	22.66		4.714	0.165	19.81		2.919	0.120	20.99
+SQ-29,548	5	75.77	7.210	176.2	7	82.08 *	7.222	199.0 *	6	86.82 *#	7.683 #$^\$$	241.4 *#
±SEM		3.725	0.139	17.27		2.855	0.102	15.66		2.929	0.112	17.28
+FURE	5	69.25	7.360	167.1	7	64.34	7.387	159.7	6	71.47	7.711	202.2
±SEM		2.888	0.124	12.77		3.030	0.143	16.53		4.186	0.195	27.60
+NS-398	5	73.82	7.582	207.5	5	61.61 #	7.277	152.7 #	5	70.36	7.624 $^\$$	190.9 *
±SEM		5.746	0.267	29.95		4.113	0.200	20.22		3.652	0.170	24.58
+INDO	5	76.61	7.564	206.6	5	67.88	7.618	182.8	5	68.88	7.540	179.8 *
±SEM		4.008	0.173	21.78		3.088	0.158	13.54		3.772	0.174	22.93

Values are based on the concentration–response curves shown in Figures 3–7. Data are expressed as means ± SEM where n represents the number of animals. * $p < 0.05$ compared with the control conditions, # $p < 0.05$ compared with the $Cu_{6.5}$ group, $^\$$ $p < 0.05$ compared with the $NP_{3.25} + Cu_{3.25}$ group as determined by one-way ANOVA followed by Tukey's post hoc test.

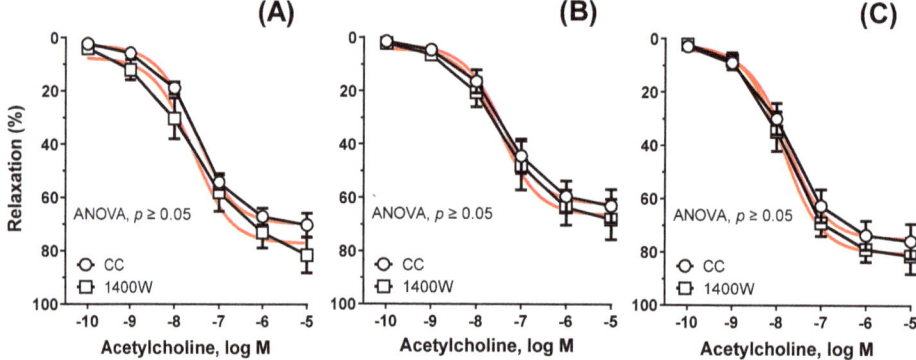

Figure 4. The influence of 1400 W on the relaxant response to acetylcholine. Aortic rings from rats supplemented with $Cu_{6.5}$ (**A**), $NP_{3.25} + Cu_{3.25}$ (**B**), and $NP_{6.5}$ (**C**) were pre-incubated with the inducible nitric oxide synthase inhibitor (1400 W, 30 min, 1 µM). Results are means ± SEM, $p > 0.05$ of $n = 5$ rats; two-way ANOVA/Sidak's. Preincubation with the selective iNOS inhibitor did not modify the vasodilation.

Preincubation with 1400 W (1 µM) did not modify the vasodilation in $Cu_{6.5}$ (AUC: ×1.13), $NP_{3.25} + Cu_{3.25}$ (AUC: ×1.04), and $NP_{6.5}$ (AUC: ×0.92), see Figure 4A–C.

Neither the selective COX-2 inhibitor (NS-398, 10 µM), nor the non-selective COX-1/2 inhibitor (indomethacin, 10 µM) changed the acetylcholine-induced response in the following groups of rats: $Cu_{6.5}$ (AUC: ×1.09, and ×1.10, respectively, Figure 5A), and $NP_{3.25} + Cu_{3.25}$ (AUC: ×0.90, and ×1.05, respectively, Figure 5B). However, a decreased response was observed in the $NP_{6.5}$ group (×0.84, and ×0.81, respectively, Figure 5C). There was no significant difference between NS-398- and indomethacin-induced response in $NP_{6.5}$ (AUC: ×1.04), opposite to some changes in $NP_{3.25} + Cu_{3.25}$ (AUC: ×0.86).

Preincubation with HET0016 (0.1 µM) potentiated vasodilation in $NP_{3.25} + Cu_{3.25}$ (AUC: ×1.39, Figure 6B), and $NP_{6.5}$ (AUC: ×1.52, Figure 6C) fed rats. This was not observed in the control group $Cu_{6.5}$ (AUC: ×1.02, Figure 6A).

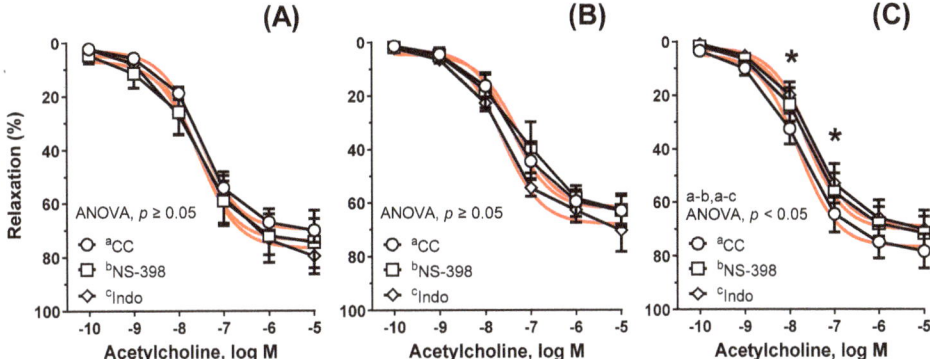

Figure 5. The influence of NS-398 and indomethacin (Indo) on the relaxant response to acetylcholine. Aortic rings from rats supplemented with $Cu_{6.5}$ (**A**), $NP_{3.25} + Cu_{3.25}$ (**B**), and $NP_{6.5}$ (**C**) were pre-incubated with the selective cyclooxygenase-2 (COX-2) inhibitor (NS-398, 30 min, 10 µM) and the non-selective COX-1/2 inhibitor (Indo, 30 min, 10 µM). Results are means ± SEM, * $p < 0.05$ of $n = 5$ rats; ANOVA/Tukey's. Preincubation with NS-398 and indomethacin attenuated vasodilation of rat thoracic aorta in the $NP_{6.5}$ group exclusively.

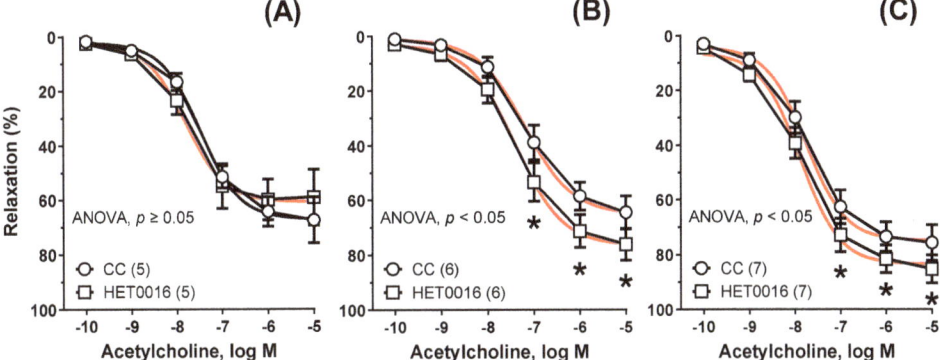

Figure 6. The influence of HET0016 on the relaxant response to acetylcholine. Aortic rings from rats supplemented with $Cu_{6.5}$ (**A**), $NP_{3.25} + Cu_{3.25}$ (**B**), and $NP_{6.5}$ (**C**) were pre-incubated with an inhibitor of 20-HETE formation (HET0016, 30 min, 0.1 µM). Results are the means ± SEM, * $p < 0.05$ two-way ANOVA/Sidak's. Number of animals is indicated in parenthesis. Preincubation with HET0016 potentiated vasodilation in $NP_{3.25} + Cu_{3.25}$, and $NP_{6.5}$ fed rats. This was not observed in the control group ($Cu_{6.5}$).

Neither the thromboxane-A_2 synthase inhibitor (furegrelate, 1 µM) nor the TP antagonist (SQ-29,548, 1 µM) changed the acetylcholine-induced response in $Cu_{6.5}$ (Figure 7A). However, in the $NP_{3.25} + Cu_{3.25}$ (AUC: ×1.38, Figure 7B) and the $NP_{6.5}$ (AUC: ×1.57, Figure 7C) groups of rats, SQ-29,548 potentiated vasodilation. Furegrelate did not modify that response (AUC: ×1.05, and ×1.03, respectively). Moreover, a significant increase was also observed between SQ-29,548 and furegrelate (AUC: ×1.31, and ×1.53, respectively) (Figure 7B,C).

The vasodilator response to acetylcholine is presented in Figures 3–7. Results are expressed as E_{max} (%), pEC_{50} and AUC, see Table 1.

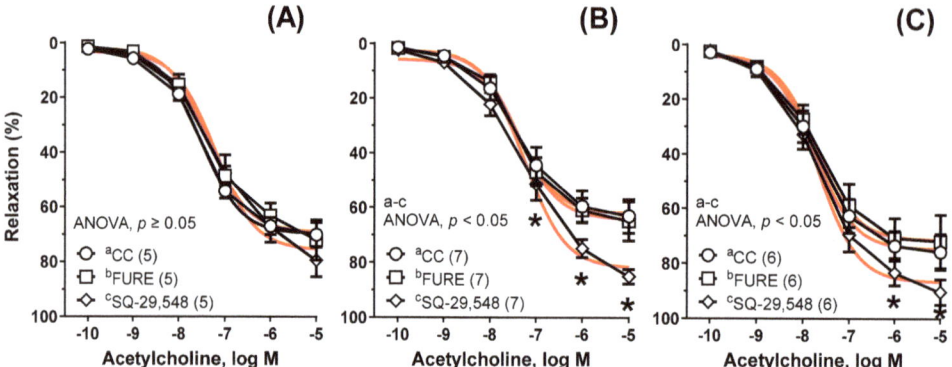

Figure 7. The influence of furegrelate and SQ-29,548 on the relaxant response to acetylcholine. Aortic rings from rats supplemented with $Cu_{6.5}$ (**A**), $NP_{3.25} + Cu_{3.25}$ (**B**), and $NP_{6.5}$ (**C**) were pre-incubated with the thromboxane-A_2 synthetase inhibitor (FURE, 30 min, 1 µM) and the thromboxane-A_2 receptor antagonist (SQ-29,548, 30 min, 1 µM). Results are means ± SEM, * $p < 0.05$; ANOVA/Tukey's. Number of animals is indicated in parenthesis. SQ-29,548 potentiated vasodilation in the $NP_{3.25} + Cu_{3.25}$ and in the $NP_{6.5}$ group of rats.

4. Discussion

Our previous studies revealed differences in the vascular tone regulation and the antioxidant status of rats supplemented with copper NPs (of 40–60 nm size) [1,2,12,17,18]. Of great importance is that in the previous experiments, both the age (either 4, 5, or 6 weeks) of Wistar Han IGS rats and the duration of feed intake (either 4 or 8 weeks) were what differentiated these studies from the one presented now, which can be described as 24 + 8 (24 weeks of age + 8 weeks of experimental feeding); and this was carried out on Wistar–Kyoto (WKY) rats, as a control for the spontaneously hypertensive rat (SHR) model which was also analyzed, but will be described elsewhere. Based on the previous results, antioxidant status and the participation of arachidonic acid metabolites were further investigated in the regulation of the vasodilator response induced by acetylcholine. Three different diets (i) standard with copper carbonate ($Cu_{6.5}$), (ii) with metal copper NPs ($NP_{6.5}$), and (iii) half dose of each ($NP_{3.25} + Cu_{3.25}$) were prepared in the form of pellets, and given daily to rats in order to study the physiological properties of dietary copper NPs.

Experimental supplementation with $NP_{6.5}$ neither modified the body weight nor the feed intake, which is in agreement with our previous results 4 + 8 (4 weeks of age + 8 weeks of experimental feeding), and 5 + 4 (5 weeks of age + 4 weeks of experimental feeding) [2,3,12,17]. However, in the $NP_{3.25} + Cu_{3.25}$ group of rats, we observed a significant increase in the daily feed intake compared to $Cu_{6.5}$ and $NP_{6.5}$, and an increase of body weight gain (not significant), which might be explained by the higher feed intake, and may become significant when more rats per group are studied. The observed increase in feed intake is difficult to explain and merits further investigation. Experimental treatment with $NP_{6.5}$ markedly reduced blood plasma Cu and increased Zn, which resulted in a decreased Cu/Zn-ratio. This is opposite to the 4 + 8 study, when Zn remained unchanged. However, in the same study, Cu and the Cu/Zn-ratio also decreased [18]. In the $NP_{3.25} + Cu_{3.25}$ group of rats, the Cu/Zn-ratio decreased significantly, which was due to a decrease in Cu and an increase in Zn (both results were not significant). There was no statistically significant difference between $NP_{3.25} + Cu_{3.25}$ and $NP_{6.5}$ in the Cu, Zn, and Cu/Zn-ratio. We have now observed, for the first time, increased activity of SOD and decreased CAT in $NP_{6.5}$ supplemented rats. This is contrary to our previous studies (4 + 8, and 6 + 8), when the activity of SOD was not modified and CAT increased [2,19]. However, another experiment from our research group (5 + 4) pointed to a decrease in CAT [12]. Increased SOD (result not significant) and decreased CAT were also observed for the $NP_{3.25} + Cu_{3.25}$ group. Increased SOD indicates an effective means of scavenging superoxide anion, whereas decreased CAT points to possible enzyme depletion in response to the increased oxidative stress and intensified scavenging of hydrogen peroxide. Another enzyme of hydrogen peroxide degradation, glutathione peroxidase, was not modified in this study, and this is opposite to a significant decrease in the 5 + 4 study [12]. Copper in the form of NPs neither modified FRAP nor MDA. These findings are not entirely in agreement with our previous results (4 + 8 and 6 + 8), when FRAP increased [2,19], and MDA either increased (5 + 4 and 7 + 8) [1,12] or was not modified (4 + 8, and 6 + 8) [2,3,19]. We previously reported that replacing $Cu_{6.5}$ with $NP_{6.5}$ and reducing the dose (from a standard 6.5 mg/kg to a 3.25 mg/kg in the diet of rats 5 + 4) had particularly unfavorable effects on the respiratory system, causing adverse changes to the lungs. Surprisingly, these treatments also had a positive effect on the redox status of the liver and brain [20]. Moreover, the addition of copper NPs into the rat diet (5 + 4 and 7 + 8) reduced protein oxidation and nitration [1,12], as well as DNA oxidation and methylation. Meanwhile, lowering the daily dose increased the oxidation of proteins and DNA methylation [12]. In our study, neither $NP_{6.5}$ nor $NP_{3.25} + Cu_{3.25}$ modified the acetylcholine-induced vasodilation compared to $Cu_{6.5}$ control. However there was a tendency to increased vasodilation in $NP_{6.5}$ supplemented rats. This stays in agreement with the 4 + 8 study [2], and is in opposition to the 7 + 8 study, when $NP_{6.5}$ potentiated the vasodilator response induced by acetylcholine in a significant way [1]. Surprisingly, in the present study, $NP_{6.5}$ potentiated that response compared to $NP_{3.25} + Cu_{3.25}$. Preincubation with NS-398 (COX-2 inhibitor) diminished that response, which was completely abolished with indomethacin (COX-1/2 inhibitor). These results suggest participation of COX-2 in NP-induced response, which is a dose dependent mechanism. In another experiment, conducted by Cendrowska-Pinkosz et al. [21], $NP_{6.5}$ in the diet of rats did not change the acetylcholinesterase level (an enzyme that catalyzes the breakdown of acetylcholine) in the blood compared to $Cu_{6.5}$ (7 + 8), so the observed changes might not be due to enzyme depletion nor surplus. Even though we did not currently report any changes in acetylcholine-induced vasodilation followed by $NP_{6.5}$ and $NP_{3.25} + Cu_{3.25}$ intake (compared to the control $Cu_{6.5}$), the contribution of nitric oxide and arachidonic acid metabolites cannot be ruled out. We observed that iNOS inhibition with 1400 W did not modify that response in aortas from all three studied groups, which is contrary to the previous study (7 + 8), when the overproduction of NO from iNOS was engaged in vascular relaxation in the $NP_{6.5}$ group of rats [1]. Considering that the sensitivity of the arteries to nitric oxide was not altered (study with an exogenous NO donor sodium nitroprusside) [2], arachidonic acid derivatives may also be responsible for the vascular tone regulation of copper NPs, as we suggested previously [18]. Preincubation with either COX-2 or COX-1/2 inhibitors attenuated the vasodilator response in $NP_{6.5}$, indicating the involvement of a vasodilatory net effect of prostanoids origin from COX-2. This was neither observed for the control ($Cu_{6.5}$) nor when the dose was reduced by half (in the $NP_{3.25} + Cu_{3.25}$ group). The results with $NP_{6.5}$ are contrary to our previous report (4 + 8), which had revealed a decreased sensitivity of the smooth muscles to prostanoids (no significant change in acetylcholine-induced response after COX-1/2 inhibition) [2]. Given these results, the participation of another vasoconstrictor agent in vascular relaxation was studied. 20-Hydroxyeicosatetraenoic acid (20-HETE) is a potent metabolite of arachidonic acid. This reaction is mediated by cytochrome P450 and can be further metabolized by COX to 20-hydroxy compounds. Preincubation with a 20-HETE inhibitor potentiated the vascular relaxation in both $NP_{6.5}$ and $NP_{3.25} + Cu_{3.25}$ groups, indicating that 20-HETE is involved in acetylcholine-induced relaxation. However, this was not observed in young rats (7 + 8) [1]. Finally, we analyzed the contribution of the potent vasoconstrictor thromboxane-A_2 in the acetylcholine-induced response. However, the present results showed that thromboxane-A_2 is not an important vasoconstrictor candidate engaged in the vascular tone regulation of supplemented rats (studies with the thromboxane-A_2 synthesis inhibitor, furegrelate). Through the activation of thromboxane-A_2 receptors (TP), prostacyclin, prostaglandins, isoprostanes, and 20-HETE participate in the endothelial dysfunction associated with cardiovascular risk factors [15]. In this study, when the TP were blocked with SQ-29,548, we observed increased vasodilation in both groups of copper NPs supplemented rats ($NP_{6.5}$ and $NP_{3.25} + Cu_{3.25}$). These data point towards a potent vasoconstrictor that acts on the TP, suggesting 20-HETE as a possible candidate. However, other vasoconstrictors should also be taken under consideration in further studies [16]. As there is an interplay between vasoconstrictor and vasodilator factors, vasodilators should also be analyzed; this will be done in another study.

These data point to some significant changes induced by metal copper NPs, which are age-dependent and are observed between younger (12-week-old) and older (32-week-old) male WKY rats. Indeed, age-related changes in blood vessels elasticity/stiffness might be exacerbated by daily diet [22]. Many recent studies have focused on dietary intervention to improve vascular health and delay the onset of vascular aging [23]. Dietary intervention may improve not only the vascular/cardiovascular impairment, but also vascular cognitive impairment and dementia. However, so far, only certain vitamins (vitamin E, folate), multi-nutrient formulations, and unsaturated fatty acids have shown some initial promise [24].

5. Conclusions

Our findings have shown that increased oxidative stress accompanies copper NP intake, which further modulates vascular relaxation with the participation of 20-HETE, through the thromboxane-A_2 receptors. When a daily dose of copper NPs was decreased by half, the interplay between COX metabolites was also modified; however, the Cu/Zn-ratio and CAT remained unchanged compared to the higher dose. Further studies should concentrate on animals with metabolic disorders.

Supplementary Materials: The following are available online at https://www.mdpi.com/article/10.3390/nu13113793/s1, Table S1: Experimental results (means with SD).

Author Contributions: Conceptualization, J.J., K.O., L.G., M.K.-W. and M.M.; methodology, J.J., K.O. and M.M.; software, M.M. and M.K.-W.; validation, M.M.; formal analysis, E.C., J.J., K.O., K.S. and M.M.; investigation, E.C., J.J., K.O., K.S. and M.M.; resources, M.M.; data curation, E.C., J.J., K.O. and M.M.; writing—original draft preparation, M.M.; writing—review and editing, M.M.; visualization, M.M.; supervision, K.O., and M.M.; project administration, M.M.; funding acquisition, M.M. All authors have read and agreed to the published version of the manuscript.

Funding: This research was funded by National Science Centre, Poland granted to M.M. (MINIATURA 2019/03/X/NZ9/00171).

Institutional Review Board Statement: All efforts were made to minimize animal suffering. Permission (number 90/2019) was granted by the Local Ethics Committee for Animal Experiments in Olsztyn, Poland. This study is in accordance to Directive 2010/63/EU which conforms to the Guide for the Care and Use of Laboratory Animals (NIH Publications No. 86–26, revised 2014), and ARRIVE guidelines and complies with the '3Rs'.

Informed Consent Statement: Not applicable.

Data Availability Statement: Data supporting reported results can be found in Supplementary Materials.

Conflicts of Interest: The authors declare no conflict of interest. The funders had no role in the design of the study; in the collection, analyses, or interpretation of data; in the writing of the manuscript, or in the decision to publish the results.

References

1. Majewski, M.; Lis, B.; Olas, B.; Ognik, K.; Juśkiewicz, J. Dietary supplementation with copper nanoparticles influences the markers of oxidative stress and modulates vasodilation of thoracic arteries in young Wistar rats. *PLoS ONE* **2020**, *15*, e0229282. [CrossRef] [PubMed]
2. Majewski, M.; Ognik, K.; Juśkiewicz, J. Copper nanoparticles modify the blood plasma antioxidant status and modulate the vascular mechanisms with nitric oxide and prostanoids involved in Wistar rats. *Pharmacol. Rep.* **2019**, *71*, 509–516. [CrossRef] [PubMed]
3. Majewski, M.; Ognik, K.; Juśkiewicz, J. The interaction between resveratrol and two forms of copper as carbonate and nanoparticles on antioxidant mechanisms and vascular function in Wistar rats. *Pharmacol. Rep.* **2019**, *71*, 862–869. [CrossRef] [PubMed]
4. Tang, H.; Xu, M.; Luo, J.; Zhao, L.; Ye, G.; Shi, F.; Lv, C.; Chen, H.; Wang, Y.; Li, Y. Liver toxicity assessments in rats following sub-chronic oral exposure to copper nanoparticles. *Environ. Sci. Eur.* **2019**, *31*, 30. [CrossRef]

5. Galhardi, C.M.; Diniz, Y.S.; Faine, L.A.; Rodrigues, H.G.; Burneiko, R.C.M.; Ribas, B.O.; Novelli, E.L. Toxicity of copper intake: Lipid profile, oxidative stress and susceptibility to renal dysfunction. *Food Chem. Toxicol.* **2004**, *42*, 2053–2060. [CrossRef]
6. Majewski, M.; Jurgoński, A.; Fotschki, B.; Juśkiewicz, J. The toxic effects of monosodium glutamate (MSG)—The involvement of nitric oxide, prostanoids and potassium channels in the reactivity of thoracic arteries in MSG-obese rats. *Toxicol. Appl. Pharmacol.* **2018**, *359*, 62–69. [CrossRef] [PubMed]
7. Majewski, M.; Kozlowska, A.; Thoene, M.; Lepiarczyk, E.; Grzegorzewski, W.J. Overview of the role of vitamins and minerals on the kynurenine pathway in health and disease. *J. Physiol. Pharmacol.* **2016**, *67*, 3–20. [PubMed]
8. Majewski, M.; Ognik, K.; Thoene, M.; Rawicka, A.; Juśkiewicz, J. Resveratrol modulates the blood plasma levels of Cu and Zn, the antioxidant status and the vascular response of thoracic arteries in copper deficient Wistar rats. *Toxicol. Appl. Pharmacol.* **2020**, *390*, 114877. [CrossRef] [PubMed]
9. Majewski, M.; Kasica, N.; Jakimiuk, A.; Podlasz, P. Toxicity and cardiac effects of acute exposure to tryptophan metabolites on the kynurenine pathway in early developing zebrafish (Danio rerio) embryos. *Toxicol. Appl. Pharmacol.* **2018**, *341*, 16–29. [CrossRef]
10. Luo, J.; Hao, S.; Zhao, L.; Shi, F.; Ye, G.; He, C.; Lin, J.; Zhang, W.; Liang, H.; Wang, X.; et al. Oral exposure of pregnant rats to copper nanoparticles caused nutritional imbalance and liver dysfunction in fetus. *Ecotoxicol. Environ. Saf.* **2020**, *206*, 111206. [CrossRef]
11. Jankowski, J.; Ognik, K.; Kozłowski, K.; Stępniowska, A.; Zduńczyk, Z. Effect of different levels and sources of dietary copper, zinc and manganese on the performance and immune and redox status of Turkeys. *Animals* **2019**, *9*, 883. [CrossRef]
12. Ognik, K.; Cholewińska, E.; Juśkiewicz, J.; Zduńczyk, Z.; Tutaj, K.; Szlązak, R. The effect of copper nanoparticles and copper (II) salt on redox reactions and epigenetic changes in a rat model. *J. Anim. Physiol. Anim. Nutr. Berl.* **2019**, *103*, 675–686. [CrossRef]
13. Majewski, M.; Lis, B.; Juśkiewicz, J.; Ognik, K.; Jedrzejek, D.; Stochmal, A.; Olas, B. The composition and vascular/antioxidant properties of Taraxacum officinale flower water syrup in a normal-fat diet using an obese rat model. *J. Ethnopharmacol.* **2021**, *265*, 113393. [CrossRef] [PubMed]
14. Żary-Sikorska, E.; Fotschki, B.; Jurgoński, A.; Kosmala, M.; Milala, J.; Kołodziejczyk, K.; Majewski, M.; Ognik, K.; Juśkiewicz, J. Protective effects of a strawberry ellagitannin-rich extract against pro-oxidative and pro-inflammatory dysfunctions induced by a high-fat diet in a rat model. *Molecules* **2020**, *25*, 5874. [CrossRef]
15. Majewski, M.; Kucharczyk, E.; Kaliszan, R.; Markuszewski, M.; Fotschki, B.; Juskiewicz, J.; Borkowska-Sztachańska, M.; Ognik, K. The characterization of ground raspberry seeds and the physiological response to supplementation in hypertensive and normotensive rats. *Nutrients* **2020**, *12*, 1630. [CrossRef] [PubMed]
16. Majewski, M.; Lepczyńska, M.; Dzika, E.; Grzegorzewski, W.; Markiewicz, W.; Mendel, M.; Chłopecka, M. Evaluation of the time stability of aortic rings in young wistar rats during an eight-hour incubation period. *J. Elementol.* **2019**, *24*, 677–686. [CrossRef]
17. Majewski, M.; Ognik, K.; Zdunczyk, P.; Juskiewicz, J. Effect of dietary copper nanoparticles versus one copper (II) salt: Analysis of vasoreactivity in a rat model. *Pharmacol. Rep.* **2017**, *69*, 1282–1288. [CrossRef] [PubMed]
18. Majewski, M.; Ognik, K.; Juśkiewicz, J. Copper nanoparticles enhance vascular contraction induced by prostaglandin F2-alpha and decrease the blood plasma cu-zn ratio in wistar rats. *J. Elementol.* **2019**, *24*, 911–922. [CrossRef]
19. Majewski, M.; Ognik, K.; Juśkiewicz, J. The antioxidant status, lipid profile, and modulation of vascular function by fish oil supplementation in nano-copper and copper carbonate fed Wistar rats. *J. Funct. Foods* **2020**, *64*, 103595. [CrossRef]
20. Ognik, K.; Cholewińska, E.; Tutaj, K.; Cendrowska-Pinkosz, M.; Dworzański, W.; Dworzańska, A.; Juśkiewicz, J. The effect of the source and dosage of dietary Cu on redox status in rat tissues. *J. Anim. Physiol. Anim. Nutr. Berl.* **2020**, *104*, 352–361. [CrossRef] [PubMed]
21. Cendrowska-Pinkosz, M.; Krauze, M.; Juśkiewicz, J.; Ognik, K. The effect of the use of copper carbonate and copper nanoparticles in the diet of rats on the level of β-amyloid and acetylcholinesterase in selected organs. *J. Trace Elem. Med. Biol.* **2021**, *67*, 126777. [CrossRef] [PubMed]
22. Logvinov, S.V.; Naryzhnaya, N.V.; Kurbatov, B.K.; Gorbunov, A.S.; Birulina, Y.G.; Maslov, L.L.; Oeltgen, P.R. High carbohydrate high fat diet causes arterial hypertension and histological changes in the aortic wall in aged rats: The involvement of connective tissue growth factors and fibronectin. *Exp. Gerontol.* **2021**, *154*, 111543. [CrossRef] [PubMed]
23. Balasubramanian, P.; DelFavero, J.; Ungvari, A.; Papp, M.; Tarantini, A.; Price, N.; de Cabo, R.; Tarantini, S. Time-restricted feeding (TRF) for prevention of age-related vascular cognitive impairment and dementia. *Ageing Res. Rev.* **2020**, *64*, 101189. [CrossRef] [PubMed]
24. Vlachos, G.S.; Scarmeas, N. Dietary interventions in mild cognitive impairment and dementia. *Dialogues Clin. Neurosci.* **2019**, *21*, 69–82. [CrossRef] [PubMed]

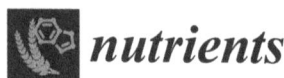

Article

Analysis of White Mulberry Leaves and Dietary Supplements, ATR-FTIR Combined with Chemometrics for the Rapid Determination of 1-Deoxynojirimycin

Agata Walkowiak-Bródka [1], Natalia Piekuś-Słomka [1], Kacper Wnuk [2] and Bogumiła Kupcewicz [1,*]

1. Department of Inorganic and Analytical Chemistry, Faculty of Pharmacy, Nicolaus Copernicus University, 85-089 Torun, Poland
2. Department of Biostatistics and Biomedical Systems Theory, Faculty of Pharmacy, Nicolaus Copernicus University, 85-067 Torun, Poland
* Correspondence: kupcewicz@cm.umk.pl

Citation: Walkowiak-Bródka, A.; Piekuś-Słomka, N.; Wnuk, K.; Kupcewicz, B. Analysis of White Mulberry Leaves and Dietary Supplements, ATR-FTIR Combined with Chemometrics for the Rapid Determination of 1-Deoxynojirimycin. *Nutrients* 2022, 14, 5276. https://doi.org/10.3390/nu14245276

Academic Editors: Bruno Trimarco and Gaetano Santulli

Received: 20 November 2022
Accepted: 7 December 2022
Published: 10 December 2022

Publisher's Note: MDPI stays neutral with regard to jurisdictional claims in published maps and institutional affiliations.

Copyright: © 2022 by the authors. Licensee MDPI, Basel, Switzerland. This article is an open access article distributed under the terms and conditions of the Creative Commons Attribution (CC BY) license (https:// creativecommons.org/licenses/by/ 4.0/).

Abstract: Diabetes mellitus is a metabolic disease affecting more people every year. The treatment of diabetes and its complications involve substantial healthcare expenditures. Thus, there is a need to identify natural products that can be used as nutraceuticals to prevent and treat early-stage diabetes. White mulberry (*Morus alba* L.) is a plant that has been used in traditional Chinese medicine for thousands of years due to its many beneficial biological properties. White mulberry leaves are a source of 1-deoxynojirimycin (DNJ), which, due to its ability to inhibit α-glucosidase, can be used to regulate postprandial glucose concentration. In addition to consuming dried white mulberry leaves as herbal tea, many functional foods also contain this raw material. The development of the dietary supplements market brings many scientific and regulatory challenges to the safety, quality and effectiveness of such products containing concentrated amounts of nutraceuticals. In the present study, the quality of 19 products was assessed by determining the content of DNJ, selected (poly)phenols and antioxidant activity (DPPH• assay). Nine of these products were herbal teas, and the other samples were dietary supplements. These results indicate the low quality of tested dietary supplements, the use of which (due to the low content of nutraceuticals) cannot bring the expected beneficial effects on health. Moreover, a method for determining the content of DNJ (the essential component for antidiabetic activity) based on ATR-FTIR spectroscopy combined with PLS regression has been proposed. This might be an alternative method to the commonly used chromatographic process requiring extraction and derivatization of the sample. It allows for a quick screening assessment of the quality of products containing white mulberry leaves.

Keywords: mulberry; *Morus alba*; 1-deoxynojirimycin; DNJ; dietary supplements; PLS regression

1. Introduction

Diabetes mellitus (DM) is one of the most prevalent metabolism-related disorders associated with impaired insulin production (type 1) or developed insulin resistance (type 2). According to the International Diabetes Federation, in 2019, nearly 10% of people aged 20–79 (463 million) were living with diabetes worldwide, and this is expected to reach 700 million by 2045 [1]. The increased prevalence of diabetes mellitus means that cardiovascular disorders, blindness, stroke, kidney failure, foot ulcers, and depression will also increase. By 2045, the annual healthcare expenditure on treating diabetes and its complications are expected to be USD 845 billion [1]. Type 2 diabetes mellitus (T2DM) accounts for approximately 90% of all diabetic patients and is strongly associated with the current obesity epidemic [2]. Oral hypoglycemic drugs are the basis of pharmacotherapy for type 2 diabetes. Among them, α-glucosidase inhibitors (e.g., acarbose, voglibose, and miglitol) are recommended as the first-line therapy [3]. The α-glucosidase is an enzyme that catalyzes the hydrolysis of glycosidic bonds in dietary carbohydrates to absorb monosaccharides in the small intestine. Inhibiting the activity of this biomolecule reduces postprandial hyperglycemia, which plays a crucial role in the treatment and prevention of diabetes mellitus and its complications [4]. Although drugs from the group of α-glucosidase inhibitors have fewer side effects than other oral hypoglycemic drugs (sulfonamides, glinides, gliptins, biguanides, and thiazolidinediones), with prolonged use, they may cause some side effects such as gastrointestinal reactions and liver damage. [3]. Therefore, the search for plants/natural products that can be used as functional food, and identifying their active compounds that could be used as nutraceuticals or drugs has drawn considerable attention.

White mulberry (*Morus alba* L.) belongs to the mulberry family (*Moraceae*) and is native to Central Asia, but nowadays it is also cultivated in Europe. It has been used in traditional Chinese medicine for thousands of years. White mulberry leaves contain various beneficial components to health such as flavonoids, alkaloids, phenolics, amino acids, and polysaccharides. Numerous studies have shown that functional components included in white mulberry possess abundant biological activities, including antidiabetic, hypolipidemic, antiatherogenic, anticancer, cardiovascular, cardioprotective, antidopaminergic, antibacterial, antioxidant, and anti-inflammatory effects [5–8]. According to research presented in [9], the entire group of compounds (flavonoids and polysaccharides) found in white mulberry leaves is responsible for antidiabetic effects.

The main active mulberry component, 1-deoxynojirimycin (DNJ), is the polyhydroxylated piperidine alkaloid (tertrahydroxy piperidine derivative) (Figure 1), which can be defined as a glucose analogue with an amine group substitution for the oxygen atom in the pyranose ring [10]. DNJ competitively inhibits intestinal α-glucosidase and thus reduces glucose absorption, leading to lower blood glucose levels. In addition to its role in modulating glucose and insulin metabolism, DNJ also exhibits lipid-regulating and anti-obesity activity [11], inhibits adipogenesis [12], and is likely to have neuroprotective effects and may be an essential factor in preventing pathological brain changes in patients with Alzheimer's disease [13].

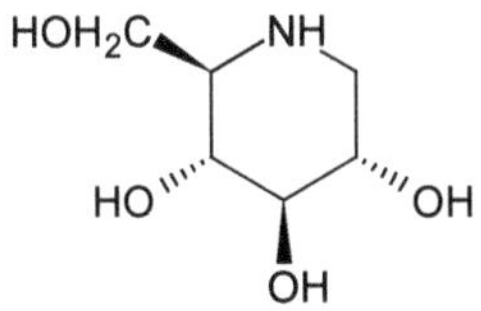

(2R,3R,4R,5S)-2-(hydroxymethyl)piperidin-1-ium-3,4,5-triol

Figure 1. Structure of 1-deoxynojirimycin (DNJ).

The mechanism of DNJs multidirectional action still needs to be characterized. Detailed proteomic studies [14] show that long-term supplementation of mulberry leaf powder could enhance metabolic regulation by modulating the expression of signaling proteins in the insulin signaling pathway. Furthermore, cited work [14] also demonstrated an improvement in the functioning of mitochondria after supplementation of DNJ from mulberry leaves. Mitochondrial dysfunction leads to a decrease in ATP production and an increase in the production of reactive oxygen species, and consequently, to the development of insulin resistance. Improving mitochondria functioning is, therefore, a crucial element in preventing and treating type 2 diabetes. Other detailed studies on the mechanism of action of mulberry leaf extract and DNJ in mice suggested that it improved insulin resistance by modulating the insulin signaling pathway in the skeletal muscle of db/db mice after mulberry leaf or DNJ supplementation [15].

Interesting sources of DNJ are culture supernatant extracts (CSE) obtained from *Bacillus* sp. and *Streptomyces* sp. According to [16], appropriately selected culture conditions of *B. amyloliquefaciens* to allow obtaining SCE with the ability to lower postprandial glucose levels were comparable to white mulberry leaf extract. The literature indicates the potential use of DNJ from microorganisms for functional purposes [16].

From an analytical point of view, DNJ is a demanding molecule. Because of its high hydrophilicity and small molecular weight, the interaction with the stationary phase of conventional reverse-phase liquid chromatography (RP-HPLC) columns is so weak that DNJ is not retained in the column. The lack of chromophores in the DNJ structure (as in many other aminoglycosides) makes it impossible to use direct ultraviolet or fluorescence detection. To use RP-HPLC with a UV detector (the most widely used quantitative analysis technique) to quantify DNJ, it is necessary to derivatize the sample [17,18]. This procedure extends the analysis time, generates costs, and degrades the sample.

It is worth noting that some DNJ analogues, such as the miglitol mentioned above (*N*-EtOH-DNJ), miglustat (*N*-Bu-DNJ), and migalastat (DGJ, stereoisomer of DNJ), are registered drugs used for the treatment of type 2 diabetes, type I Gaucher disease or Niemann–Pick type C lysosomal storage diseases, and Fabry disease, respectively [19]. Importantly, research [20] suggests that miglitol can restore the counterregulatory response to hypoglycemia following antecedent hypoglycemia. In addition, data are available on other possible applications of these drugs, e.g., the treatment of cystic fibrosis [21], cancer [22], or COVID-19 [23]. In addition, the compound *N*-(5-adamantane-1-yl-methoxypentyl)-deoxynojirimycin (AMP-DNM) seems to be promising in the treatment of diabetes and obesity by promoting satiety, activating brown adipose tissue [24], and the effect on sterol regulatory element-binding proteins [25].

White mulberry leaves are most often consumed in teas or dietary supplements (tablets, capsules) containing extracts or powdered dried raw material. The global dietary supplements market size was USD 61.20 billion in 2020, estimated to be USD 128.64 billion in 2028 [26]. The increasing interest in a healthy lifestyle and well-being is expected to be a key driving factor for the dietary supplements market. The much lower requirements for the production process and quality control of dietary supplements compared to drugs, such as the fact that plant raw materials are not subject to standardization, with the high complexity of herbs and extracts that may cause severe problems with their quality and may be a potential threat to the consumer [27]. The diversification of the chemical composition of plant products may result from the origin of the plant, the time and place of harvesting, the drying process, extraction, the presence of impurities, or deliberate forgery. Therefore, the quality control of plant-origin samples presents several challenges for modern analytical chemistry.

There are various spectroscopic techniques for a characteristic chemical profile of a plant or a fingerprint analysis. Fourier-transform infrared spectroscopy (FTIR) combined with multivariate data analysis is an effective tool for extracting specific chemical information. This approach has become a standard procedure for herbal species analysis. The application of attenuated total reflectance—Fourier transform infrared spectroscopy (ATR-FTIR) is strongly encouraged because it is rapid, non-destructive, and inexpensive compared to other analytical methods. The IR spectrum contains information on the biochemical composition of the sample, chemical bonds, and functional groups of the compounds. It allows for detecting differences between samples based on their chemical fingerprints [28,29].

This study aimed to quantify DNJ in white mulberry dry leaves (teas) and dietary supplements. To the best of our knowledge, there are no available data on determining the content of DNJ in products sold as dietary supplements. Moreover, the quality assessment of dietary supplements was based on determining the content of chlorogenic acid (CGA), neochlorogenic acid (nCGA), and rutin. Additionally, the DPPH• radical scavenging activity was evaluated to measure antioxidant properties.

This work also presents the potential application of mid-infrared spectroscopy with ATR sampling combined with chemometric tools for relatively fast and non-destructive quantification of DNJ in white mulberry leaf products.

2. Materials and Methods

2.1. Materials

All chemicals and solvents used in this study were purchased from Sigma–Aldrich (Saint Louis, MO, USA). The solvents (acetonitrile, water, methanol, and formic acid) used in this study were all analytical and HPLC grade. 2,2-diphenyl-1-picrylhydrazil (DPPH$^\bullet$) was used to prepare the solution with an absorbance value of about 1. 1-deoxynojirimycin (DNJ), chlorogenic acid, neochlorogenic acid, and rutin were used as analytical standards. Sodium borate buffer (pH 8.5), glycine, acetic acid, and 9-fluorenylmethyl chloroformate (FMOC-Cl) were used in the derivatization process of DNJ in samples.

The study analyzed 19 herbal products containing white mulberry leaves or extracts. Ten of them (S1–S10) were dietary supplements. The other samples were herbal teas (T1–T9). The commercial products were purchased from local pharmacies and markets (Bydgoszcz, Poland) and online pharmacies.

2.2. HPLC Analysis

High-performance liquid chromatography with a photodiode array detector (HPLC-DAD), (Shimadzu Corp., Kyoto, Japan) was used for the the quantitative analysis of 1-deoxynojirimycin, chlorogenic acid, neochlorogenic acid, and rutin in white mulberry leaves and dietary supplements samples.

For the preparation of samples for the determination of (poly)phenolic compounds (rutin, chlorogenic acid, neochlorogenic acid), about 500 mg of dried leaves or dietary supplement products (crushed in a mortar) were added to 15 mL of the methanol-water mixture (50:50), vortexed for 30 min, and then centrifuged (22,000 g) for 10 min (MPW-352RH centrifuge, MPW MED. INSTRUMENTS, Warsaw, Poland). The obtained extracts were filtered through a syringe filter with a pore diameter of 0.45 μm and subjected to further analysis.

A Kinetex® column (150 mm × 4.6 mm, 5 μm) was used to separate (poly)phenolic compounds. The analysis was carried out using reverse-phase high-performance liquid chromatography (RP-HPLC). The mobile phase consisted of 0.2% formic acid in water (phase A) and acetonitrile (phase B). At a flow rate of 0.7 mL/min, the gradient was as follows: 0–2 min 10% B, 2–6 min 10–24% B, 6–11 min 10–24% B, 11–16 min 24–10% B and 16–25 min 10% B. UV detection wavelength of 325 and 350 nm and the injection volume of 20 μL was applied. Injection of each sample was performed in triplicate. The concentrations of rutin, chlorogenic acid, and neochlorogenic acid in samples were calculated from the calibration curves equation based on the peak area and recounted as the content in 1 g of dried white mulberry leaves.

The methods were validated for linearity, precision, accuracy, recovery, detection (LOD), and quantification (LOQ) limits according to ICH guideline ICH Q2 (R2) [30]. The detection limit was expressed as LOD = $(3.3 \cdot \sigma)/S$, and the quantitation limit was defined as LOQ = $(10 \cdot \sigma)/S$ (where σ is the standard deviation of the response (n = 6), S is the slope of the calibration curve). The slope (S) was estimated from the calibration curve of the analyte, and σ based on the standard deviation of the blank. Recovery tests were completed by adding a known amount of the standard to the raw materials at two concentration levels. Then, the materials mixed with standards were prepared and analyzed under optimized conditions. Linearity was carried out on sets of standard solutions with different concentrations. The regression equations and regression coefficient (R^2) values were calculated. Finally, precision was expressed as the relative standard deviation (%RSD).

The extraction and derivatization of samples for DNJ determination were carried out using the method described in [31]. About 500 mg of dried leaves or dietary supplement products (crushed in a mortar) wer added to 15 mL aqueous 0.05 M HCl, vortexed for 30 min, and centrifuged (22,000 g) for 10 min and subsequently filtered with a PTFE filter (0.45 μm pore size). The obtained extract was used for subsequent derivatization. Ten microliters of the extract was mixed with the same amount of 0.4 M sodium borate buffer (pH 8.5) in a microtube. Twenty microliters of 5 mM FMOC-Cl in acetonitrile was added with rapid mixing for 20 min at 20 °C. To terminate the reaction by quenching the remaining FMOC-Cl, 10 µL of 0.1 M glycine was added. The mixture was diluted with 950 mL of 0.1% aqueous acetic acid (17.5 mM) to stabilize the DNJ-FMOC and filtered through a syringe filter (0.45 µm pore size).

DNJ was analyzed using a Kinetex® column (150 mm × 4.6 mm, 5 µm) after derivatization with FMOC-Cl. Each peak was identified from a separate reaction with DNJ, glycine, or water. The detection wavelength was 265 nm. The samples were eluted with a mobile phase of 0.2% formic acid in water (phase A) and acetonitrile (phase B) with a ratio of 70:30 at a flow rate of 0.8 mL/min for 25 min. The injection of each sample was performed in triplicate. Method validation was performed analogously to the methods for (poly)phenolic compounds. The DNJ concentration in samples was calculated from the calibration curve equation based on the peak area and recounted as the content in 1 g of dried white mulberry leaves. The chromatograms of the derivatized standard DNJ and exemplary derivatized samples extracted from a dietary supplement and from mulberry leaves are shown in Figure S1 (Supplementary Material).

2.3. Antioxidant Activity

This study used the DPPH• radical (2,2-diphenyl-1-picrylhydrazyl) to assess antioxidant activity. The methanolic DPPH solution (0.05 M) was prepared and stored in darkness before the experiments. A volume of 150 µL methanolic-aqueous extracts (prepared as described in 2.2) was mixed with 1 mL DPPH• methanolic solution. The mixture was shaken and incubated at 25 °C in the dark. Absorbance was measured after 30 min, at λ = 517 nm, against a blank. A Shimadzu model UV-VIS spectrophotometer (UV-1800) equipped with a quartz cell (10 mm optical path) was employed for the spectral measurements. Assays were performed in triplicate.

The EC_{50} (concentration of sample required to scavenge 50% of the DPPH• free radicals) values were derived from the dose-response curve and recalculated to dry mulberry leaves.

2.4. ATR-FTIR Spectroscopy

The ATR-FTIR experiments were carried out with a Ge-based ATR accessory (Pike Technologies, Madison, WI, USA) and a Shimadzu 8400 s spectrometer (Shimadzu Corp., Kyoto, Japan). Before the analysis, the solid samples (dry leaves, tablets, and capsules) were ground to a fine powder in a mortar. Next, a small portion of each sample was applied onto the surface of the ATR crystal and pressed by the clamp with constant pressure. The spectra (40 scans each) were measured in absorbance mode, within a 750–4000 cm^{-1} wavenumber range at a resolution of 4 cm^{-1}. Each sample was measured in triplicate.

2.5. Chemometric Analysis

The PLS (Partial Least Square) regression model with interval variable selection was constructed for a quantitative alternative to RP-HPLC and fast analysis of DNJ in samples.

The data set was split using the Kennard–Stone algorithm into a calibration (15 products) and a test set (four products). Preprocessing was used, including baseline correction (weighted least squares baseline function) integrated with the standard normal variate method (SNV) and autoscaling. Variables were selected based on the interval PLS algorithm (iPLS), which is very useful for spectral data analysis [32]. The following three intervals were chosen: 1101–1196 cm^{-1}, 1333–1427 cm^{-1}, and 1603–1697 cm^{-1}. Variable selection was processed in stepwise forward mode (size of interval = 30, variable step = 10, number of intervals = auto).

The accuracy of the constructed model was assessed based on validation parameters: determination coefficient of calibration (R^2_{CAL}) and root mean square error of calibration ($RMSE_{CAL}$). Cross-validation was employed as an internal validation using the leave-one-out method to assess how well the model described the relationships within the calibration data. Statistical outputs were calculated as follows: coefficient of determination of cross-validation (R^2_{CV}) and root mean square error of cross-validation ($RMSE_{CV}$).

To evaluate the predictive ability of the model, an external test set was used, consisting of samples from four products (two dietary supplements and two teas). Using the test set, validation parameters were calculated, such as the determination coefficient of prediction (R^2_{PRED}) and root mean square error of prediction ($RMSE_{PRED}$). Additionally, based on the William's plot (distribution of studentized residuals against the leverage), the models applicability domain (AD) was determined. Furthermore, the Y-randomization test examined the verification of model robustness with a 100-response permutation.

All the calculations were performed using PLS-Toolbox 7.5 (Eigenvector Research, Inc., Manson, WA, USA) and MATLAB software version R2020b (The MathWorks, Inc., Natick, MA, USA).

3. Results and Discussion

The use of functional food, including dietary supplements, can bring the expected beneficial effects only if their good quality is ensured. The lack of uniform unambiguous requirements for this type of nutrition is associated with a high risk of low-quality products in the market. For the above reasons, to assess the quality of products containing white mulberry leaves (in the form of herbal teas and dietary supplements), the content of DNJ (the essential biomolecule for the antidiabetic activity), (poly)phenolic compounds (chlorogenic acid, neochlorogenic acid, and rutin), and general antioxidant activity were determined.

3.1. Determination of DNJ, CGA, nCGA, and Rutin

In our study, we have used the HPLC-DAD technique to obtain a quantitative evaluation of DNJ, CGA, nCGA, and rutin content in white mulberry leaves and dietary supplements. The methods developed for this purpose are of high quality, as evidenced by the values of validation parameters presented in Table 1.

Table 1. Validation metrics of RP-HPLC methods.

Parameter	DNJ	CGA	nCGA	Rutin
Range (µg/mL)	3.14–157.14	10.00–140.00	5.00–80.00	5.00–50.00
Regression equation	y = 88.68x − 0.06	y = 44.56x − 0.17	y = 52.56x − 0.10	y = 24.48x − 0.02
Regression coefficient (R^2)	0.999 ± 0.001	0.995 ± 0.002	0.999 ± 0.001	0.999 ± 0.001
Recovery (%)	90.4 ± 1.7	96.2 ± 1.2	94.1 ± 0.6	93.8 ± 1.1
Precision (%RSD)	7.5	5.6	6.7	6.2
LOD (ng/mL)	9.1	3.52	2.82	4.07
LOQ (ng/mL)	27.7	10.67	8.55	12.33

Abbreviations: CGA, chlorogenic acid; DNJ, 1-deoxynojirimycin; LOD, limit of detection; LOQ, limit of quantification; nCGA, neochlorogenic acid; RSD, relative standard deviation.

The optimization of an analytical method with adequate validation parameters is particularly important in quantifying DNJ due to the need to derivatize the sample. The calculated metrics demonstrate the high efficiency of derivatization and extraction processes.

Figure 2 shows the results of DNJ determination, recalculated to the content (µg) per 1 g of dry leaves in white mulberry dietary supplements (S1–S10) and herbal teas (T1–T9). Since the DNJ values differ significantly, a gap on the scale was used for better visualization and comparison of the results (the gap was marked with the red dotted line).

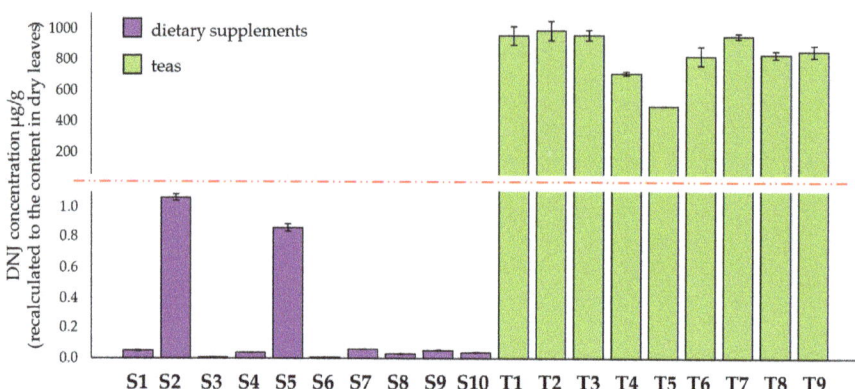

Figure 2. DNJ content in samples expressed in μg/g (recalculated to the content in dry leaves). The red dotted line indicates the gap on the scale (for DNJ concentration between 1.2–100 μg/g).

DNJ concentrations in dietary supplements (S1–S10) and leaves (T1–T9) (expressed as the content of DNJ in 1 g of dried leaves) were found to vary from 0.006 to 992.314 μg/g. The DNJ content in teas was similar and fluctuated in the range of 503.405 to 992.314 μg/g. These results are comparable with the literature [31,33–35]. An extremely low amount of DNJ was observed in the samples of dietary supplements (from 0.006 to 1.064 μg/g). Two products (S2 and S5) with the highest content of DNJ (but still very low) in the group of dietary supplements comprised of powdered white mulberry leaves. Other dietary supplements are produced using extracts of varying concentrations (drug extract ratio, DER from 4:1 to 20:1). There are many possible explanations for the low content of DNJ in dietary supplements. One of them is the low efficiency of the extraction process. The extraction yield is influenced by many factors, such as preparation of the raw material, type of solvent used, and duration and temperature of the process [36]. Inadequately selected conditions for extraction may lead to limited isolation of active substances or, on the other hand, their degradation. Lack of optimization of the extraction method may result in poor quality of the produced dietary supplements. Likewise, the formulation of dietary supplement tablets or capsules can negatively affect the active ingredient content. A disturbing possible explanation for the obtained results is the use of a lower amount of raw material than what was declared.

The literature has provided information on the recommended amounts of DNJ to lower postprandial glucose levels [37–39]. Suggested doses are in the range of 6–18 mg three times a day. Using 30 mg as a recommended dietary intake (RDI) and considering the number of tablets/capsules proposed by manufacturers, we calculated the percentage of the daily amount satisfied by taking dietary supplements (Figure 3).

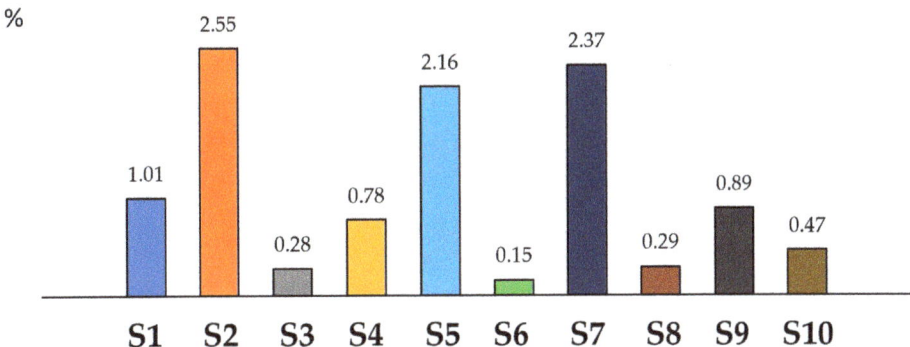

Figure 3. The percentage of recommended dietary intake of DNJ, which is covered by the dose of dietary supplements (S1–S10) suggested by manufacturers.

As seen in Figure 3, the use of any analyzed supplement, as suggested by the manufacturer, does not provide even 3% of the recommended dietary intake of DNJ.

The contents of (poly)phenolic compounds in the studied products are shown in Figure 4. The results are consistent with those obtained for DNJ determinations. In products with the status of dietary supplements, the content of (poly)phenolic compounds, responsible mainly for the antioxidant properties of white mulberry leaves, is negligible.

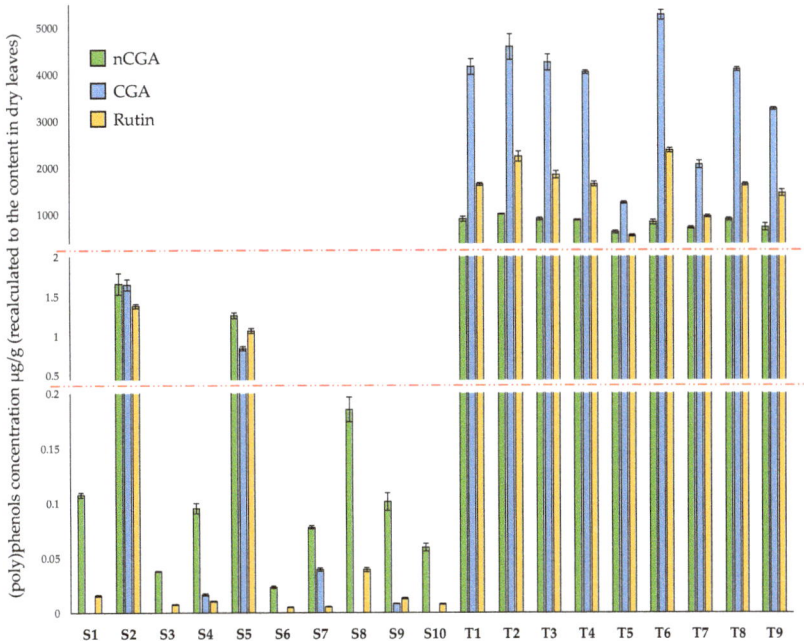

Figure 4. Chlorogenic acid (CGA), neochlorogenic acid (nCGA), and rutin content in samples expressed in µg/g (recalculated to the content in dry leaves). The red dotted lines indicate the gaps on the scale, for (poly)phenols concentration between 0.2–0.5 µg/g and between 2–400 µg/g).

The available literature [40–44] indicate high variability in dried white mulberry leaf CGA, nCGA, and rutin content. As the authors emphasize, this is due to the differences between raw materials from various crops and the considerable influence of the type of extractant used. Nevertheless, the analysis performed in this study for tea products is consistent with previously published data, even for T5 and T7 products with the lowest (poly)phenol content.

Besides the very low content of CGA, nCGA, and rutin in studied dietary supplements, attention is also drawn to their changed proportion compared to tea samples. Half of the tested dietary supplements practically do not contain CGA, while in the case of teas, this compound was present in the largest amount among those determined. A relatively low content of rutin is also noticeable and is very similar in all tested dietary supplements containing the extract (S1, S3, S4, S6–S10). The above observations suggest a particular sensitivity of rutin and CGA to inappropriate extraction conditions (e.g., using too much ethanol, because it is easier to evaporate than water).

The chromatographic analyses indicate the low quality of the tested dietary supplements. Significant differences between the content of the active substances (DNJ, CGA, nCGA, and rutin) between teas and dietary supplements suggest using a smaller amount of the raw material than declared. On the other hand, higher contents of the active compounds were in only two dietary supplements (S2 and S5), which composed of dried white mulberry leaves. These results indicate an inaccurate optimization method for obtaining plant extracts (which are components of other dietary supplements).

3.2. DPPH• Assay

Oxidative stress plays a critical role in diabetes and many other serious conditions, including aging, cancer, chronic inflammation, neurodegenerative diseases, atherosclerosis, etc. Therefore, plant materials showing antioxidant activity arouse the interest of researchers. Naturally occurring nutrients with potent antioxidant properties are (poly)phenols [45] found in dried white mulberry leaves. A commonly used method in assessing antioxidant properties (as free radical scavenging) is the DPPH• assay. The results of the evaluation of free radical scavenging capacity for white mulberry dietary supplements and teas are presented in Figure 5. The lower the EC_{50} value, the greater the antioxidant capacity of the product. Since the EC_{50} values differ significantly, gaps on the scale were used for better visualization and comparison of the results (the gaps were marked with the red dotted lines).

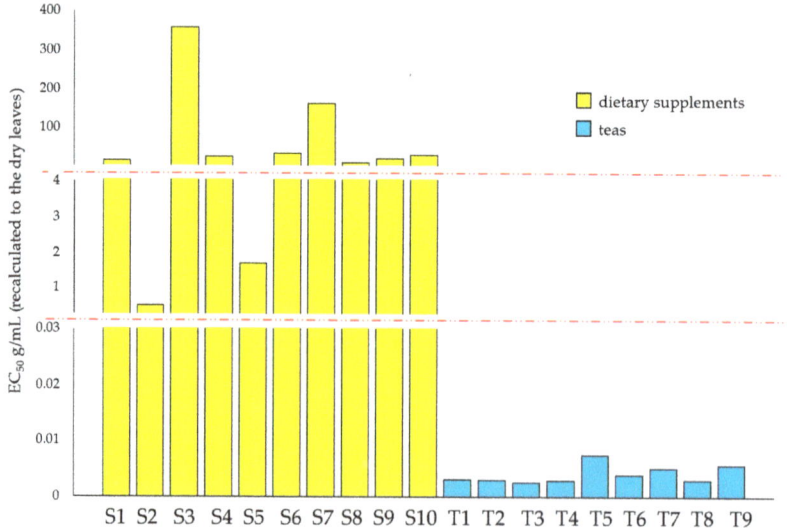

Figure 5. Results of DPPH• assays (as EC_{50}) of white mulberry teas and dietary supplements (recalculated to the dry leaves). The red dotted lines indicate the gaps on the scale, for EC50 values between 0.03–0.1 g/mL and between 4–10 g/mL).

As can be seen in Figure 4, the free radical scavenging activity of teas (T1–T9) significantly exceeds other tested products (S1–S10). Among the dietary supplements, samples S2 and S5 exhibited greater antioxidant capacity than the others (middle part of Figure 5). These results are consistent with the content of nCGA, CGA, and rutin (Figure 4). The highest amounts of rutin and phenolic acids among dietary supplements were found in S2 and S5 products. As noted, these two dietary supplements contain powdered dried leaves of white mulberry, not an extract as in the others.

3.3. ATR-FTIR Spectra

The ATR-FTIR spectra of the investigated food products (Figure 6) displayed typical vibrational patterns of plant constituents, such as sugars, proteins, and lipids. White mulberry leaves contain about 15–30% proteins, 2–8% lipids, 10–40% carbohydrates, and 10–37% neutral dietary fiber [46]. The ATR-FTIR spectra of the mulberry leaves (blue) and dietary supplements containing extract from leaves (red) showed the broad and intense band at 2790–3570 cm^{-1} assigned to the stretch vibration of O-H and C-H, and it was not helpful in this work because all spectra were very similar in this range. In this region, 900–1700 cm^{-1} signals of the flavonoid molecules and DNJ can be found [47], which is confirmed by the spectra of rutin, chlorogenic acid, and DNJ analytical standards. The vibrations observed in 1650–1580 cm^{-1} can be attributed to N-H of amines. The peaks at 1572 and 1541 cm^{-1} are assigned to the aromatic ring (C-C) skeletal vibrations. The band at 1410 cm^{-1} was assigned to C-H bending vibration. Absorptions between 1300 and 1000 cm^{-1} showed stretching vibrations of the pyranose ring [31]. The absorption at 935 and 1205 cm^{-1} were assigned to C-C, C-O stretching, and C-O-H, C-O-C deformation modes of oligo- and polysaccharides modes [48]. The distinctive band at 1047 cm^{-1} can be assigned to the vibrational frequency of -CH$_2$OH groups of carbohydrates [49]. Bands in the range of 1300–1492 cm^{-1} are associated with O-C-H, C-C-H, and C-O-H bending modes.

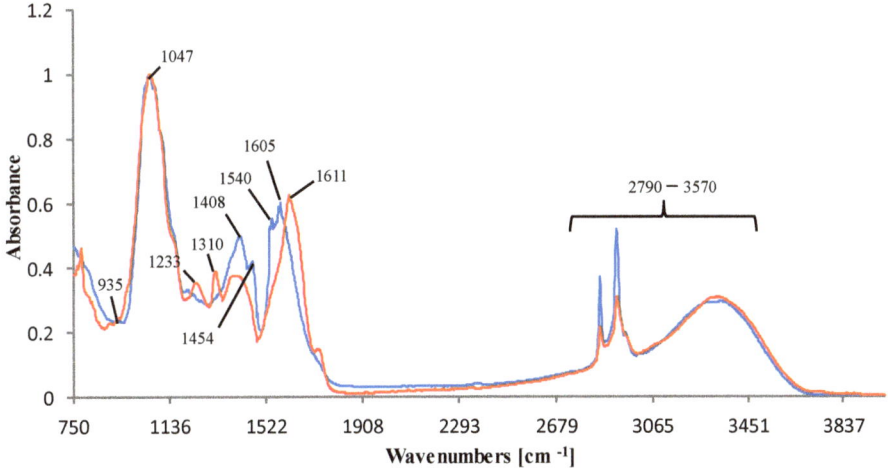

Figure 6. Normalized ATR-FTIR spectra of exemplary samples: white mulberry leaves (blue) and dietary supplement (red).

3.4. iPLS Model

The low content of DNJ, the essential component of white mulberry leaves, in the tested dietary supplements proves how important their quality control is. The relatively complicated and time-consuming procedure of quantitative analysis of DNJ (extraction and derivatization) prompted us to search for an alternative method based on spectroscopic techniques combined with chemometrics.

We decided to calculate the interval partial least squares (iPLS) regression model to predict DNJ content in samples containing white mulberry leaves based on the ATR-FTIR spectra. Figure S2 shows the average spectrum of tested samples (dietary supplements and teas) and the DNJ spectrum after preprocessing using the SNV with highlighted intervals used to build the iPLS model. The model was built by employing three intervals (1101–1196 cm^{-1}, 1333–1427 cm^{-1}, and 1603–1697 cm^{-1}) from the fingerprint region of FTIR spectra 850–1800 cm^{-1}. Figure 7 presents the relationships between measured and predicted values of DNJ concentration using the model. The model, constructed with six latent variables (LV), had good validation metrics: $RMSE_{CAL} = 0.025$; $RMSE_{CV} = 0.095$; $RMSE_{PRED} = 0.016$; $R^2_{cal} = 0.995$, $R^2_{cv} = 0.925$ without overfitting. The permutation test (Y randomization) confirms the models good quality (all three tests: Wilcoxon, sign test, and Rand t-test, were passed, $p < 0.05$). Therefore, ATR-FTIR spectra combined with PLS regression can be an efficient tool for the prediction of DNJ in white mulberry leaf products (teas and dietary supplements).

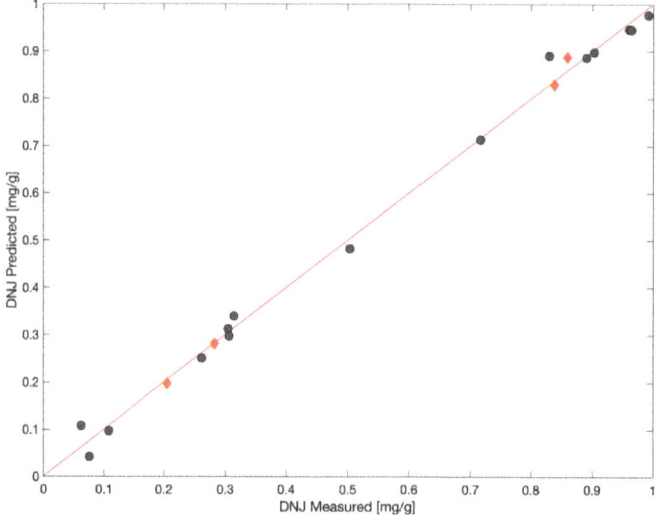

Figure 7. Results of iPLS model. Relationships between measured and predicted values of DNJ concentration using the model (●—calibration set, ♦—test set). LV number = 6; cross-validation method: leave-one-out; $RMSE_{CAL} = 0.025$; $RMSE_{CV} = 0.095$; $RMSE_{PRED} = 0.016$; $R^2_{CAL} = 0.995$.

4. Conclusions

The results of the quantitative chromatographic analysis indicated that dietary supplements with white mulberry leaf extract contained a negligible quantity of active substances, such as (poly)phenols and DNJ (α-glucosidase inhibitor), compared to the declared amount of raw material (dried leaves). These observations confirm the need to increase plant-based functional food quality control.

Herein, we propose an alternative to the chromatographic method for quantifying DNJ in food samples based on ATR-FTIR spectroscopy combined with PLS regression. This methodology does not require sample extraction and derivatization. Furthermore, it is relatively simple, non-destructive, inexpensive, and in line with green chemistry. Following the global need for appropriate regulation of dietary supplements, the method developed in the present study can be considered promising for routine quality control of dietary supplements containing white mulberry leaves.

Supplementary Materials: The following supporting information can be downloaded at: https://www.mdpi.com/article/10.3390/nu14245276/s1. Figure S1: Chromatograms of derivatized standard—DNJ (blue line) and exemplary derivatized samples: extract from a dietary supplement (pink line) and from dry Mulberry leaves (green line); Figure S2: The average spectrum of tested samples: dietary supplements and teas (green line) and the DNJ spectrum (grey line). Spectra were preprocessed by SNV. The red boxes indicate spectral intervals used to build the iPLS model for DNJ prediction.

Author Contributions: Conceptualization, A.W.-B. and B.K.; methodology, data curation, A.W.-B., K.W., N.P.-S. and B.K.; writing—original draft preparation, A.W-B. and N.P.-S.; writing—review and editing, B.K. All authors have read and agreed to the published version of the manuscript.

Funding: This research was funded by the Nicolaus Copernicus University in Toruń, Collegium Medicum in Bydgoszcz, grant MN-SDF/7/WF/2019 to Agata Walkowiak.

Institutional Review Board Statement: Not applicable.

Informed Consent Statement: Not applicable.

Data Availability Statement: Not applicable.

Conflicts of Interest: The author declare no conflict of interest.

References

1. International Diabetes Federation. *IDF Diabetes Atlas*, 9th ed.; International Diabetes Federation: Brussels, Belgium, 2019.
2. Ndjaboue, R.; Farhat, I.; Ferlatte, C.-A.; Ngueta, G.; Guay, D.; Delorme, S.; Ivers, N.; Shah, B.R.; Straus, S.; Yu, C.; et al. Predictive models of diabetes complications: Protocol for a scoping review. *Syst. Rev.* **2020**, *9*, 137. [CrossRef] [PubMed]
3. Liu, Y.; Zhou, X.; Zhou, D.; Jian, Y.; Jia, J.; Ge, F. Isolation of Chalcomoracin as a Potential α-Glycosidase Inhibitor from Mulberry Leaves and Its Binding Mechanism. *Molecules* **2022**, *27*, 5742. [CrossRef] [PubMed]
4. Kwon, R.-H.; Thaku, N.; Timalsina, B.; Park, S.-E.; Choi, J.-S.; Jung, H.-A. Inhibition Mechanism of Components Isolated from *Morus alba* Branches on Diabetes and Diabetic Complications via Experimental and Molecular Docking Analyses. *Antioxidants* **2022**, *11*, 383. [CrossRef] [PubMed]
5. Zhou, Q.Y.-J.; Liao, X.; Kuang, H.-M.; Li, J.-Y.; Zhang, S.-H. LC-MS Metabolite Profiling and the Hypoglycemic Activity of *Morus alba* L. Extracts. *Molecules* **2022**, *27*, 5360. [CrossRef]
6. Gao, T.; Chen, J.; Xu, F.; Wang, Y.; Zhao, P.; Ding, Y.; Han, Y.; Yang, J.; Tao, Y. Mixed Mulberry Fruit and Mulberry Leaf Fermented Alcoholic Beverages: Assessment of Chemical Composition, Antioxidant Capacity In Vitro and Sensory Evaluation. *Foods* **2022**, *11*, 3125. [CrossRef]
7. Ma, G.; Chai, X.; Hou, G.; Zhao, F.; Meng, Q. Phytochemistry, bioactivities and future prospects of mulberry leaves: A review. *Food Chem.* **2021**, *372*, 131335. [CrossRef]
8. Lange, E.; Kęszycka, P.K.; Pałkowska-Goździk, E.; Billing-Marczak, K. Comparison of Glycemic Response to Carbohydrate Meals without or with a Plant-Based Formula of Kidney Bean Extract, White Mulberry Leaf Extract, and Green Coffee Extract in Individuals with Abdominal Obesity. *Int. J. Environ. Res. Public Heal.* **2022**, *19*, 12117. [CrossRef]
9. Lv, Q.; Lin, J.; Wu, X.; Pu, H.; Guan, Y.; Xiao, P.; He, C.; Jiang, B. Novel active compounds and the anti-diabetic mechanism of mulberry leaves. *Front. Pharmacol.* **2022**, *13*, 986931. [CrossRef]
10. Zhang, W.; Mu, W.; Wu, H.; Liang, Z. An overview of the biological production of 1-deoxynojirimycin: Current status and future perspective. *Appl. Microbiol. Biotechnol.* **2019**, *103*, 9335–9344. [CrossRef]
11. Tsuduki, T.; Kikuchi, I.; Kimura, T.; Nakagawa, K.; Miyazawa, T. Intake of mulberry 1-deoxynojirimycin prevents diet-induced obesity through increases in adiponectin in mice. *Food Chem.* **2013**, *139*, 16–23. [CrossRef]
12. Wang, G.Q.; Zhu, L.; Ma, M.L.; Chen, X.C.; Gao, Y.; Yu, T.Y.; Yang, G.S.; Pang, W.J. Mulberry 1-Deoxynojirimycin Inhibits Adipogenesis by Repression of the ERK/PPARγ Signaling Pathway in Porcine Intramuscular Adipocytes. *J. Agric. Food Chem.* **2015**, *63*, 6020–6212. [CrossRef]
13. Chen, Z.; Du, X.; Yang, Y.; Cui, X.; Zhang, Z.; Li, Y. Comparative study of chemical composition and active components against α-glucosidase of various medicinal parts of *Morus alba* L. *Biomed. Chromatogr.* **2018**, *32*, e4328. [CrossRef] [PubMed]
14. Fongsodsri, K.; Thaipitakwong, T.; Rujimongkon, K.; Kanjanapruthipong, T.; Ampawong, S.; Reamtong, O.; Aramwit, P. Mulberry-Derived 1-Deoxynojirimycin Prevents Type 2 Diabetes Mellitus Progression via Modulation of Retinol-Binding Protein 4 and Haptoglobin. *Nutrients* **2022**, *14*, 4538. [CrossRef] [PubMed]
15. Kang, C.W.; Park, M.; Lee, H.J. Mulberry (*Morus alba* L.) Leaf Extract and 1-Deoxynojirimycin Improve Skeletal Muscle Insulin Resistance via the Activation of IRS-1/PI3K/Akt Pathway in db/db Mice. *Life* **2022**, *12*, 1630. [CrossRef] [PubMed]
16. Takasu, S.; Parida, I.S.; Onose, S.; Ito, J.; Ikeda, R.; Yamagishi, K.; Higuchi, O.; Tanaka, F.; Kimura, T.; Miyazawa, T.; et al. Evaluation of the anti-hyperglycemic effect and safety of microorganism 1-deoxynojirimycin. *PLoS ONE* **2018**, *13*, e0199057. [CrossRef]

17. Gao, K.; Zheng, C.; Wang, T.; Zhao, H.; Wang, J.; Wang, Z.; Zhai, X.; Jia, Z.; Chen, J.; Zhou, Y.; et al. 1-Deoxynojirimycin: Occurrence, Extraction, Chemistry, Oral Pharmacokinetics, Biological Activities and In Silico Target Fishing. *Molecules* **2016**, *21*, 1600. [CrossRef]
18. Marchetti, L.; Saviane, A.; Montà, A.; Paglia, G.; Pellati, F.; Benvenuti, S.; Bertelli, D.; Cappellozza, S. Determination of 1-Deoxynojirimycin (1-DNJ) in Leaves of Italian or Italy-Adapted Cultivars of Mulberry (*Morus* sp.pl.) by HPLC-MS. *Plants* **2021**, *10*, 1553. [CrossRef]
19. Zamoner, L.O.B.; Aragão-Leoneti, V.; Carvalho, I. Iminosugars: Effects of Stereochemistry, Ring Size, and N-Substituents on Glucosidase Activities. *Pharmaceuticals* **2019**, *12*, 108. [CrossRef]
20. Jokiaho, A.J.; Winchester, M.; Donovan, C.M. N-Hydroxyethyl-1-Deoxynojirimycin (Miglitol) Restores the Counterregulatory Response to Hypoglycemia Following Antecedent Hypoglycemia. *Diabetes* **2022**, *71*, 1063–1072. [CrossRef]
21. Noël, S.; Wilke, M.; Bot, A.G.M.; De Jonge, H.R.; Becq, F. Parallel Improvement of Sodium and Chloride Transport Defects by Miglustat (*n*-Butyldeoxynojirimycin) in Cystic Fibrosis Epithelial Cells. *J. Pharmacol. Exp. Ther.* **2008**, *325*, 1016–1023. [CrossRef]
22. Jennemann, R.; Volz, M.; Bestvater, F.; Schmidt, C.; Richter, K.; Kaden, S.; Müthing, J.; Gröne, H.-J.; Sandhoff, R. Blockade of Glycosphingolipid Synthesis Inhibits Cell Cycle and Spheroid Growth of Colon Cancer Cells In Vitro and Experimental Colon Cancer Incidence In Vivo. *Int. J. Mol. Sci.* **2021**, *22*, 10539. [CrossRef] [PubMed]
23. Rajasekharan, S.; Bonotto, R.M.; Alves, L.N.; Kazungu, Y.; Poggianella, M.; Martinez-Orellana, P.; Skoko, N.; Polez, S.; Marcello, A. Inhibitors of Protein Glycosylation Are Active against the Coronavirus Severe Acute Respiratory Syndrome Coronavirus SARS-CoV-2. *Viruses* **2021**, *13*, 808. [CrossRef] [PubMed]
24. Chao, D.H.M.; Wang, Y.; Foppen, E.; Ottenhoff, R.; van Roomen, C.; Parlevliet, E.T.; van Eijk, M.; Verhoek, M.; Boot, R.; Marques, A.R.; et al. The Iminosugar AMP-DNM Improves Satiety and Activates Brown Adipose Tissue Through GLP1. *Diabetes* **2019**, *68*, 2223–2234. [CrossRef]
25. Bijl, N.; Scheij, S.; Houten, S.; Boot, R.G.; Groen, A.K.; Aerts, J.M.F.G. The Glucosylceramide Synthase Inhibitor*N*-(5-Adamantane-1-yl-methoxy-pentyl)-deoxynojirimycin Induces Sterol Regulatory Element-Binding Protein-Regulated Gene Expression and Cholesterol Synthesis in HepG2 Cells. *J. Pharmacol. Exp. Ther.* **2008**, *326*, 849–855. [CrossRef]
26. Fortune Business Insights. Dietary Supplements Market Size, Share & COVID-19 Impact Analysis, By Type (Vitamins, Minerals, Enzymes, Fatty Acids, Proteins, and Others), Form (Tablets, Capsules, Liquids, and Powders), and Regional Forecasts, 2021–2028. Available online: https://www.fortunebusinessinsights.com/dietary-supplements-market-102082 (accessed on 15 October 2022).
27. Dwyer, J.T.; Coates, P.M.; Smith, M.J. Dietary Supplements: Regulatory Challenges and Research Resources. *Nutrients* **2018**, *10*, 41. [CrossRef] [PubMed]
28. Kharbach, M.; Marmouzi, I.; El Jemli, M.; Bouklouze, A.; Heyden, Y.V. Recent advances in untargeted and targeted approaches applied in herbal-extracts and essential-oils fingerprinting—A review. *J. Pharm. Biomed. Anal.* **2020**, *177*, 112849. [CrossRef] [PubMed]
29. Durak, T.; Depciuch, J. Effect of plant sample preparation and measuring methods on ATR-FTIR spectra results. *Environ. Exp. Bot.* **2020**, *169*, 103915. [CrossRef]
30. European Medicines Agency. *ICH Q2(R2) Validation of Analytical Procedures*; European Medicines Agency: Amsterdam, The Netherlands, 2022.
31. Kim, J.-W.; Kim, S.-U.; Lee, H.S.; Kim, I.; Ahn, M.Y.; Ryu, K.S. Determination of 1-deoxynojirimycin in Morus alba L. leaves by derivatization with 9-fluorenylmethyl chloroformate followed by reversed-phase high-performance liquid chromatography. *J. Chromatogr. A* **2003**, *1002*, 93–99. [CrossRef]
32. Nørgaard, L.; Saudland, A.; Wagner, J.; Nielsen, J.P.; Munck, L.; Engelsen, S.B. Interval Partial Least-Squares Regression (*i*PLS): A Comparative Chemometric Study with an Example from Near-Infrared Spectroscopy. *Appl. Spectrosc.* **2000**, *54*, 413–419. [CrossRef]
33. Hu, X.-Q.; Jiang, L.; Zhang, J.-G.; Deng, W.; Wang, H.-L.; Wei, Z.-J. Quantitative determination of 1-deoxynojirimycin in mulberry leaves from 132 varieties. *Ind. Crop. Prod.* **2013**, *49*, 782–784. [CrossRef]
34. Ji, T.; Li, J.; Su, S.-L.; Zhu, Z.-H.; Guo, S.; Qian, D.-W.; Duan, J.-A. Identification and Determination of the Polyhydroxylated Alkaloids Compounds with α-Glucosidase Inhibitor Activity in Mulberry Leaves of Different Origins. *Molecules* **2016**, *21*, 206. [CrossRef] [PubMed]
35. Guo, N.; Jiang, Y.-W.; Kou, P.; Liu, Z.-M.; Efferth, T.; Li, Y.-Y.; Fu, Y.-J. Application of integrative cloud point extraction and concentration for the analysis of polyphenols and alkaloids in mulberry leaves. *J. Pharm. Biomed. Anal.* **2019**, *167*, 132–139. [CrossRef] [PubMed]
36. Chen, C.; Razali, U.M.; Saikim, F.; Mahyudin, A.; Noor, N.M. Morus alba L. Plant: Bioactive Compounds and Potential as a Functional Food Ingredient. *Foods* **2021**, *10*, 689. [CrossRef] [PubMed]
37. Thaipitakwong, T.; Supasyndh, O.; Rasmi, Y.; Aramwit, P. A randomized controlled study of dose-finding, efficacy, and safety of mulberry leaves on glycemic profiles in obese persons with borderline diabetes. *Complement. Ther. Med.* **2019**, *49*, 102292. [CrossRef]
38. Asai, A.; Nakagawa, K.; Higuchi, O.; Kimura, T.; Kojima, Y.; Kariya, J.; Miyazawa, T.; Oikawa, S. Effect of mulberry leaf extract with enriched 1-deoxynojirimycin content on postprandial glycemic control in subjects with impaired glucose metabolism. *J. Diabetes Investig.* **2011**, *2*, 318–323. [CrossRef]

39. Chung, H.I.; Kim, J.; Kim, J.Y.; Kwon, O. Acute intake of mulberry leaf aqueous extract affects postprandial glucose response after maltose loading: Randomized double-blind placebo-controlled pilot study. *J. Funct. Foods* **2013**, *5*, 1502–1506. [CrossRef]
40. Zhang, D.-Y.; Wan, Y.; Hao, J.-Y.; Hu, R.-Z.; Chen, C.; Yao, X.-H.; Zhao, W.-G.; Liu, Z.-Y.; Li, L. Evaluation of the alkaloid, polyphenols, and antioxidant contents of various mulberry cultivars from different planting areas in eastern China. *Ind. Crop. Prod.* **2018**, *122*, 298–307. [CrossRef]
41. Polumackanycz, M.; Wesolowski, M.; Viapiana, A. Morus alba L. and Morus nigra L. Leaves as a Promising Food Source of Phenolic Compounds with Antioxidant Activity. *Plant Foods Hum. Nutr.* **2021**, *76*, 458–465. [CrossRef]
42. Sánchez-Salcedo, E.M.; Mena, P.; García-Viguera, C.; Hernández, F.; Martínez, J.J. (Poly)phenolic compounds and antioxidant activity of white (*Morus alba*) and black (*Morus nigra*) mulberry leaves: Their potential for new products rich in phytochemicals. *J. Funct. Foods* **2015**, *18*, 1039–1046. [CrossRef]
43. Radojković, M.; Zeković, Z.; Mašković, P.; Vidović, S.; Mandić, A.; Mišan, A.; Đurović, S. Biological activities and chemical composition of Morus leaves extracts obtained by maceration and supercritical fluid extraction. *J. Supercrit. Fluids* **2016**, *117*, 50–58. [CrossRef]
44. Przeor, M.; Flaczyk, E.; Kmiecik, D.; Buchowski, M.S.; Staniek, H.; Tomczak-Graczyk, A.; Kobus-Cisowska, J.; Gramza-Michałowska, A.; Foksowicz-Flaczyk, J. Functional Properties and Antioxidant Activity of *Morus alba* L. Leaves var. Zolwinska Wielkolistna (WML-P)—The Effect of Controlled Conditioning Process. *Antioxidants* **2020**, *9*, 668. [CrossRef]
45. Lim, S.H.; Choi, C.-I. Pharmacological Properties of *Morus nigra* L. (Black Mulberry) as A Promising Nutraceutical Resource. *Nutrients* **2019**, *11*, 437. [CrossRef]
46. Gryn-Rynko, A.; Bazylak, G.; Olszewska-Slonina, D. New potential phytotherapeutics obtained from white mulberry (*Morus alba* L.) leaves. *Biomed. Pharmacother.* **2016**, *84*, 628–636. [CrossRef]
47. Adiana, M.; Mazura, M. Study on Senna alata and its different extracts by Fourier transform infrared spectroscopy and two-dimensional correlation infrared spectroscopy. *J. Mol. Struct.* **2011**, *991*, 84–91. [CrossRef]
48. Hu, Y.; Pan, Z.J.; Liao, W.; Li, J.; Gruget, P.; Kitts, D.D.; Lu, X. Determination of antioxidant capacity and phenolic content of chocolate by attenuated total reflectance-Fourier transformed-infrared spectroscopy. *Food Chem.* **2016**, *202*, 254–261. [CrossRef] [PubMed]
49. Biancolillo, A.; Marini, F.; D'Archivio, A.A. Geographical discrimination of red garlic (*Allium sativum* L.) using fast and non-invasive Attenuated Total Reflectance-Fourier Transformed Infrared (ATR-FTIR) spectroscopy combined with chemometrics. *J. Food Compos. Anal.* **2020**, *86*, 103351. [CrossRef]

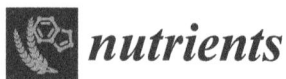

Systematic Review

Astaxanthin Influence on Health Outcomes of Adults at Risk of Metabolic Syndrome: A Systematic Review and Meta-Analysis

Leona Yuen-Ling Leung [1,2,3], Sidney Man-Ngai Chan [4], Hon-Lon Tam [5,6,*] and Emily Sze-Wan Wong [4,*]

1. The Ronin Institute, Montclair, NJ 07043, USA; leonaleung@ronininstitute.org
2. Hong Kong Food Science and Technology Association, Hong Kong, China
3. Canadian Academy of Independent Scholars, Vancouver, BC V6B 5K3, Canada
4. School of Science and Technology, Hong Kong Metropolitan University, Hong Kong, China; mnchan@hkmu.edu.hk
5. Education Department, Kiang Wu Nursing College of Macau, Macau 999078, China
6. School of Nursing, The Hong Kong Polytechnic University, Hung Hom, Hong Kong, China
* Correspondence: alantam@kwnc.edu.mo (H.-L.T.); eswwong@hkmu.edu.hk (E.S.-W.W.)

Abstract: The use of medication is effective in managing metabolic syndrome (MetS), but side effects have led to increased attention on using nutraceuticals and supplements. Astaxanthin shows positive effects in reducing the risk of MetS, but results from individual studies are inconclusive. This systematic review summarizes the latest evidence of astaxanthin in adults with risk factors of MetS. A systematic search of English and Chinese randomized controlled trials in 14 electronic databases from inception to 30 June 2021 was performed. Two reviewers independently screened the titles and abstracts, and conducted full-text review, quality appraisal, and extraction of data. Risk of bias was assessed by PEDro. A total of 7 studies met the inclusion criteria with 321 participants. Six studies were rated to have excellent methodological quality, while the remaining one was rated at good. Results show marginal effects of astaxanthin on reduction in total cholesterol and systolic blood pressure, and a significant attenuating effect on low-density lipoprotein cholesterol. Further robust evidence is needed to examine the effects of astaxanthin in adults at risk of MetS.

Keywords: astaxanthin; cardiometabolic disease; metabolic syndrome; systematic review; meta-analysis

Citation: Leung, L.Y.-L.; Chan, S.M.-N.; Tam, H.-L.; Wong, E.S.-W. Astaxanthin Influence on Health Outcomes of Adults at Risk of Metabolic Syndrome: A Systematic Review and Meta-Analysis. *Nutrients* **2022**, *14*, 2050. https://doi.org/10.3390/nu14102050

Academic Editors: Gaetano Santulli and Bruno Trimarco

Received: 25 April 2022
Accepted: 10 May 2022
Published: 13 May 2022

Publisher's Note: MDPI stays neutral with regard to jurisdictional claims in published maps and institutional affiliations.

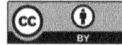

Copyright: © 2022 by the authors. Licensee MDPI, Basel, Switzerland. This article is an open access article distributed under the terms and conditions of the Creative Commons Attribution (CC BY) license (https://creativecommons.org/licenses/by/4.0/).

1. Introduction

Metabolic syndrome (MetS) is also known as syndrome X or the deadly quartet. A Swedish physician establshed the concept in the 1920s. The meaning of MetS was modified and revised by various scholars and professional organizations [1,2] for over 70 years. Until 1998, there existed a unified operational definition of MetS coined by World Health Organisation (WHO) [1,2]. In subsequent years, at least seven professional bodies further revised the definition with risk factors of cardiovascular and metabolic diseases, such as hypertension, dyslipidemia, obesity, and hyperglycemia (Table 1) [3]. Individuals with at least 3 or more criteria of the above risk factors are diagnosed as MetS. The global prevalence of MetS ranges from 10% to 84%, mostly affecting developed countries [4]. For example, a recent significant health concern in Japan is that half of the males and one-fifth of females aged 40 to 74 years suffer from MetS or pre-MetS [5]. MetS increases the risk of sudden cardiac death by 70% [6], the risk of cardiovascular events by twofold, and the risk of Type 2 diabetes mellitus (T_2DM) by fivefold [3], thus raising healthcare costs [7].

Single or combination use of medications, regular physical activities, and/or dietary management are imperative in managing risk factors of MetS [5,7,8]. However, numerous adverse effects and the high cost of medication treatment [9], failing to meet the minimal recommended level of physical exercise [8], hard-to-follow diet regime [5], and requiring strong mind control to change the mindset and control thoughts [9] were reported. Therefore, cost-effective approaches on using bioactive compounds [10], nutraceuticals and supplements on prevention and treatment of various chronic diseases such as T_2DM emerged. In addition, there are increased concerns about the use of bioactive compounds [10], nutraceuticals, and supplements for managing MetS [11].

Astaxanthin (AST), a natural carotenoid, shows a very strong antioxidant effect that is 14, 65, and 54 times higher than that of vitamin E, C, and ß-carotene, respectively [12]. The compound is commonly found in various aquatic animals, including salmon, shrimp, and crustaceans. Moreover, the most abundance source of AST is microalgal species *Haematococcus pluvialis* [13]. Donoso et al. [14] revealed that AST has numerous beneficial effects such as protecting the cardiovascular system, maintaining healthy vision, enhancing the immune system, improving skin condition, managing diabetic problems, and protecting the nervous system. Hence, the compound is commonly used globally as a supplement, including in Japan, South Korea, Sweden, and the US with global market size of more than USD 110 million in 2018 [15]. In addition, there is an exponential increase in the number of studies related to AST on health, beauty, and safety issues. Brendler and Williamson [15] reviewed the safety issues of 87 AST clinical trials on humans, and no serious adverse effects were reported, even at very high dosage (i.e., 45 mg daily which is about 2 times of the highest daily recommended dosage). However, there is a lack of systematic review (SR) and meta-analysis on investigating the effectiveness of AST in managing the risk factors of MetS on various dosages and durations.

This SR focuses on the use of AST in adults with risk factors of MetS. The objectives were to (i) discuss the effects of physiological (primary) outcomes on the use of AST; (ii) evaluate the effects of various dosages, durations, and frequencies of AST administration; and (iii) report on the adherence rate (secondary outcome).

Table 1. Comparing criteria of metabolic syndrome of seven professional institutions.

Risk Factor	WHO (1998) [16]	EGIR (1999) [16]	AACE (2003) [1]	CDS (2004) [17]	IDF (2005) [16]	NCEP-ATP III (2005 Revision) [16]	JCDCG (2007) [18]
Core element	Insulin resistance (IGT, IFG, T$_2$DM or other evidence of IR)	Hyperinsulinemia (plasma insulin > 75th percentile)	Insulin resistance (IGT, IFG)	None	Central obesity (WC): ≥90 cm (M), ≥80 cm (F)	None	None
Criteria	IR or diabetes, plus two of the five criteria below	Hyperinsulinemia, plus two of the four criteria below	IR, final diagnosis is left to physician discretion	Any three of the four criteria below	Obesity, plus two of the four criteria below	Any three of the five criteria below	Any four of the five criteria below
Obesity	Waist/hip ratio: >0.90 (M), >0.85 (F); or BMI >30 kg/m^2	WC: ≥94 cm (M), ≥80 cm (F)	BMI >25 kg/m^2 or WC: >40 inches (M), >35 inches (F)	BMI > 25 kg/m^2	Central obesity already required	WC: >40 inches (M), >35 inches (F)	WC: ≥90 cm (M), ≥85 cm (F)
Hyper-glycemia	IR already required	IR already required	IR already required	Fasting glucose ≥ 110 mg/dL or Tx	Fasting glucose ≥ 100 mg/dL	Fasting glucose ≥ 100 mg/dL or Tx	Fasting glucose ≥ 110 mg/dL or with a history of T$_2$DM
Dys-lipidemia	TG ≥150 mg/dL or HDL-C: <35 mg/dL (M), <39 mg/dL (F)	TG ≥117 mg/dL or HDL-C <39 mg/dL	TG ≥150 mg/dL or HDL-C: <40 mg/dL (M), <50 mg/dL (F)	TG ≥150 mg/dL or HDL-C: <35 mg/dL (M), <39 mg/dL (F)	TG ≥150 mg/dL or Tx	TG ≥150 mg/dL or Tx	TG ≥150 mg/dL
Dyslipidemia (second separate criteria)	-	-	-	-	HDL-C: <40 mg/dL (M), <50 mg/dL (F); or Tx	HDL-C: <40 mg/dL (M), <50 mg/dL (F); or Tx	HDL-C: <40 mg/dL
Hyper-tension	≥140/90 mmHg	≥140/90 mmHg or Tx	>130/85 mmHg	≥140/90 mmHg or Tx	>130/85 mmHg or Tx	>130/85 mmHg or Tx	≥130/85 mmHg or Tx
Other criteria	Microalbuminuria	-	Other features of IR				

BMI: body mass index; F: female; HDL-C: high-density lipoprotein cholesterol; IFG: impaired fasting glucose; IGT: impaired glucose tolerance; IR: insulin resistance; M: male; Tx: treatment; T$_2$DM: Type 2 diabetes mellitus; TG: triglyceride; WC: waist circumference.

2. Materials and Methods

This SR and meta-analysis was registered with the International Prospective Register of Systematic Review (PROSPERO) (CRD42020215881), established with reference to the Preferred Reporting Items for Systematic Review and Meta-Analysis Protocols (PRISMA-P) guideline.

2.1. Search Strategy

Medical subject heading (MeSH) and keywords were used to identify relevant studies: "astaxanthin (蝦紅素/青素)" or "metabolic syndrome (代謝綜合症/代合征)" or "cardiometabolic disease (心臟代謝疾病)" or "blood pressure (血壓/血)" or "blood sugar (血糖)" or "body mass index (身體質量指數/身体量指)" or "waist circumference (腰圍)". Fourteen electronic databases were searched for eligible studies, including eight English databases: the Cochrane Library (Cochrane Database of Systematic Reviews (CDSR), Cochrane Central Register of Controlled Trials (CENTRAL), Cochrane Methodology Register (CMR)), Cumulative Index to Nursing and Allied Health Literature (CINAHL), EMBASE, Google Scholar, MEDLINE, OvidSP, ProQuest, ScienceDirect; as well as six Chinese databases: Capital Medical University Library (Beijing, China), China National Knowledge Infrastructure (CNKI), Chinese Biomedical Literature database (CBM), Chinese Medical Current Content (CMCC), Union Search, and WangFang were searched from inception to 30 June 2021. ClinicalTrials.gov (accessed on 30 June 2021), and University Hospital Medical Information Network Clinical Trials Registry (UMIN-CTR) were searched for relevant and ongoing studies. In addition, hand searching was also performed to identify the reference list of related literatures or reviews. A sample search for PubMed is available as supporting information (Supplementary File S1).

2.2. Selection Criteria

Studies that fulfilled the following criteria were included in the current review: (1) Study design: randomized controlled trials (RCTs). (2) Participants: Mean age ≥ 18 years, irrespective of race and gender, and fulfilling any one of the risk factors of MetS defined by the WHO European Group for the Study of Insulin Resistance (EGIR), American Association of Clinical Endocrinology (AACE), Chinese Diabetes Society (CDS), International Diabetes Federation (IDF), National Cholesterol Education Program (NCEP), Adult Treatment Panel III (ATPIII), Chinese Joint Committee for Developing Chinese Guidelines (JCDGC) were regarded as the baseline of the study. Studies conducted on animals, children, and adolescents, and those that were still recruiting participants were excluded in this review. (3) Intervention: studies examined the use of AST in any dosage and regime, and the control group included the use of placebo that did not contain AST or did not receive any intervention. (4) Outcome measures: Studies involving at least one measure of the risk factors of MetS: (i) waist circumference (WC), body mass index (BMI), blood pressure (systolic and diastolic blood pressure) (BP), glycosylated hemoglobin level (HbA1c), fasting blood glucose (FBG), lipid profile (total cholesterol (TC), triglyceride, high-density lipoprotein cholesterol (HDL-C), low-density lipoprotein cholesterol (LDL-C)), insulin resistance level, and (ii) adherence rate were included. We also contacted the authors for clarification of some unpublished data.

2.3. Selection Process

All selected studies were extracted and imported to Rayyan QCRI web tool [19], and checked for duplicates. Two independent reviewers (L.L.Y.L. and H.L.T.) assessed the titles and abstracts of all potential studies identified by search strategy. Full texts were obtained if the abstract had provided adequate information regarding inclusion and exclusion criteria. Next, the full text of all retrieved studies was evaluated on the basis of participants, interventions, outcomes measures, and type of study. Decisions to include studies in the review were by the same independent reviewers. Two independent reviewers employed the self-designed eligibility verification checklist (Supplementary File S2) to conduct the selection process. Disagreements between the two reviewers were resolved by discussion. Disputes were resolved by a third reviewer (E.S.-W.W.) through discussion.

2.4. Data Collection Process and Data Extraction

Data extraction was performed on a pilot-tested standardized form (Supplementary File S3) modified from the JBI data extraction form for experimental or observational studies [20] on Microsoft Excel by the first and third authors, and the accuracy of the information was checked by the second and fourth authors. Two reviewers independently performed the data extraction process by employing a three-step approach to select studies that potentially met the inclusion criteria. The following information was extracted: first author's name, study location, year of publication, sample size, participant information, intervention details, outcome measures (all time points), and authors' conclusions.

2.5. Data Synthesis and Statistical Analysis

Meta-analysis was performed when at least two studies had evaluated the same outcome. All quantitative data from selected studies were pooled in statistical meta-analysis by using RevMan 5.4. All results were subjected to double data entry. Mean difference (MD) and its corresponding 95% confidence interval (CI) for each study were used to estimate the pooled effects of the included studies on each continuous variable measured on the same instrument. Unit conversions performed on those outcome measures are presented in different units (e.g., mmol/L to mg/dL). Heterogeneity was statistically assessed by using I^2, taking >75%, 50%, and <25% for high, moderate, and low heterogeneity, respectively [21,22]. The random effect was applied to count effect sizes to provide more balance on individual study weight; hence, the summary effect was more conservative [23,24].

2.6. Risk of Bias in Individual Studies

Two reviewers (L.L.-Y.L. and H.-L.T.) independently assessed the risk of bias (RoB) of the included studies. All studies were appraised by using the Physiotherapy Evidence Database (PEDro) [25]. It included a total of 11 items, and each satisfied item contributed 1 point to the total score except the first item. Only items 2 to 10 were rated, and the total score ranged between 0 and 10 points. The included studies were rated as "poor", "fair", "good" or "excellent" with scores < 4, 4 to 5, 6 to 8, or 9 to 10, respectively. The items used for the assessment of the included studies were as follows: eligibility criteria and source; random allocation; concealed allocation; baseline comparability; blinding of participants, therapists and assessors; adequate follow-up; intention-to-treat analysis; between-group statistical comparisons; and reporting of point measures of variability (Supplementary File S4). Disagreements between the two reviewers were resolved by discussion and recommendations from the third reviewer (E.S.-W.W.).

3. Results

3.1. Study Selection

The flow of the literature search and the selection process are summarized in Figure 1. A total of 190 records in English and Chinese were identified from electronic databases and other sources. The full-text screening identified 7 studies (317 subjects completed the trials) eligible for inclusion, and a total of 183 papers were excluded due to non-RCT studies, combined intervention, and duplicate records. The list of excluded studies is presented in Supplementary File S5. For interventional studies involving animals or humans and studies that required ethical approval, the corresponding ethical approval authorities and ethical approval code are listed.

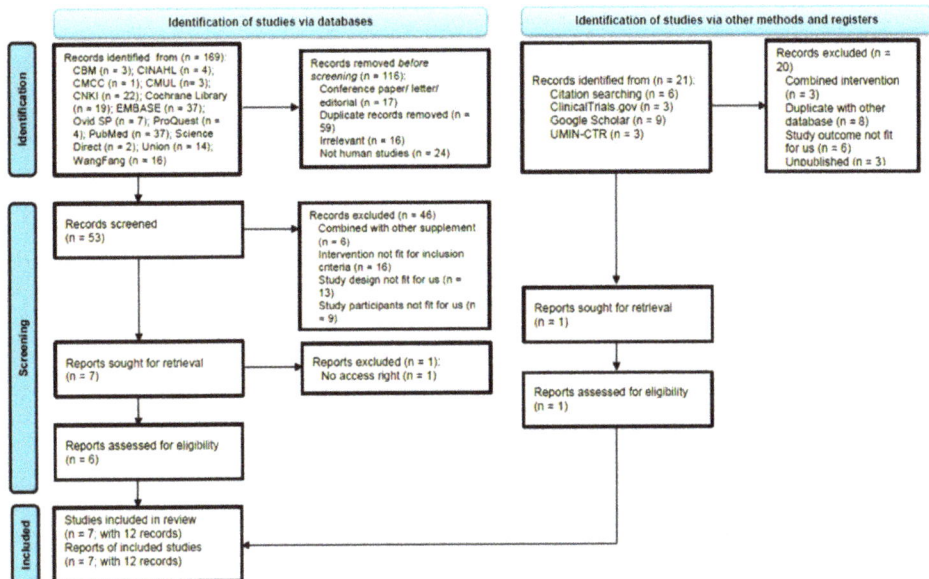

Figure 1. PRISMA flow diagram of searching and selection of the articles. Note. CBM: Chinese Biomedical Literature Database; CINAHL = Cumulative Index of Nursing and Allied Health Literature; CMCC = Chinese Medical Current Content; CMUL = Capital Medical University Library; CNKI: China National Knowledge; EMBASE: Excerpta Medica database; UMIN-CTR: University Hospital Medical Information Network Clinical Trials Registry.

3.2. Study Characteristics

The overall characteristics of the included RCTs are presented in Table 2. All studies were double-blind and published in English. The included studies were published between 2009 and 2018. Two were conducted in Japan [26,27], and the rest were conducted in Iran [28], Finland [29], Korea [30], Australia [31], and Canada [32]. The included studies comprised 17 treatment arms with a total of 321 participants (185 participants in the AST arm and 136 participants in the control arm). The sample sizes varied from 27 [30] to 63 [32]. The daily dosage of AST varied from 0.16 [29] to 20 mg [30]. Two studies reported outcomes in terms of different dosages of AST [26,27]. The range of intervention periods was from 8 weeks [28,29] to 12 months [31]. Participant characteristics included carpal tunnel syndrome (CTS), T2DM, obesity, mild and moderate hypertension, and having undergone renal transplantation. Reported outcomes included the risk factors of MetS: systolic blood pressure (SBP), diastolic blood pressure (DBP), body mass index (BMI), fasting blood glucose (FBG), lipid profile (e.g., total cholesterol (TC), high-density lipoprotein cholesterol (HDL-C), low-density lipoprotein cholesterol (LDL-C), triglyceride (TG)) and waist circumference (WC).

3.3. Quality of the Included Studies

The methodological quality of included studies was assessed with the PEDro scale as shown in Table 3. Scores of all included studies ranged from 8 to 10 with an average score of 9.29. The overall quality of the included studies was good to excellent. All included studies performed randomization, concealed allocation, blinding of participants, between-group comparison, point measure and measures of variability with similar baseline characteristics and more than 85% retention. Six out of the seven included studies [26,28–32] involved the blinding of the therapists, and only four [28,29,31,32] included the blinding of assessors throughout.

Table 2. Review characteristics of included studies (n = 7).

	Design, Country, No. Study Site	Number of Participants (% Female)	Mean Age in Years (SD)	Study Population	Primary Aim	Outcomes	Attrition Rate (%)	ITT	Protocol
Choi et al. (2011) [30]	Double-blind RCT • Korea • 1 study site	27 (n = 4, 14.81%)	Placebo 30.1 ± 9.5; Ix 31.1 ± 9.4	Overweight adults (aged 20–55 years; BMI > 25.0 kg/m²); and overweight (BMI > 25.0 kg/m²)	Evaluate positive effects of AST on LPs and OS state in overweight adults	At baseline and week 12: anthropometric data, LPs, apolipidprotein A1, apolipidprotein B MDA, 15-isoprostane F2t (ISP; also known as 8-epi-PGF2α, 8-iso-PGF2α, or 8-isoprostane), SOD, TAC measured to evaluate OS at baseline and at 4, 8, and 12 weeks	Adherence rate: Ix 93.4 and placebo 92.9%	27	No information
Coombes et al. (2016) [31]	Double-blind RCT • Australia • 2 study sites	33 (n = 16, 26%)	All 49.9 ± 12.2; (Placebo 50.9 ± 13.4; Ix 49.1 ± 11.2)	Age > 18 and <85 y and having undergone renal transplantation	Assess the effect of AST on arterial stiffness, OS, and inflammation in renal transplant recipients	Primary outcomes: PWV, OS (total F2-isoprostanes), and inflammation (pentraxin-3) Secondary outcomes: Vascular function, CIMT, Aix, CBP, SERV, and additional measures of OS and inflammation	3 (4.92%)	58	No information
MacDermid et al. (2012) [32]	Double-blind RCT • Canada • 1 study site	63 (n = 18, 28.57%)	Control 49 ± 9; Ix 49 ± 7	CTS clinically diagnosed by hand surgeons and supported by electrophysiological abnormality; competent to comply with treatment and complete study evaluations; aged 18–65 years	Evaluate effectiveness of food additive AST as adjunct in management of CTS	Primary outcome: severity of symptoms of CTS (symptom severity scale) Secondary outcomes: physical impairments, disability and health status measures	0 (0%)	63	No information
Mashhadi et al. (2018) [28]	Double-blind RCT • Iran • 1 study site	44 (n = 27, 61.36%)	Placebo 54 ± 8; Ix 51 ± 9.7	Adults aged 30–60 years; definitive diagnosis of T2DM with no insulin therapy; no pregnancy or lactation; absence of self-reported specific diseases and malignancies, kidney failure, heart disease, thyroid, and other inflammatory diseases; not taking vitamin and antioxidant supplements during the last 6 months; and no smoking or drinking	Investigate potential effects of AST on participants with T2DM	Adiponectin concentration, lipid peroxidation, glycemic control, insulin sensitivity, and anthropometric indices	1 (2.38%)	43	Yes
Nakagawa et al. (2011) [27]	Double-blind RCT • Japan • 1 study site	30 (n = 15, 50%)	All 56.3 ± 5.3; (Control 56.6 ± 4.4; 6 mg/day 56.3 ± 6.6; 12 mg/day; 56.1 ± 5.1)	Healthy subjects (fifteen men and fifteen women), between 50 and 69 years of age, with a BMI of 27.5 (SD 2.1) kg/m²	Assess the efficacy of 12-week AST (6 or 12 mg/d) on both AST and PLOOH levels in the erythrocytes of thirty middle-aged and senior subjects	Erythrocyte AST, phospholipid hydroperoxides, blood biochemical	0 (0%)	30	No information

Table 2. Cont.

	Design, Country, No. Study Site	Number of Participants (% Female)	Mean Age in Years (SD)	Study Population	Primary Aim	Outcomes	Attrition Rate (%)	ITT	Protocol
Sarkkinen et al. (2018) [29]	Double-blind RCT • Finland • 2 study sites	35 (n = 17, 48.57%)	All 55.4 ± 8.6 (Placebo 55.3 ± 8.4; 1x 55.5 ± 9.0)	(1) age 18–65 years, (2) overweight female or male (BMI between 25 and 30 kg/m^2), (3) mildly or moderately elevated BP (systolic 140–159/ diastolic 90–99 mmHg)	Compare the amount and the type of adverse events during 8-week follow-up after ingestion of krill powder preparation in comparison to ingestion of respective amount of placebo in overweight study subjects with mildly or moderately elevated BP	• Anthropometric data, BP • Routine clinical chemistry and haematology (day 0 and 56) • Plasma total and lipoprotein lipids; total TGs and TC with enzymatic, colorimetric test and LDL-C and HDL-C concentrations with homogenous enzymatic colorimetric method	0 (0%)	35	Yes
Yoshida et al. (2010) [26]	Double-blind RCT • Japan • 1 study site	61 (n = 20, 32.79%)	All 44 ± 8 (18 mg/day 43.8 ± 10.4; 12 mg/day 42.8 ± 8.8; 6 mg/day 47.0 ± 7.0; 0 mg/day 44.3 ± 7.0)	Healthy subjects (41 men and 20 women) with TG levels of 120–200 mg/dL	Investigate AST consumption ameliorates dyslipidemia and the association with an increase in serum adiponectin levels	FPG, TC, TG, LDL-C, and HDL-C	0 (0%)	61	No information

Aix: augmentation index; AST: astaxanthin; BMI: body mass index; BP: blood pressure; CBP: central blood pressure; CIMT: carotid artery intima-media thickness; CTS: carpal tunnel syndrome; FPG: Fasting plasma glucose; HDL-C: high-density lipoprotein cholesterol; LDL-C: low-density lipoprotein cholesterol; LPs: lipid profiles; MDA: malondialdehyde; OS: oxidative stress; PLOOH: phospholipid hydroperoxides; PWV: aortic pulse wave velocity; RCT: randomized controlled trial; SERV: sub-endocardial viability ratio; SOD: superoxide dismutase; TAC: total antioxidant capacity; T$_2$DM: Type 2 diabetes mellitus; TC: total cholesterol; TG: triglyceride.

Table 3. Results of PEDro Scale (n = 7).

Items	Choi et al. (2011) [30]	Coombes et al. (2016) [31]	MacDermid et al. (2012) [32]	Mashhadi et al. (2018) [28]	Nakagawa et al. (2011) [27]	Sarkkinen et al. (2018) [29]	Yoshida et al. (2010) [26]
1. Eligibility criteria were specified	Y	Y	Y	Y	Y	Y	Y
2. Subjects were randomly allocated to groups (in a crossover study, subjects were randomly allocated an order in which treatments were received)	Y	Y	Y	Y	Y	Y	Y
3. Allocation was concealed	Y	Y	Y	Y	Y	Y	Y

Table 3. Cont.

Items	Choi et al. (2011) [30]	Coombes et al. (2016) [31]	MacDermid et al. (2012) [32]	Mashhadi et al. (2018) [28]	Nakagawa et al. (2011) [27]	Sarkkinen et al. (2018) [29]	Yoshida et al. (2010) [26]
4. The groups were similar at baseline regarding the most important prognostic indicators	N	Y	Y	Y	Y	Y	Y
5. There was blinding of all subjects	Y	Y	Y	Y	Y	Y	Y
6. There was blinding of all therapists who administered the therapy	Y	Y	Y	Y	N	Y	Y
7. There was blinding of all assessors who measured at least one key outcome	N	Y	Y	Y	N	Y	N
8. Measures of at least one key outcome were obtained from more than 85% of the subjects initially allocated to groups	Y	Y	Y	Y	Y	Y	Y
9. All subjects for whom outcome measures were available received the treatment or control condition as allocated or, where this was not the case, data for at least one key outcome was analysed by "intention to treat"	Y	Y	Y	Y	Y	Y	Y
10. The results of between-group statistical comparisons are reported for at least one key outcome	Y	Y	Y	Y	Y	Y	Y

Table 3. Cont.

Items	Choi et al. (2011) [30]	Coombes et al. (2016) [31]	MacDermid et al. (2012) [32]	Mashhadi et al. (2018) [28]	Nakagawa et al. (2011) [27]	Sarkkinen et al. (2018) [29]	Yoshida et al. (2010) [26]
11. The study provides both point measures and measures of variability for at least one key outcome	Y	Y	Y	Y	Y	Y	Y
Overall score	8	10	10	10	8	10	9
Quality	Good	Excellent	Excellent	Excellent	Good	Excellent	Excellent

N: not fulfilling the criteria; Y: fulfilling the criteria; overall score (only items 2–11 were counted) < 4: poor; 4–5: fair; 6–8: good; and 9–10: excellent [25].

3.4. Meta-Analsysis Results—Primary Outcomes

3.4.1. Body Mass Index (BMI)

Four studies [26–28,30] evaluated the effects of AST on body mass index (BMI). These studies involved 162 subjects (AST group = 102, control group = 60). Figure 2 indicates that AST did not reduce BMI (MD = −0.55; 95% CI = −1.59, 0.50; I^2 = 47%; p = 0.31), Supplementary File S6 Figure S2a,b indicate the subgroup analysis on different dosage and duration of AST, respectively.

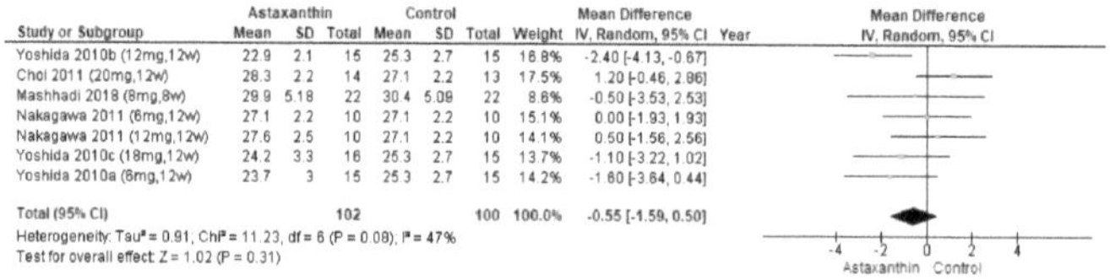

Figure 2. Forest plot of effect of astaxanthin on body mass index [26–28,30]. Bold means total data.

3.4.2. Fasting Blood Glucose (FBG)

Three studies [26–28] evaluated the effects of AST on FBG. The pooled result showed no significant effects of AST on FBG reduction (MD = −1.30; 95% CI = −4.50, 1.90; I^2 = 0%; p = 0.43; Figure 3), Supplementary File S6 Figure S3a,b indicate the subgroup analysis on different dosage and duration of AST, respectively.

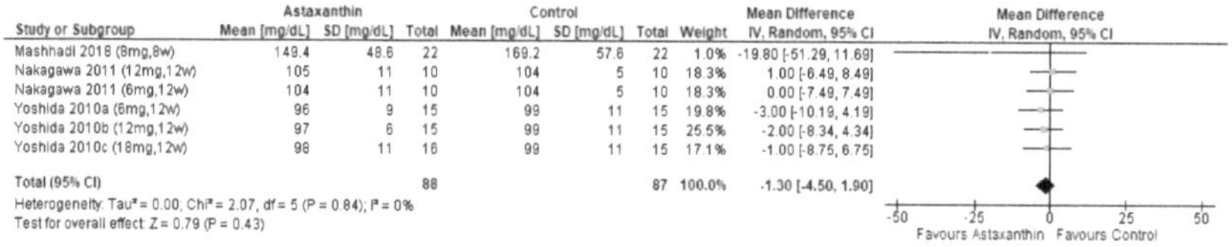

Figure 3. Forest plot of the effect of astaxanthin on fasting blood glucose [26–28]. Bold means total data.

3.4.3. Systolic Blood Pressure (SBP)

Four studies [26–28,31] included 297 subjects (AST group = 154 subjects, control group = 143) were pooled for analysis. The result showed AST had marginally significant effect on SBP reduction (MD = −4.15; 95% CI = −8.34, 0.04; I^2 = 0%; p = 0.05; Figure 4). Subgroup analysis exhibited that the SBP was reduced significantly when AST was administered for more than 8 weeks (MD = −4.69; 95% CI = −9.23, −0.16; I^2 = 0%; p = 0.04) (Supplementary File S6 Figure S4a). Supplementary File S6 Figure S4a,b indicate the subgroup analysis on different dosage and duration of AST.

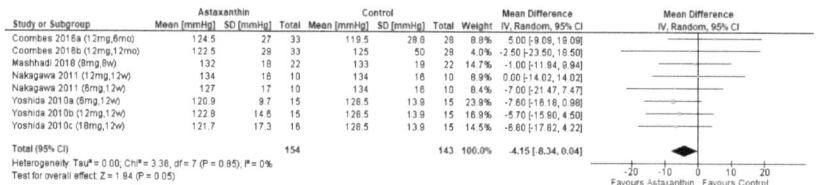

Figure 4. Forest plot of the effect of astaxanthin on systolic blood pressure [26–28,31]. Bold means total data.

3.4.4. Diastolic Blood Pressure (DBP)

The outcome of DBP was reported in four studies [26–28,31], which involved 297 subjects (AST group = 154 subjects, control group = 143). However, the pooled result did not reveal any significant DBP reduction after the administration of AST (MD = −2.09; 95% CI

= −4.87, 0.69; I^2 = 10%; p = 0.14; Figure 5), Supplementary File S6 Figure S5a,b indicate the subgroup analysis on different dosage and duration of AST, respectively.

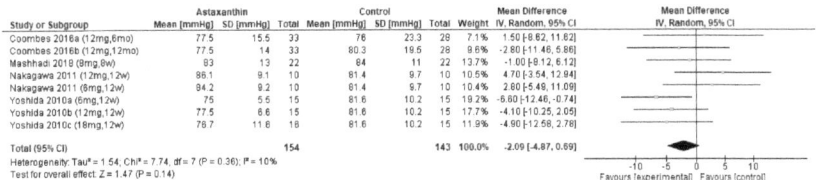

Figure 5. Forest plot of the effect of astaxanthin on diastolic blood pressure [26–28,31]. Bold means total data.

3.4.5. Total Cholesterol (TC)

The pooled result of seven studies [26–32] involving 450 subjects showed marginal significant difference between AST and the control group (MD = 0.66; 95% CI = 0.01, 1.32; I^2 = 31%; p = 0.05; Figure 6) on TC reduction. Moreover, significant differences were found in TC for subjects consumed AST more than 8 weeks and dosages ranging from ≤6 mg/day on reducing of TC (Supplementary File S6 Figure S6a,b).

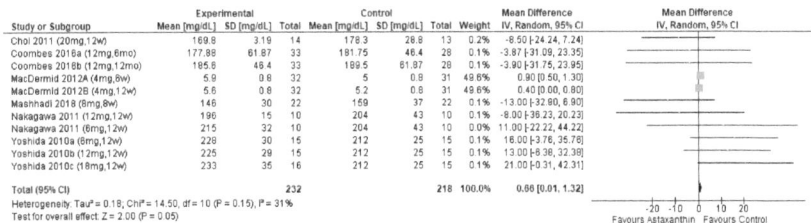

Figure 6. Forest plot of the effect of astaxanthin on total cholesterol [26–28,30–32]. Bold means total data.

3.4.6. High-density Lipoprotein Cholesterol (HDL-C)

No significant pooled effects on HDL-C reduction were found in seven studies [26–32], regardless the various subgroup analysis on different dosages and durations (MD = 0.55; 95% CI = −0.26, 0.36; I^2 = 29%; p = 0.77; Figure 7) (Supplementary File S6 Figure S7a,b).

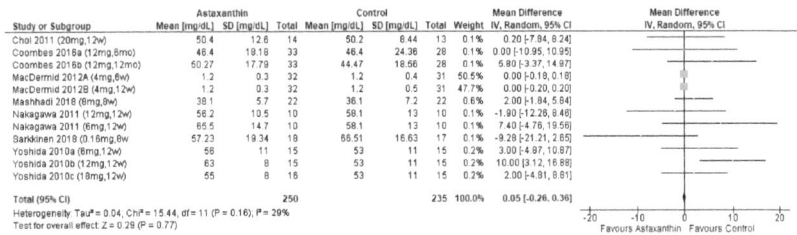

Figure 7. Forest plot of the effect of astaxanthin on high-density lipoprotein cholesterol [26–32]. Bold means total data.

3.4.7. Low-density Lipoprotein Cholesterol (LDL-C)

The outcome of LDL-C was reported in seven studies [26–32], involving 485 subjects. However, AST significantly increased the level of LDL-C (MD = 0.64; 95% CI = 0.64, 0.89; I^2 = 0%; p < 0.00001; Figure 8), regardless the duration of consumption and dosage of administration (Supplementary File S6 Figure S8a,b).

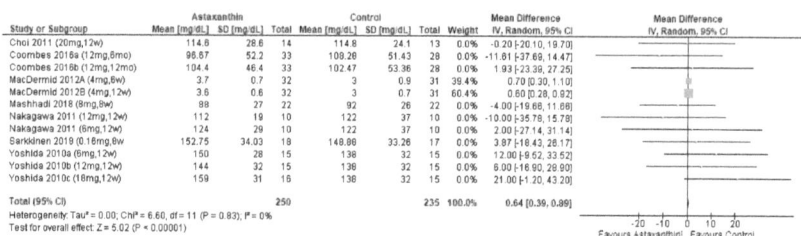

Figure 8. Forest plot of the effect of astaxanthin on low-density lipoprotein cholesterol [26–32]. Bold means total data.

3.4.8. Triglyceride (TG)

Six studies [26,28–32] evaluated the effects of AST on TG with a total of 445 subjects. The results showed no significant difference (MD = −0.34; 95% CI = −1.76, 1.08; I^2 = 48%; p = 0.64; Figure 9) between the AST group (n = 230) and the control group (n = 215). However, subgroup analysis indicated significant attenuating effects of AST on TG for consumption more than 8 weeks (MD = −15.25; 95% CI = −29.75, −0.75; I^2 = 46%; p = 0.04) and the dosage between 7 and 12 mg/day (MD = −30.08; 95% CI = −51.80, 8.36; I^2 = 0%; p = 0.007) (Supplementary File S6 Figure S9a,b).

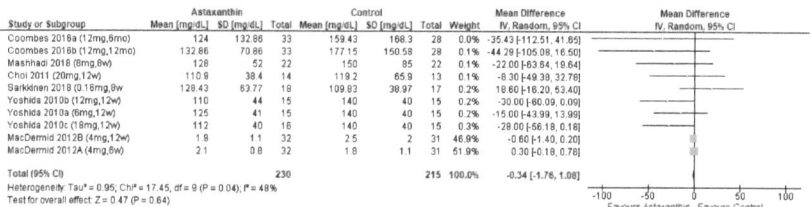

Figure 9. Forest plot of the effect of astaxanthin on triglyceride [26,28–32]. Bold means total data.

3.4.9. Waist Circumference (WC)

Only one study [30] involving 27 participants (AST group = 14, control group = 13) reported that the use of AST could significantly reduce WC at week 12. However, the sample size of the study was very small.

3.5. Secondary Outcome

Adherence was the secondary outcome of this review. Only one study [30] reported this outcome. The result showed that the adherence rate at week 12 was 93.4% and 92.9% for the AST and control groups, respectively.

4. Discussion

In this systematic review, an extensive database search was conducted, and a validated appraisal tool was used to evaluate the effectiveness of AST in alleviating the risk factors of MetS. Results indicate that AST was effective in reducing SBP, TC, and LDL-C, where the former two had marginal statistical significant results (p = 0.05), and the latter showed statistical significance (p < 0.05). Subjects' SBP decreased when dosed with AST for more than 8 weeks. AST induced attenuating effects on TC for using AST at the dosages of ≤6 mg/day for less than 8 weeks. Consuming AST at the dosages of ≤6 mg/day showed statistically significant effects on LDL-C for more than 8 weeks but not less than 8 weeks. In addition, AST was effective in the reduction of TG when subjects consumed dosage between 7 and 12 mg/day for more than 8 weeks.

Yanai, et al. [33] supported our findings of AST reducing SBP, as AST was associated with the enhancement of superoxide scavenging and vasorelaxation. For the lipid profile, a study conducted by Choi et al. [30] revealed that AST aided in improving the lipid profile by speeding the process of dissolution and controlling the production of LDL. On the other hand, contradictory studies to the results in this SR were also found. Xia et al. [34] reported that AST indicated improvement in HDL but not other lipid profiles, blood pressure, and serum glucose. Another related SR conducted by Ursoniu et al. [12] concluded that there was no significant effect of AST on lipid profile and serum glucose. However, these two reviews [12,34] were focused on the effects on physical biomarkers, while the present study was disease-based with a focus on MetS. In addition, there was a 12-week study [30] reported an adherence rate of over 92% in both groups; however, there was no information on the strategies on sustained adherence rate.

4.1. Reporting Biases

Publication bias may occur since results of some clinical trials conducted by pharmaceutical or health products companies that are registered in WHO International Clinical Trial Registry Platform, and UMIN-CTR Clinical Trial, were not published. This type of publication bias may lead to spurious beneficial treatment effects or missing some important adverse effects. To deal with this bias, we searched the gray literature and those potential studies. However, the clinical trials studying this topic are still very limited. Among the seven included studies, only one [29] mentioned the allocation concealment of subjects in the trial, while the six other studies [26–28,30–32] only briefly mentioned that the trials belong to RCTs, which may have led to randomization bias. Three studies [26,27,30] did not delineate the blinding of the outcome assessors, since the outcome assessors might alter the assessment intentionally, and measurement bias might occur [35].

4.2. Strengths

This is the first SR to investigate the effects of AST on risk factors of MetS with a registered SR protocol. Subgroup analyses, and changes between before and after intervention treatments had been performed to explore the effectiveness of AST with different dosages and duration. An extensive and comprehensive search strategy was adopted to identify studies in multiple databases. In addition, in this SR, study selection and data extraction were separately conducted by two independent reviewers, and a third reviewer was consulted if necessary to minimize errors and potential bias [24]. All included studies had good-to-excellent quality in terms of methodology (PEDro = 8 to 10).

4.3. Limitations

There were several limitations of this SR. First, variations across the included studies with different dosages and different health conditions led to moderate heterogeneity in some results. Second, the dietary patterns and activities of subjects in some individual studies were not mentioned. Moreover, there is no definitive dosage and duration of AST for adults at risk of MetS. The total number of participants was small, which could have led to wide confidence intervals and worse result precision [24]. The covered identified studies were only those in English and Chinese, which may have led to publication bias, language bias, and missing studies published in other languages. However, the search of 14 databases may have reduced this bias.

4.4. Implication for Future Studies

There are several implications for future studies. First, different intervals of intervention outcomes can be measured for the better identification of the effects and progress of AST, such as increasing the duration of all included studies to more than 8 weeks. Intervention outcome measurements can be extended to 1 month or longer after the completion of the intervention to assess the sustainable effect of AST. Furthermore, a more rigorous RCT with a large sample is needed to further confirm findings. In addition, dietary and medication records should be properly kept for the identification of any confounding factors affecting outcomes.

5. Conclusions

This SR indicated the potential effects of AST on improving SBP, TC, and LDL, although the effectiveness of AST on managing risk factors of MetS was still inconclusive because of the limited number of included studies. Rigorous large-scale RCT on human subjects should be conducted to further confirm the effectiveness of AST on adults at risk of MetS.

Supplementary Materials: The following supporting information can be downloaded at: https://www.mdpi.com/article/10.3390/nu14102050/s1, File S1: Sample search strategy for PubMed; File S2: Study eligibility verification form; File S3: Data extraction sheet for systematic review; File S4: PEDro appraisal tool; File S5: List of excluded SRs; File S6: Meta-analysis results.

Author Contributions: Study concept and design: L.Y.-L.L. and S.M.-N.C. Literature search and selection: L.Y.-L.L. and H.-L.T. Data collection, extraction, analysis and interpretation: L.Y.-L.L. and H.-L.T. Validation of data analysis and data interpretation: S.M.-N.C. and E.S.-W.W. Writing—original draft: L.Y.-L.L. and H.-L.T. Writing—review and editing: L.Y.-L.L., H.-L.T., S.M.-N.C. and E.S.-W.W. All authors have read and agreed to the published version of the manuscript.

Funding: This research received no external funding.

Institutional Review Board Statement: Not applicable.

Informed Consent Statement: Not applicable.

Data Availability Statement: Not applicable.

Conflicts of Interest: The authors declare no conflict of interest.

References

1. Grundy, S.M.; Cleeman, J.I.; Daniels, S.R.; Donato, K.A.; Eckel, R.H.; Franklin, B.A.; Gordon, D.J.; Krauss, R.M.; Savage, P.J.; Smith, S.C., Jr.; et al. Diagnosis and management of the metabolic syndrome: An American Heart Association/National Heart, Lung, and Blood Institute Scientific Statement. *Circulation* **2005**, *112*, 2735–2752. [CrossRef] [PubMed]
2. Cornier, M.A.; Dabelea, D.; Hernandez, T.L.; Lindstrom, R.C.; Steig, A.J.; Stob, N.R.; Van Pelt, R.E.; Wang, H.; Eckel, R.H. The metabolic syndrome. *Endocr. Rev.* **2008**, *29*, 777–822. [CrossRef] [PubMed]
3. Alberti, K.G.; Eckel, R.H.; Grundy, S.M.; Zimmet, P.Z.; Cleeman, J.I.; Donato, K.A.; Fruchart, J.C.; James, W.P.; Loria, C.M.; Smith, S.C., Jr.; et al. Harmonizing the metabolic syndrome: A joint interim statement of the International Diabetes Federation Task Force on Epidemiology and Prevention; National Heart, Lung, and Blood Institute; American Heart Association; World Heart Federation; International Atherosclerosis Society; and International Association for the Study of Obesity. *Circulation* **2009**, *120*, 1640–1645. [CrossRef] [PubMed]
4. Regufe, V.M.G.; Pinto, C.; Perez, P. Metabolic syndrome in type 2 diabetic patients: A review of current evidence. *Porto Biomed. J.* **2020**, *5*, 101. [CrossRef]
5. Shirouchi, B.; Matsuoka, R. Alleviation of Metabolic Syndrome with Dietary Egg White Protein. *J. Oleo Sci.* **2019**, *68*, 517–524. [CrossRef]
6. Hess, P.L.; Al-Khalidi, H.R.; Friedman, D.J.; Mulder, H.; Kucharska-Newton, A.; Rosamond, W.R.; Lopes, R.D.; Gersh, B.J.; Mark, D.B.; Curtis, L.H.; et al. The Metabolic Syndrome and Risk of Sudden Cardiac Death: The Atherosclerosis Risk in Communities Study. *J. Am. Heart Assoc.* **2017**, *6*, 006103. [CrossRef]
7. Swarup, S.; Goyal, A.; Grigorova, Y.; Zeltser, R. Metabolic Syndrome. In *Treasure Island*; StatPearls: Tampa, FL, USA, 2022.
8. Zhang, Y.; Mei, S.; Yang, R.; Chen, L.; Gao, H.; Li, L. Effects of lifestyle intervention using patient-centered cognitive behavioral therapy among patients with cardio-metabolic syndrome: A randomized, controlled trial. *BMC Cardiovasc. Disord.* **2016**, *16*, 227. [CrossRef]
9. Mallappa, R.H.; Rokana, N.; Duary, R.K.; Panwar, H.; Batish, V.K.; Grover, S. Management of metabolic syndrome through probiotic and prebiotic interventions. *Indian J. Endocrinol. Metab.* **2012**, *16*, 20–27. [CrossRef]
10. Haswell, C.; Ali, A.; Page, R.; Hurst, R.; Rutherfurd-Markwick, K. Potential of Beetroot and Blackcurrant Compounds to Improve Metabolic Syndrome Risk Factors. *Metabolites* **2021**, *11*, 338. [CrossRef]
11. Vergara, D.; Scoditti, E.; Aziz, A.A.; Giudetti, A.M. Editorial: Dietary Antioxidants and Metabolic Diseases. *Front. Nutr.* **2021**, *8*, 617859. [CrossRef]
12. Ursoniu, S.; Sahebkar, A.; Serban, M.C.; Banach, M. Lipid profile and glucose changes after supplementation with astaxanthin: A systematic review and meta-analysis of randomized controlled trials. *Arch. Med. Sci. AMS* **2015**, *11*, 253–266. [CrossRef] [PubMed]
13. Davinelli, S.; Nielsen, M.E.; Scapagnini, G. Astaxanthin in Skin Health, Repair, and Disease: A Comprehensive Review. *Nutrients* **2018**, *10*, 522. [CrossRef] [PubMed]

14. Donoso, A.; Gonzalez-Duran, J.; Munoz, A.A.; Gonzalez, P.A.; Agurto-Munoz, C. Therapeutic uses of natural astaxanthin: An evidence-based review focused on human clinical trials. *Pharmacol. Res.* **2021**, *166*, 105479. [CrossRef] [PubMed]
15. Brendler, T.; Williamson, E.M. Astaxanthin: How much is too much? A safety review. *Phytother. Res. PTR* **2019**, *33*, 3090–3111. [CrossRef]
16. Huang, P.L. A comprehensive definition for metabolic syndrome. *Dis. Models Mech.* **2009**, *2*, 231–237. [CrossRef]
17. Metabolic Syndrome Study Group of the Chinese Diabetes Society. Metabolic syndrome: Chinese Diabetes Society consultation. *Chin. J. Diabetes* **2004**, *12*, 156–161.
18. Hou, X.; Lu, J.; Weng, J.; Ji, L.; Shan, Z.; Liu, J.; Tian, H.; Ji, Q.; Zhu, D.; Ge, J.; et al. Impact of waist circumference and body mass index on risk of cardiometabolic disorder and cardiovascular disease in Chinese adults: A national diabetes and metabolic disorders survey. *PLoS ONE* **2013**, *8*, 57319. [CrossRef]
19. Ouzzani, M.; Hammady, H.; Fedorowicz, Z.; Elmagarmid, A. Rayyan-a web and mobile app for systematic reviews. *Syst. Rev.* **2016**, *5*, 210. [CrossRef]
20. Pearson, A.; Field, J.; Jordan, Z. *Evidence-Based Clinical Practice in Nursing and Health Care: Assimilating Research, Experience and Expertise*; Blackwell Publishing: Malden, MA, USA, 2006.
21. Aromataris, E.; Munn, Z. *JBI Manual for Evidence Synthesis*; JBI: Adelaide, Australia, 2020.
22. Higgins, J.P.; Thompson, S.G.; Deeks, J.J.; Altman, D.G. Measuring inconsistency in meta-analyses. *BMJ* **2003**, *327*, 557–560. [CrossRef]
23. Chen, H.; Manning, A.K.; Dupuis, J. A method of moments estimator for random effect multivariate meta-analysis. *Biometrics* **2012**, *68*, 1278–1284. [CrossRef]
24. Higgins, J.P.T.; Thomas, J.; Chandler, J.; Cumpston, M.; Li, T.; Page, M.J.; Welch, V.A. *Cochrane Handbook for Systematic Reviews of Interventions*, 2nd ed.; The Cochrane Collaboration and John Wiley & Sons: Hoboken, NJ, USA, 2019.
25. Cashin, A.G.; McAuley, J.H. Clinimetrics: Physiotherapy Evidence Database (PEDro) Scale. *J. Physiother.* **2020**, *66*, 59. [CrossRef] [PubMed]
26. Yoshida, H.; Yanai, H.; Ito, K.; Tomono, Y.; Koikeda, T.; Tsukahara, H.; Tada, N. Administration of natural astaxanthin increases serum HDL-cholesterol and adiponectin in subjects with mild hyperlipidemia. *Atherosclerosis* **2010**, *209*, 520–523. [CrossRef] [PubMed]
27. Nakagawa, K.; Kiko, T.; Miyazawa, T.; Burdeos, G.C.; Kimura, F.; Satoh, A.; Miyazawa, T. Antioxidant effect of astaxanthin on phospholipid peroxidation in human erythrocytes. *Br. J. Nutr.* **2011**, *105*, 1563–1571. [CrossRef]
28. Mashhadi, N.S.; Zakerkish, M.; Mohammadiasl, J.; Zarei, M.; Mohammadshahi, M.; Haghighizadeh, M.H. Astaxanthin improves glucose metabolism and reduces blood pressure in patients with type 2 diabetes mellitus. *Asia Pac. J. Clin. Nutr.* **2018**, *27*, 341–346. [CrossRef] [PubMed]
29. Sarkkinen, E.S.; Savolainen, M.J.; Taurio, J.; Marvola, T.; Bruheim, I. Prospective, randomized, double-blinded, placebo-controlled study on safety and tolerability of the krill powder product in overweight subjects with moderately elevated blood pressure. *Lipids Health Dis.* **2018**, *17*, 287. [CrossRef]
30. Choi, H.D.; Kim, J.H.; Chang, M.J.; Kyu-Youn, Y.; Shin, W.G. Effects of astaxanthin on oxidative stress in overweight and obese adults. *Phytother. Res.* **2011**, *25*, 1813–1818. [CrossRef] [PubMed]
31. Coombes, J.S.; Sharman, J.E.; Fassett, R.G. Astaxanthin has no effect on arterial stiffness, oxidative stress, or inflammation in renal transplant recipients: A randomized controlled trial (the XANTHIN trial). *Am. J. Clin. Nutr.* **2016**, *103*, 283–289. [CrossRef] [PubMed]
32. MacDermid, J.C.; Vincent, J.I.; Gan, B.S.; Grewal, R. A blinded placebo-controlled randomized trial on the use of astaxanthin as an adjunct to splinting in the treatment of carpal tunnel syndrome. *Hand* **2012**, *7*, 1–9. [CrossRef]
33. Yanai, H.; Ito, K.; Yoshida, H.; Tada, N. Antihypertensive effects of astaxanthin. *Integr. Blood Press. Control.* **2008**, *1*, 1–3. [CrossRef]
34. Xia, W.; Tang, N.; Kord-Varkaneh, H.; Low, T.Y.; Tan, S.C.; Wu, X.; Zhu, Y. The effects of astaxanthin supplementation on obesity, blood pressure, CRP, glycemic biomarkers, and lipid profile: A meta-analysis of randomized controlled trials. *Pharmacol. Res.* **2020**, *161*, 105113. [CrossRef]
35. Probst, P.; Grummich, K.; Heger, P.; Zaschke, S.; Knebel, P.; Ulrich, A.; Buchler, M.W.; Diener, M.K. Blinding in randomized controlled trials in general and abdominal surgery: Protocol for a systematic review and empirical study. *Syst. Rev.* **2016**, *5*, 48. [CrossRef]

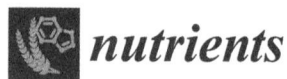

Review

Functional Role of Taurine in Aging and Cardiovascular Health: An Updated Overview

Gaetano Santulli [1,2,*], Urna Kansakar [1], Fahimeh Varzideh [2], Pasquale Mone [2], Stanislovas S. Jankauskas [1] and Angela Lombardi [1]

1. Department of Medicine, Fleischer Institute for Diabetes and Metabolism (FIDAM), Einstein-Mount Sinai Diabetes Research Center (ES-DRC), Einstein Institute for Aging Research, Albert Einstein College of Medicine, New York, NY 10461, USA; urna.kansakar@einsteinmed.edu (U.K.); stanislovas.jankauskas@einsteinmed.edu (S.S.J.); angela.lombardi@einsteinmed.edu (A.L.)
2. Department of Molecular Pharmacology, Division of Cardiology, Wilf Family Cardiovascular Research Institute, Albert Einstein College of Medicine, New York, NY 10461, USA; fahimeh.varzideh@einsteinmed.edu (F.V.); drpasquale.mone@gmail.com (P.M.)
* Correspondence: gsantulli001@gmail.com

Abstract: Taurine, a naturally occurring sulfur-containing amino acid, has attracted significant attention in recent years due to its potential health benefits. Found in various foods and often used in energy drinks and supplements, taurine has been studied extensively to understand its impact on human physiology. Determining its exact functional roles represents a complex and multifaceted topic. We provide an overview of the scientific literature and present an analysis of the effects of taurine on various aspects of human health, focusing on aging and cardiovascular pathophysiology, but also including athletic performance, metabolic regulation, and neurological function. Additionally, our report summarizes the current recommendations for taurine intake and addresses potential safety concerns. Evidence from both human and animal studies indicates that taurine may have beneficial cardiovascular effects, including blood pressure regulation, improved cardiac fitness, and enhanced vascular health. Its mechanisms of action and antioxidant properties make it also an intriguing candidate for potential anti-aging strategies.

Keywords: aging; 2-aminoethanesulfonic acid; cardiovascular risk; energy drinks; inflammation; metabolism; oxidative stress; supplements; tauric acid; taurine

1. Introduction

Taurine (2-aminoethanesulfonic acid, also known as tauric acid) is a non-protein amino acid found in various animal tissues, especially in the brain, heart, and skeletal muscles. It is also present in several foods, such as meat, fish, dairy products, and energy drinks.

The main aim of this review is to summarize the key functional roles played by taurine in aging and in cardiovascular pathophysiology, especially based on the most recent findings in these fields. Specifically, taurine has been linked to, antioxidant activity, anti-inflammatory effects, and blood pressure regulation, with major implications for human health.

2. Nomenclature, Chemistry, and Biochemistry

The name taurine derives from the Latin taurus (cognate to Ancient Greek ταῦρος, "taûros") meaning bull or ox: indeed, taurine was first isolated from the bile of the ox, *Bos taurus*, in 1827 by the German scientists Leopold Gmelin and Friedrich Tiedemann [1]. Early studies focused on its presence in animal tissues, where it was found in high concentrations in the brain, heart, and skeletal muscles. Later on, in 1846, the English chemist Edmund Ronalds confirmed the presence of taurine in human bile [2]. Taurine is detected in high concentrations in oxidative tissues, characterized by a high number of mitochondria,

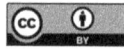

and in lower concentrations in glycolytic tissues [3–6]. The taurine content in various human tissues is reported in Table 1; over the years, researchers have explored its role in various physiological processes, leading to an increased understanding of its significance in human health.

Table 1. Taurine content in human tissues (data from Refs. [7–11]).

Tissue	Content in μmol/L (Liquid) or μmol/g (Solid)
Bile	~200
Plasma	50–100
Leukocytes and platelets	10–50
Retina	30–40
Heart	6–25
Brain	0.8–20
Skeletal muscle	2.2–5.4
Kidney	1.4–1.8
Liver	0.3–2
Erythrocytes	0.05–0.08

Chemically, taurine is classified as a beta-amino acid, and its molecular formula is $C_2H_7NO_3S$ (Molecular Weight, MW: 125.15). Structurally, it is characterized by an amino group (NH_2), a carboxyl group (COOH), and a sulfonic acid group (SO_3H) attached to the beta carbon (Figure 1); unlike other amino acids, taurine lacks a chiral center, meaning it is optically inactive; its relatively simple structure allows it to perform diverse functions within the body.

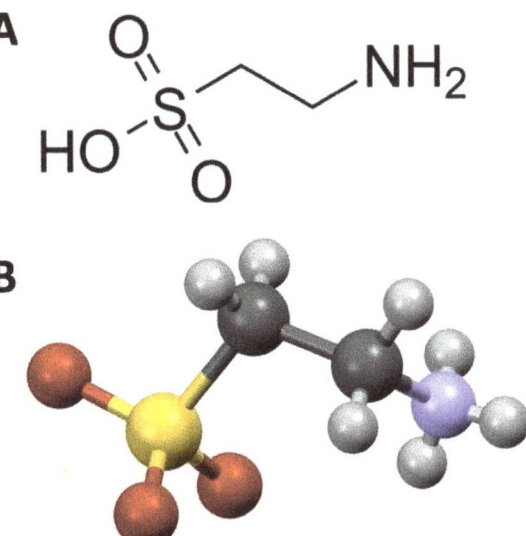

Figure 1. Chemical structure (**A**) and call-and-stick model (**B**) of taurine.

While the human body can synthesize taurine to some extent, dietary intake is essential to maintain optimal levels. Foods rich in taurine include meat, fish, poultry, and dairy products. Vegetarians and vegans may have a lower taurine intake due to their dietary restrictions [12], but the significance of this in terms of deficiency remains unclear.

Taurine is synthesized in humans in the liver mainly via the "cysteine sulfinic pathway" (Figure 2). Cysteine dioxygenase oxidizes cysteine to form cysteine sulfinic acid, which is then decarboxylated by cysteine sulfinic acid decarboxylase to obtain hypotaurine, which is then oxidized by hypotaurine dioxygenase to form taurine [13–18]. An alternative pathway is trans-sulfuration, in which homocysteine is converted into cystathionine, which is then transformed into hypotaurine by cystathionine gamma-lyase, cysteine dioxygenase, and cysteine sulfinic acid decarboxylase, and finally oxidized to form taurine [19–21].

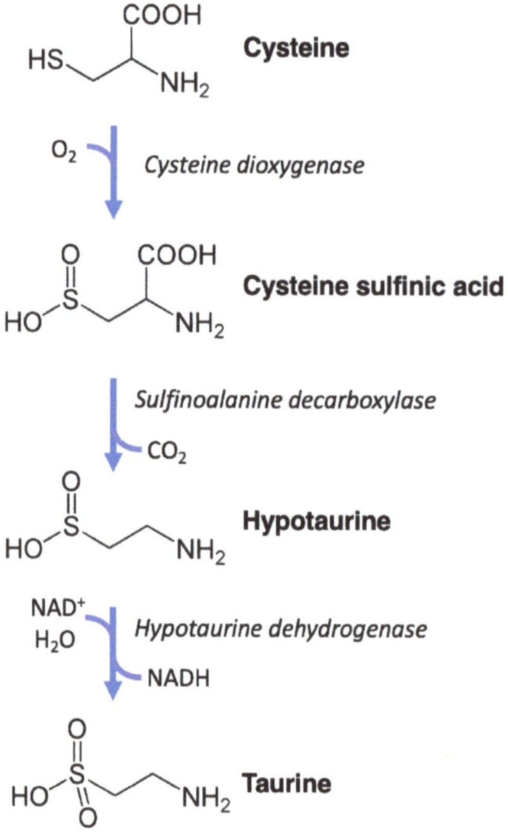

Figure 2. Representation of the chemical reactions of the cysteine sulfinic pathway leading to taurine synthesis.

Taurine has been extensively studied to determine its effects on human health. In terms of cellular function, taurine is primarily found in the intracellular fluid of many tissues, where it plays a vital role in a number of physiological processes [22–28]. It acts as an osmolyte, regulating cell volume and maintaining cell integrity [29,30]. In the liver, taurine is conjugated with bile acids, forming bile salts that aid in fat digestion and absorption in the intestines [31–34]. These processes are crucial for lipid metabolism and absorption of fat-soluble vitamins [35].

Taurine has also been shown to be involved in calcium (Ca^{2+}) signaling, modulation of ion channels, and neurotransmission, affecting neural excitability and synaptic transmission. Intriguingly, this amino acid exhibits important antioxidant properties, protecting cells from oxidative and nitrosative stress by scavenging free radicals and reactive oxygen species (ROS) [36–44]. These antioxidant actions certainly contribute to its potential benefits in terms of neuroprotection and cardiovascular health [45]. In fact, taurine is highly concentrated in the brain and several studies indicate that taurine might act as a neurotransmitter or neuromodulator, influencing neurotransmitter release and receptor function, affecting cognitive processes, mood, behavior, memory, learning, and anxiety regulation [46–51].

Taurine has been thought to be essential for the development and survival of neural cells and to protect them under cell-damaging conditions, indeed in the brain stem taurine regulates vital functions, including cardiovascular control and arterial blood pressure. Its neuroprotective effects involve also reducing neuronal apoptosis and inflammation [46], making it a subject of interest in research on neurodegenerative diseases and brain injuries and offering benefits during stroke recovery [52–56]. Premature infants are vulnerable to taurine deficiency because they lack some of the enzymes needed to synthesize cysteine and taurine. However, human breast milk contains high levels of taurine which is sufficient for newborns; formula milk is often supplemented with taurine, although evidence is mixed as to whether this strategy is actually beneficial or not [57–62]. Nevertheless, further studies are needed to fully understand taurine's neurological effects.

As we will discuss below in a dedicated paragraph, taurine has been associated with several benefits especially on the cardiovascular system, including blood pressure regulation, anti-inflammatory effects, and improvements in endothelial function; overall, these properties contribute to its potential in reducing the risk of cardiovascular diseases [63–65].

3. Taurine and Cardiovascular Health

Taurine plays a crucial role in cardiovascular physiology. Numerous studies have investigated the potential cardioprotective effects of taurine, focusing on its impact on blood pressure, cardiac contractility, and vascular function. It may help reduce blood pressure in individuals with hypertension and improve endothelial function, leading to enhanced vascular health. Its antioxidant properties may also reduce the risk of cardiovascular diseases such as atherosclerosis and heart failure [66,67].

As we will see in detail in the paragraphs below, the main cardiovascular effects of taurine are attributed to a number of underlying mechanisms. For instance, its modulation of ion channels, including Ca^{2+} and potassium (K^+) channels, influences cardiac electrical activity and vascular tone. Its role in Ca^{2+} homeostasis also impacts myocardial contractility and relaxation. Additionally, the antioxidant properties of taurine, for which the exact underlying mechanisms remain unclear, might help protect against oxidative stress, a factor involved in the pathophysiology of cardiovascular disease. Interestingly, two taurine-containing modified uridines, 5-taurinomethyluridine ($\tau m^5 u$) and 5-taurinomethyl-2-thiouridine ($\tau m^5 s^2 u$) have been identified in mitochondrial tRNA: these conjugates could be associated with the actions of taurine as an antioxidant [68–71]. Another proposed mechanism is the stabilization of intracellular levels of antioxidant enzymes like superoxide dismutase (SOD) and glutathione [72,73].

Taurine has been also implicated in metabolic regulation, particularly in relation to glucose and lipid metabolism [74,75]. Various studies indicate that taurine might help improve insulin sensitivity, making it beneficial for individuals with type 2 diabetes (T2D) or those at risk of developing the condition [76–79]. A recent preclinical study has shown that taurine can rescue pancreatic β-cell stress by stimulating α-cell trans-differentiation [80]. Additionally, taurine may aid in reducing triglyceride levels and improving lipid profiles [81–85], potentially lowering the risk of cardiovascular diseases and metabolic syndrome.

Preclinical investigations have provided valuable insights into the cardiovascular effects of taurine. In models of hypertension, heart failure, and atherosclerosis, taurine supplementation has consistently been shown to improve cardiac function, reduce blood pressure, and enhance vascular health. At the same time, human studies investigating taurine's cardiovascular effects have also yielded promising results. Clinical trials have demonstrated its potential to reduce blood pressure, improve left ventricular function, and enhance exercise capacity in individuals with heart failure.

3.1. Taurine and Cardiac Function

Taurine accounts for ~50% of the total free amino acids in the heart; it has been shown to enhance cardiac contractility and improve heart function in both human and animal models. Animal studies have revealed that taurine deficiency induces atrophic cardiac remodeling [86], whilst taurine supplementation can increase myocardial contractility, stroke volume, and cardiac output [87–93]. In humans, taurine has been associated with improvements in the left ventricular function and exercise tolerance [94–98]. Notably, in 1985 taurine was approved as treatment for patients with heart failure in Japan [96].

The beneficial effects of taurine on Ca^{2+} and sodium (Na^+) handling [89,90,99–103], myocardial energetics [104,105], and cellular signaling pathways (including glucose transport, 3-phosphoinositide-dependent protein kinase-1, AKT, sirtuin 1 (SIRT1), FOXO3, p38, NFkappaB, and others) [106–121] are thought to underlie its major cardioprotective effects. Other mechanisms include the promotion of natriuresis and diuresis, most likely via an osmoregulatory activity in the kidney, a regulation of vasopressin release, and a modulation of the atrial natriuretic factor secretion [122–125]. In addition, taurine has been shown to attenuate the actions of angiotensin II on its downstream signaling pathways, on Ca^{2+} transport, and on protein synthesis [113].

3.2. Taurine and Vascular Function

The endothelium, a single layer of cells lining the blood vessels, plays a crucial role in vascular health. Taurine has been shown to improve the endothelial function by promoting nitric oxide (NO) production and reducing endothelial dysfunction [126]. Enhanced endothelial function contributes to better vascular relaxation, reduced inflammation, and improved blood flow, which may benefit cardiovascular health and reduce the risk of atherosclerosis and cardiovascular events [127–130].

The ability of taurine to regulate ion channels [131,132], modulate Ca^{2+} homeostasis [133–135], and enhance endothelial function [136–140] may contribute to its antihypertensive properties. Additionally, its antioxidant activity [54,126,141–143] may help protect blood vessels from oxidative stress, further contributing to its beneficial effects on blood pressure regulation.

Both human and animal studies have demonstrated that taurine supplementation can lead to a modest reduction in blood pressure [144–147]. Despite the fact that the effects of taurine on a healthy endothelium remain controversial, with some investigators showing an enhancement of the endothelium-dependent relaxation in response to acetylcholine [148] and other reports not confirming these findings [145,149], its beneficial action on a dysfunctional endothelium is more consistent [130,140,144]. A synergistic action in terms of cell survival has been experimentally shown [150] when combining taurine with another well-established enhancer of vascular function, i.e., L-arginine [129,151–153].

Strikingly, in a recent clinical trial, 120 patients with T2D were randomly allocated to take either 1 g of taurine or placebo three times per day for an 8-week period; taurine-supplemented patients displayed a significant decrease in serum insulin and HOMA-IR (Homeostatic Model Assessment for Insulin Resistance) compared to the placebo group accompanied by a significant decline in several markers of inflammation, oxidative stress, and endothelial dysfunction [154]. A meta-analysis published in 2018 concluded that the ingestion of taurine can reduce blood pressure to a clinically relevant magnitude, without any major adverse side effects [155]. However, future studies are warranted to establish the exact effects of oral taurine supplementation on targeted pathologies and the optimal supplementation doses and periods.

3.3. Taurine and Athletic Performance

The presence of taurine in many energy drinks and sports supplements (~750–1000 mg in a can of 240 mL) is most likely due to its purported role in enhancing athletic performance. However, these energy drinks also contain caffeine, which has been previously linked to perceived energy boosts [156,157].

Some studies suggest that taurine may improve exercise capacity, reduce muscle damage, and alleviate exercise-induced oxidative stress. Its potential to increase muscle contractility and decrease fatigue has garnered interest among athletes. Nevertheless, conflicting findings warrant caution in interpreting these claims and several concerns on the use and abuse of energy drinks have been raised [158–163].

4. Taurine and Aging

4.1. Taurine and Longevity

Levels of taurine have been shown to decline as we age, and offsetting this loss with a taurine supplement might delay the development of age-related health problems [164–167]. Indeed, as shown in a *Science* paper recently published, when mice received taurine supplements, their lifespans increased by approximately 10% compared to the control group [168]. Mice in the taurine group also seemed healthier, with improvements in muscle endurance and strength. Researchers fed mice between 15 and 30 mg of taurine per day depending on their age. These doses would be equivalent to 3 to 6 g of taurine for an 80-kg body weight, which is within the safe limits according to European Food Safety Authority recommendations [169,170].

Taurine was also shown to shape the gut microbiota of mice and positively affect the restoration of intestinal homeostasis [171], suggesting that it could be harnessed to re-establish a normal microenvironment and to treat or prevent gut dysbiosis.

Beneficial effects on some hallmarks of aging were observed in *Caenorhabditis elegans* worms and middle-aged rhesus monkeys (*Macaca mulatta*) [172]. The taurine-fed worms lived longer and were healthier than the controls. The monkeys had lower body weights, reduced signs of liver damage, and denser bones [168].

Consistent with these data, a previous study conducted using data from the *Korea National Health and Nutrition Examination Survey* (KNHANES) had shown that taurine supplementation can decrease the cardiometabolic risk in male elderly subjects aged 75 and older [173]. Similarly, a double-blind study conducted in 24 women randomly assigned to receive taurine (1.5 g) or placebo (1.5 g of starch) for 16 weeks revealed that taurine supplementation prevented the decrease in SOD plasma levels [141], suggesting taurine as a potential strategy to control oxidative stress during the aging process.

4.2. Taurine and Cell Senescence

Cell senescence represents one of the fundamental mechanisms of aging [174,175]. Senescent cells are characterized by the cell cycle arrest, decreased susceptibility to apoptosis, and release of a particular set of cytokines, known as senescence-associated secretory phenotype (SASP) [176–178]. Despite preventing malignant transformation, accumulation of senescent cells negatively affects tissue functionality [179,180].

Multiple evidence demonstrates that the age-dependent decrease in the taurine content is associated with cell senescence. For instance, metabolomic analyses of human umbilical vein endothelial cells (HUVECs) at different passages have revealed a correlation between lower levels of taurine and HUVECs senescence [181].

In vitro, taurine mitigated replicative aging of bone marrow-derived multipotent stromal cells and restored their osteogenic differentiation potential at late passages [182]. Deletion of *Slc6a6* (sodium- and chloride-dependent taurine transporter) resulted in a drastic shortening of the lifespan of mice [168,183]; specifically, *Slc6a6* knockout mice exhibited a high expression of senescence markers p16 and p21, mirrored by a high expression of senescence-associated beta-galactosidase (SA-β-Gal) activity in the bones and liver. Treatment of *Slc6a6* knockout mice with senolytics increased their lifespan, suggesting a causative link between cell senescence and taurine deficiency [168]. In line with these results, taurine supplementation for 10 months in aged *wild type* mice led to a reduction of senescent cells by a factor of two in the brain, gut and muscle, and almost by a factor of three in the liver and fat [168]. Some investigators indicate that taurine deficiency may induce cell senescence via activation of SMAD3 and β-catenin [184].

4.3. Taurine and Unfolded Protein Response

Loss of proteostasis is one of the hallmarks of aging. The burden of misfolded proteins increases with age due to the accumulation of somatic mutations, dysregulation of splicing, loss of chaperone activity, and malfunctioning autophagy [174,185]. Accumulation of misfolded proteins in the endoplasmic reticulum (ER) triggers an unfolded protein response (UPR) and ER stress, eventually resulting in cell death [186].

Knockout of *Slc6a6* triggers UPR in the murine skeletal muscle, as demonstrated by unbiased RNA sequencing and by the direct measurement of ER stress-associated proteins content [183]. In drosophila, taurine's beneficial effects on lifespan were totally abrogated by the silencing of *Ero1* or *Xbp1* genes; the products of these genes play crucial role in resolving ER stress [187]. Taurine cotreatment also prevented detrimental consequences of UPR during glucose deprivation or cisplatin toxicity [188,189].

4.4. Taurine and Telomere Attrition

Telomere attrition limits cell ability to proliferate endlessly [190–192]. The enzyme telomerase reverse transcriptase (TERT) prevents critical shortening of telomere length [174]. In vitro studies have shown that taurine can increase the TERT expression in dental-pulp-derived stem cells, thus maintaining their chondrogenic differentiation potential [193]. In line with this observation, a correlation was reported between the liver telomere length and the plasma levels of taurine in mice [194]. Taurine was also shown to mitigate detrimental consequences of telomere attrition; for instance, taurine supplementation prevented premature death of *D. rerio* with *Tert* deficiency [168].

4.5. Taurine and Sirtuins

Sirtuins are a family of proteins that possess either mono-ADP-ribosyltransferase or deacetylase activity [195,196]. Sirtuins regulate many signaling pathways, mostly connecting them with a metabolic state of the organism [197,198]. Their expression is decreased with age and their activation or overexpression is associated with increased longevity [199,200].

Taurine was shown to activate cytoplasmic SIRT1 in the liver, heart, and brain [121,201–204]. In these tissues, taurine-mediated upregulation of SIRT1 activity was associated with the prevention of organ dysfunction. For instance, in the heart, taurine promoted p53 inhibition via its deacetylation by SIRT1, resulting in a diminished apoptosis rate; of note, the protective effects of taurine were lost after cotreatment with a specific SIRT1 inhibitor [202].

Molecular docking modeling suggests that taurine activates SIRT1 via direct interaction with the protein; interestingly, taurine was predicted to bind another region of SIRT1 compared to the SIRT1 potent agonist resveratrol. Although the latter binds to the 289–304 amino acid sequence, taurine requires a pocket formed by amino acid 441–445 [121].

4.6. Taurine and Stem Cells

Depletion of stem cell pools is notably associated with aging and age-related disorders, leading to a gradual decline in organ functions and their healing capacities after damage [174,205–207]. Mounting data show that taurine increases the survival of stem cells, increases their regenerative capacity, and maintains stemness [208]. Notably, knocking out *Slc6a6* abrogates the development of embryonic stem cells, again pointing to the crucial role of taurine [209]. Several studies demonstrate the beneficial effects of taurine treatment on neural stem cells and stem cells involved in bone and cartilage development [193,210–214]; moreover, it has also been suggested that taurine may promote development of skeletal muscles [215].

5. Recommended Intake and Safety Concerns

Currently, there are no established dietary reference intakes (DRIs) for taurine [216]. However, it is generally believed that the typical Western diet provides sufficient taurine for most people [217,218]. Specific populations, such as vegetarians or vegans, may have a lower taurine intake, but evidence of deficiency remains limited [219,220].

The normal dietary levels of taurine can vary depending on an individual's diet and specific food choices. Taurine is a naturally occurring amino acid found in various foods [219,221–224], including seaweed, fish, meat, and some dairy products (Table 2); the average daily intake of taurine from the typical diet is estimated to be around 40 to 400 milligrams (mg) per day in adults.

Table 2. Taurine content in foods.

Food	Average Content in mg/100 g
Pyropia tenera (red algae, seaweed, dried)	979
Scallops (raw)	827
Mussels (raw)	655
Porphyra haitanensis (seaweed, dried)	646
Clams (raw)	520
Oysters (raw)	507
Octopus (raw)	388
Squid (raw)	356
Turkey (raw), dark meat	306
Chicken (raw), dark meat	169
White fish (raw)	151
Pork (raw)	61
Salami (cured)	59
Ham (baked)	50
Lamb (raw), dark meat	47
Beef (raw)	43
Tuna (canned)	42
Shrimps (raw)	39
Goat's milk (pasteurized)	6.8
Egg yolk	3.7
Yogurt	3.3
Cow's milk (pasteurized)	2.4
Ice cream	1.9

Foods that contain the highest levels of taurine come from the sea and include seaweed and shellfish; for instance, taurine represents ~80% of the total amino acid content of pacific oyster (*Crassostrea gigas*) [225].

Regarding standard supplemental doses, taurine supplements are available in various forms, including capsules, tablets, and energy drinks. The recommended dosage of taurine as a dietary supplement might vary based on the specific product and its intended use. In general, most taurine supplements are available in doses ranging from 500 mg to 2000 mg per serving. It is important to note that individual responses to dietary supplements can differ, and the appropriate dose for a person may depend on various factors, including age, weight, overall health status, and underlying medical conditions. For this reason, it is advisable to follow the recommended dosage provided on the supplement's packaging or as advised by a healthcare professional.

Overall, taurine is considered generally safe for most individuals when consumed in moderate amounts, as found in the average diet. However, as with any dietary supplement, moderation is key, and excessive consumption of taurine supplements beyond recommended doses may lead to potential side effects, including gastrointestinal disturbances (such as nausea, vomiting, and diarrhea) and neurological symptoms (dizziness, tremors, and headache) [226–228]. Moreover, caution should be used because of the potential interactions between taurine supplements and certain medications, particularly those having analogous effects (e.g., lowering blood pressure), targeting similar signaling pathways (e.g., Ca^{2+}, angiotensin), and used to modulate heart or central nervous system functions. medications or [49,50,229]. Pregnant and lactating women, as well as individuals with specific health conditions, such as bipolar disorder, epilepsy, or kidney problems, should exercise caution and consult healthcare professionals before taking taurine supplements.

A risk assessment study conducted by Shao and colleagues, based on toxicological evidence from several clinical trials testing taurine supplementation, established the upper level of taurine supplementation at 3 g per day [230]. The only adverse effects noted in this study after consuming a 3 g dose of taurine were gastrointestinal disorders. Notably, the minimum dose used in these trials was 3 g/day, much greater than the usual intake of taurine from a normal diet (<0.4 g/day).

6. Conclusions

Taurine has a diverse array of functions in human health. From its origins in animal tissues to its roles in aging, cardiovascular health, neuroprotection, and cellular function, taurine continues to capture the attention of researchers and health professionals alike. Recent findings specifically suggest that taurine is a promising cardioprotective agent, offering potential benefits for cardiovascular health in both human and animal studies. However, its role in reducing cardiovascular risk warrants further investigation, including large-scale clinical trials, making it an intriguing subject for ongoing research and potential therapeutic applications. Further research is also needed to fully elucidate its mechanisms of action and confirm its efficacy in different settings including longevity. An adequate dietary intake of taurine through a balanced diet is recommended, and caution should be exercised when considering taurine supplementation, especially at high doses.

Author Contributions: Conceptualization, G.S.; methodology, U.K. and P.M.; writing—original draft preparation, U.K., F.V., P.M. and S.S.J.; writing—review and editing, A.L. and G.S.; supervision, G.S.; funding acquisition, U.K., F.V., S.S.J. and G.S. All authors have read and agreed to the published version of the manuscript.

Funding: The Santulli's Lab is currently supported in part by the National Institutes of Health (NIH): National Heart, Lung, and Blood Institute (NHLBI: R01-HL164772, R01-HL159062, R01-HL146691, T32-HL144456), National Institute of Diabetes and Digestive and Kidney Diseases (NIDDK: R01-DK123259, R01-DK033823), National Center for Advancing Translational Sciences (NCATS: UL1-TR002556-06, UM1-TR004400) to G.S., by the Diabetes Action Research and Education Foundation (to G.S.), and by the Monique Weill-Caulier and Irma T. Hirschl Trusts (to G.S.). U.K. is supported in part by a postdoctoral fellowship of the American Heart Association (AHA-23POST1026190). F.V. is supported in part by a postdoctoral fellowship of the American Heart Association (AHA-22POST915561). S.S.J. is supported in part by a postdoctoral fellowship of the American Heart Association (AHA-21POST836407).

Institutional Review Board Statement: Not applicable.

Informed Consent Statement: Not applicable.

Data Availability Statement: Not applicable.

Acknowledgments: We thank Xujun Wang, for his helpful discussion.

Conflicts of Interest: The authors declare that they have no conflict of interest.

References

1. Tiedemann, F.; Gmalin, L. Einige neue Bestandtheile der Galle des Ochsen. *Ann. Phys.* **1827**, *85*, 326–337. [CrossRef]
2. Garrod, A. Lectures on the Chemistry of Pathology and Therapeutics: Showing the Application of the Science of Chemistry to the Discovery, Treatment, and Cure of Disease. *Lancet* **1848**, *52*, 333–336.
3. Baliou, S.; Adamaki, M.; Ioannou, P.; Pappa, A.; Panayiotidis, M.I.; Spandidos, D.A.; Christodoulou, I.; Kyriakopoulos, A.M.; Zoumpourlis, V. Protective role of taurine against oxidative stress (Review). *Mol. Med. Rep.* **2021**, *24*, 605. [CrossRef]
4. Jong, C.J.; Sandal, P.; Schaffer, S.W. The Role of Taurine in Mitochondria Health: More Than Just an Antioxidant. *Molecules* **2021**, *26*, 4913. [CrossRef] [PubMed]
5. Hansen, S.H.; Andersen, M.L.; Cornett, C.; Gradinaru, R.; Grunnet, N. A role for taurine in mitochondrial function. *J. Biomed. Sci.* **2010**, *17* (Suppl. S1), S23. [CrossRef] [PubMed]
6. De Luca, A.; Pierno, S.; Camerino, D.C. Taurine: The appeal of a safe amino acid for skeletal muscle disorders. *J. Transl. Med.* **2015**, *13*, 243. [CrossRef] [PubMed]
7. Jacobsen, J.G.; Smith, L.H. Biochemistry and physiology of taurine and taurine derivatives. *Physiol. Rev.* **1968**, *48*, 424–511. [CrossRef]
8. Hayes, K.C.; Sturman, J.A. Taurine in metabolism. *Annu. Rev. Nutr.* **1981**, *1*, 401–425. [CrossRef]
9. Sole, M.J.; Jeejeebhoy, K.N. Conditioned nutritional requirements and the pathogenesis and treatment of myocardial failure. *Curr. Opin. Clin. Nutr. Metab. Care* **2000**, *3*, 417–424. [CrossRef]
10. Hansen, S.H. The role of taurine in diabetes and the development of diabetic complications. *Diabetes Metab. Res. Rev.* **2001**, *17*, 330–346. [CrossRef]
11. Wojcik, O.P.; Koenig, K.L.; Zeleniuch-Jacquotte, A.; Costa, M.; Chen, Y. The potential protective effects of taurine on coronary heart disease. *Atherosclerosis* **2010**, *208*, 19–25. [CrossRef]
12. Laidlaw, S.A.; Shultz, T.D.; Cecchino, J.T.; Kopple, J.D. Plasma and urine taurine levels in vegans. *Am. J. Clin. Nutr.* **1988**, *47*, 660–663. [CrossRef] [PubMed]
13. Weinstein, C.L.; Haschemeyer, R.H.; Griffith, O.W. In vivo studies of cysteine metabolism. Use of D-cysteinesulfinate, a novel cysteinesulfinate decarboxylase inhibitor, to probe taurine and pyruvate synthesis. *J. Biol. Chem.* **1988**, *263*, 16568–16579. [CrossRef] [PubMed]
14. Drake, M.R.; De La Rosa, J.; Stipanuk, M.H. Metabolism of cysteine in rat hepatocytes. Evidence for cysteinesulphinate-independent pathways. *Biochem. J.* **1987**, *244*, 279–286. [CrossRef] [PubMed]
15. Chang, Y.C.; Ding, S.T.; Lee, Y.H.; Wang, Y.C.; Huang, M.F.; Liu, I.H. Taurine homeostasis requires de novo synthesis via cysteine sulfinic acid decarboxylase during zebrafish early embryogenesis. *Amino Acids* **2013**, *44*, 615–629. [CrossRef]
16. Zhang, D.; Fan, J.; Liu, H.; Qiu, G.; Cui, S. Testosterone enhances taurine synthesis by upregulating androgen receptor and cysteine sulfinic acid decarboxylase expressions in male mouse liver. *Am. J. Physiol. Gastrointest. Liver Physiol.* **2023**, *324*, G295–G304. [CrossRef]
17. Magnusson, K.R.; Madl, J.E.; Clements, J.R.; Wu, J.Y.; Larson, A.A.; Beitz, A.J. Colocalization of taurine- and cysteine sulfinic acid decarboxylase-like immunoreactivity in the cerebellum of the rat with monoclonal antibodies against taurine. *J. Neurosci.* **1988**, *8*, 4551–4564. [CrossRef]
18. Sharma, S.; Sahoo, B.M.; Banik, B.K. Biological Effects and Mechanisms of Taurine in Various Therapeutics. *Curr. Drug Discov. Technol.* **2023**, *online ahead of print*. [CrossRef]
19. Sbodio, J.I.; Snyder, S.H.; Paul, B.D. Regulators of the transsulfuration pathway. *Br. J. Pharmacol.* **2019**, *176*, 583–593. [CrossRef]
20. Simmons, C.R.; Liu, Q.; Huang, Q.; Hao, Q.; Begley, T.P.; Karplus, P.A.; Stipanuk, M.H. Crystal structure of mammalian cysteine dioxygenase. A novel mononuclear iron center for cysteine thiol oxidation. *J. Biol. Chem.* **2006**, *281*, 18723–18733. [CrossRef]
21. Park, E.; Park, S.Y.; Cho, I.S.; Kim, B.S.; Schuller-Levis, G. A Novel Cysteine Sulfinic Acid Decarboxylase Knock-Out Mouse: Taurine Distribution in Various Tissues with and without Taurine Supplementation. *Adv. Exp. Med. Biol.* **2017**, *975 Pt 1*, 461–474. [CrossRef]
22. Li, Y.; Peng, Q.; Shang, J.; Dong, W.; Wu, S.; Guo, X.; Xie, Z.; Chen, C. The role of taurine in male reproduction: Physiology, pathology and toxicology. *Front. Endocrinol.* **2023**, *14*, 1017886. [CrossRef]
23. Wen, C.; Li, F.; Zhang, L.; Duan, Y.; Guo, Q.; Wang, W.; He, S.; Li, J.; Yin, Y. Taurine is Involved in Energy Metabolism in Muscles, Adipose Tissue, and the Liver. *Mol. Nutr. Food Res.* **2019**, *63*, e1800536. [CrossRef]
24. Spriet, L.L.; Whitfield, J. Taurine and skeletal muscle function. *Curr. Opin. Clin. Nutr. Metab. Care* **2015**, *18*, 96–101. [CrossRef] [PubMed]
25. Wu, G. Important roles of dietary taurine, creatine, carnosine, anserine and 4-hydroxyproline in human nutrition and health. *Amino Acids* **2020**, *52*, 329–360. [CrossRef]
26. Oja, S.S.; Saransaari, P. Taurine and epilepsy. *Epilepsy Res.* **2013**, *104*, 187–194. [CrossRef]
27. Rosca, A.E.; Vladareanu, A.M.; Mirica, R.; Anghel-Timaru, C.M.; Mititelu, A.; Popescu, B.O.; Caruntu, C.; Voiculescu, S.E.; Gologan, S.; Onisai, M.; et al. Taurine and Its Derivatives: Analysis of the Inhibitory Effect on Platelet Function and Their Antithrombotic Potential. *J. Clin. Med.* **2022**, *11*, 666. [CrossRef]
28. Dong, Y.; Li, X.; Liu, Y.; Gao, J.; Tao, J. The molecular targets of taurine confer anti-hyperlipidemic effects. *Life Sci.* **2021**, *278*, 119579. [CrossRef] [PubMed]

29. Schousboe, A.; Pasantes-Morales, H. Role of taurine in neural cell volume regulation. *Can. J. Physiol. Pharmacol.* **1992**, *70*, S356–S361. [CrossRef]
30. Zhou, J.; Du, X.; Li, J.; Yamagata, N.; Xu, B. Taurine Boosts Cellular Uptake of Small D-Peptides for Enzyme-Instructed Intracellular Molecular Self-Assembly. *J. Am. Chem. Soc.* **2015**, *137*, 10040–10043. [CrossRef] [PubMed]
31. Falany, C.N.; Johnson, M.R.; Barnes, S.; Diasio, R.B. Glycine and taurine conjugation of bile acids by a single enzyme. Molecular cloning and expression of human liver bile acid CoA:amino acid N-acyltransferase. *J. Biol. Chem.* **1994**, *269*, 19375–19379. [CrossRef] [PubMed]
32. Murakami, S.; Fujita, M.; Nakamura, M.; Sakono, M.; Nishizono, S.; Sato, M.; Imaizumi, K.; Mori, M.; Fukuda, N. Taurine ameliorates cholesterol metabolism by stimulating bile acid production in high-cholesterol-fed rats. *Clin. Exp. Pharmacol. Physiol.* **2016**, *43*, 372–378. [CrossRef]
33. Bellentani, S.; Pecorari, M.; Cordoma, P.; Marchegiano, P.; Manenti, F.; Bosisio, E.; De Fabiani, E.; Galli, G. Taurine increases bile acid pool size and reduces bile saturation index in the hamster. *J. Lipid Res.* **1987**, *28*, 1021–1027. [CrossRef]
34. Batta, A.K.; Salen, G.; Shefer, S.; Tint, G.S.; Dayal, B. The effect of tauroursodeoxycholic acid and taurine supplementation on biliary bile acid composition. *Hepatology* **1982**, *2*, 811–816. [CrossRef]
35. de Aguiar Vallim, T.Q.; Tarling, E.J.; Edwards, P.A. Pleiotropic roles of bile acids in metabolism. *Cell Metab.* **2013**, *17*, 657–669. [CrossRef]
36. Ibrahim, M.A.; Eraqi, M.M.; Alfaiz, F.A. Therapeutic role of taurine as antioxidant in reducing hypertension risks in rats. *Heliyon* **2020**, *6*, e03209. [CrossRef] [PubMed]
37. Degim, Z.; Celebi, N.; Sayan, H.; Babul, A.; Erdogan, D.; Take, G. An investigation on skin wound healing in mice with a taurine-chitosan gel formulation. *Amino Acids* **2002**, *22*, 187–198. [CrossRef]
38. Chang, C.Y.; Shen, C.Y.; Kang, C.K.; Sher, Y.P.; Sheu, W.H.; Chang, C.C.; Lee, T.H. Taurine protects HK-2 cells from oxidized LDL-induced cytotoxicity via the ROS-mediated mitochondrial and p53-related apoptotic pathways. *Toxicol. Appl. Pharmacol.* **2014**, *279*, 351–363. [CrossRef]
39. Wen, C.; Li, F.; Guo, Q.; Zhang, L.; Duan, Y.; Wang, W.; Li, J.; He, S.; Chen, W.; Yin, Y. Protective effects of taurine against muscle damage induced by diquat in 35 days weaned piglets. *J. Anim. Sci. Biotechnol.* **2020**, *11*, 56. [CrossRef]
40. Kim, S.H.; Seo, H.; Kwon, D.; Yuk, D.Y.; Jung, Y.S. Taurine Ameliorates Tunicamycin-Induced Liver Injury by Disrupting the Vicious Cycle between Oxidative Stress and Endoplasmic Reticulum Stress. *Life* **2022**, *12*, 354. [CrossRef] [PubMed]
41. Niknahad, H.; Mehrabani, P.S.; Arjmand, A.; Alidaee, S.; Mazloomi, S.; Ahmadi, P.; Abdoli, N.; Saeed, M.; Rezaei, M.; Ommati, M.M.; et al. Cirrhosis-induced oxidative stress in erythrocytes: The therapeutic potential of taurine. *Clin. Exp. Hepatol.* **2023**, *9*, 79–93. [CrossRef] [PubMed]
42. Guo, Q.; Zhang, L.; Yin, Y.; Gong, S.; Yang, Y.; Chen, S.; Han, M.; Duan, Y. Taurine Attenuates Oxidized Fish Oil-Induced Oxidative Stress and Lipid Metabolism Disorder in Mice. *Antioxidants* **2022**, *11*, 1391. [CrossRef] [PubMed]
43. Ali, S.N.; Arif, A.; Ansari, F.A.; Mahmood, R. Cytoprotective effect of taurine against sodium chlorate-induced oxidative damage in human red blood cells: An ex vivo study. *Amino Acids* **2022**, *54*, 33–46. [CrossRef] [PubMed]
44. Askwith, T.; Zeng, W.; Eggo, M.C.; Stevens, M.J. Taurine reduces nitrosative stress and nitric oxide synthase expression in high glucose-exposed human Schwann cells. *Exp. Neurol.* **2012**, *233*, 154–162. [CrossRef] [PubMed]
45. Faghfouri, A.H.; Seyyed Shoura, S.M.; Fathollahi, P.; Shadbad, M.A.; Papi, S.; Ostadrahimi, A.; Faghfuri, E. Profiling inflammatory and oxidative stress biomarkers following taurine supplementation: A systematic review and dose-response meta-analysis of controlled trials. *Eur. J. Clin. Nutr.* **2022**, *76*, 647–658. [CrossRef]
46. Rafiee, Z.; Garcia-Serrano, A.M.; Duarte, J.M.N. Taurine Supplementation as a Neuroprotective Strategy upon Brain Dysfunction in Metabolic Syndrome and Diabetes. *Nutrients* **2022**, *14*, 1292. [CrossRef]
47. Ochoa-de la Paz, L.D.; Martinez-Davila, I.A.; Miledi, R.; Martinez-Torres, A. Modulation of human GABArho1 receptors by taurine. *Neurosci. Res.* **2008**, *61*, 302–308. [CrossRef]
48. Hilgier, W.; Oja, S.S.; Saransaari, P.; Albrecht, J. Taurine prevents ammonia-induced accumulation of cyclic GMP in rat striatum by interaction with GABAA and glycine receptors. *Brain Res.* **2005**, *1043*, 242–246. [CrossRef]
49. Frosini, M.; Sesti, C.; Dragoni, S.; Valoti, M.; Palmi, M.; Dixon, H.B.; Machetti, F.; Sgaragli, G. Interactions of taurine and structurally related analogues with the GABAergic system and taurine binding sites of rabbit brain. *Br. J. Pharmacol.* **2003**, *138*, 1163–1171. [CrossRef]
50. Hashimoto-Kitsukawa, S.; Okuyama, S.; Aihara, H. Enhancing effect of taurine on the rat caudate spindle. I: Interaction of taurine with the nigro-striatal dopamine system. *Pharmacol. Biochem. Behav.* **1988**, *31*, 411–416. [CrossRef]
51. Kontro, P.; Oja, S.S. Release of taurine, GABA and dopamine from rat striatal slices: Mutual interactions and developmental aspects. *Neuroscience* **1988**, *24*, 49–58. [CrossRef]
52. Jakaria, M.; Azam, S.; Haque, M.E.; Jo, S.H.; Uddin, M.S.; Kim, I.S.; Choi, D.K. Taurine and its analogs in neurological disorders: Focus on therapeutic potential and molecular mechanisms. *Redox Biol.* **2019**, *24*, 101223. [CrossRef]
53. Ramirez-Guerrero, S.; Guardo-Maya, S.; Medina-Rincon, G.J.; Orrego-Gonzalez, E.E.; Cabezas-Perez, R.; Gonzalez-Reyes, R.E. Taurine and Astrocytes: A Homeostatic and Neuroprotective Relationship. *Front. Mol. Neurosci.* **2022**, *15*, 937789. [CrossRef]
54. Seol, S.I.; Kim, H.J.; Choi, E.B.; Kang, I.S.; Lee, H.K.; Lee, J.K.; Kim, C. Taurine Protects against Postischemic Brain Injury via the Antioxidant Activity of Taurine Chloramine. *Antioxidants* **2021**, *10*, 372. [CrossRef] [PubMed]

55. Oh, S.J.; Lee, H.J.; Jeong, Y.J.; Nam, K.R.; Kang, K.J.; Han, S.J.; Lee, K.C.; Lee, Y.J.; Choi, J.Y. Evaluation of the neuroprotective effect of taurine in Alzheimer's disease using functional molecular imaging. *Sci. Rep.* **2020**, *10*, 15551. [CrossRef]
56. Liu, K.; Zhu, R.; Jiang, H.; Li, B.; Geng, Q.; Li, Y.; Qi, J. Taurine inhibits KDM3a production and microglia activation in lipopolysaccharide-treated mice and BV-2 cells. *Mol. Cell Neurosci.* **2022**, *122*, 103759. [CrossRef]
57. Verner, A.; Craig, S.; McGuire, W. Effect of taurine supplementation on growth and development in preterm or low birth weight infants. *Cochrane Database Syst. Rev.* **2007**, *2007*, CD006072. [CrossRef] [PubMed]
58. Wharton, B.A.; Morley, R.; Isaacs, E.B.; Cole, T.J.; Lucas, A. Low plasma taurine and later neurodevelopment. *Arch. Dis. Child. Fetal. Neonatal Ed.* **2004**, *89*, F497–E498. [CrossRef] [PubMed]
59. Cao, S.L.; Jiang, H.; Niu, S.P.; Wang, X.H.; Du, S. Effects of Taurine Supplementation on Growth in Low Birth Weight Infants: A Systematic Review and Meta-Analysis. *Indian J. Pediatr.* **2018**, *85*, 855–860. [CrossRef]
60. Dhillon, S.K.; Davies, W.E.; Hopkins, P.C.; Rose, S.J. Effects of dietary taurine on auditory function in full-term infants. *Adv. Exp. Med. Biol.* **1998**, *442*, 507–514. [CrossRef]
61. Gaull, G.E. Taurine in human milk: Growth modulator or conditionally essential amino acid? *J. Pediatr. Gastroenterol. Nutr.* **1983**, *2* (Suppl. S1), S266–S271. [CrossRef]
62. Furukawa, T.; Fukuda, A. Maternal taurine as a modulator of Cl^- homeostasis as well as of glycine/GABA(A) receptors for neocortical development. *Front. Cell Neurosci.* **2023**, *17*, 1221441. [CrossRef]
63. Yamori, Y.; Sagara, M.; Arai, Y.; Kobayashi, H.; Kishimoto, K.; Matsuno, I.; Mori, H.; Mori, M. Taurine Intake with Magnesium Reduces Cardiometabolic Risks. *Adv. Exp. Med. Biol.* **2017**, *975 Pt 2*, 1011–1020. [CrossRef] [PubMed]
64. Sagara, M.; Murakami, S.; Mizushima, S.; Liu, L.; Mori, M.; Ikeda, K.; Nara, Y.; Yamori, Y. Taurine in 24-h Urine Samples Is Inversely Related to Cardiovascular Risks of Middle Aged Subjects in 50 Populations of the World. *Adv. Exp. Med. Biol.* **2015**, *803*, 623–636. [CrossRef] [PubMed]
65. Zulli, A.; Lau, E.; Wijaya, B.P.; Jin, X.; Sutarga, K.; Schwartz, G.D.; Learmont, J.; Wookey, P.J.; Zinellu, A.; Carru, C.; et al. High dietary taurine reduces apoptosis and atherosclerosis in the left main coronary artery: Association with reduced CCAAT/enhancer binding protein homologous protein and total plasma homocysteine but not lipidemia. *Hypertension* **2009**, *53*, 1017–1022. [CrossRef]
66. Oudit, G.Y.; Trivieri, M.G.; Khaper, N.; Husain, T.; Wilson, G.J.; Liu, P.; Sole, M.J.; Backx, P.H. Taurine supplementation reduces oxidative stress and improves cardiovascular function in an iron-overload murine model. *Circulation* **2004**, *109*, 1877–1885. [CrossRef]
67. Swiderski, J.; Sakkal, S.; Apostolopoulos, V.; Zulli, A.; Gadanec, L.K. Combination of Taurine and Black Pepper Extract as a Treatment for Cardiovascular and Coronary Artery Diseases. *Nutrients* **2023**, *15*, 2562. [CrossRef] [PubMed]
68. Wada, T.; Shimazaki, T.; Nakagawa, S.; Otuki, T.; Kurata, S.; Suzuki, T.; Watanabe, K.; Saigo, K. Chemical synthesis of novel taurine-containing uridine derivatives. *Nucleic Acids Res. Suppl.* **2002**, *2*, 11–12. [CrossRef]
69. Suzuki, T.; Suzuki, T.; Wada, T.; Saigo, K.; Watanabe, K. Taurine as a constituent of mitochondrial tRNAs: New insights into the functions of taurine and human mitochondrial diseases. *EMBO J.* **2002**, *21*, 6581–6589. [CrossRef]
70. Fakruddin, M.; Wei, F.Y.; Suzuki, T.; Asano, K.; Kaieda, T.; Omori, A.; Izumi, R.; Fujimura, A.; Kaitsuka, T.; Miyata, K.; et al. Defective Mitochondrial tRNA Taurine Modification Activates Global Proteostress and Leads to Mitochondrial Disease. *Cell Rep.* **2018**, *22*, 482–496. [CrossRef]
71. Kirino, Y.; Goto, Y.; Campos, Y.; Arenas, J.; Suzuki, T. Specific correlation between the wobble modification deficiency in mutant tRNAs and the clinical features of a human mitochondrial disease. *Proc. Natl. Acad. Sci. USA* **2005**, *102*, 7127–7132. [CrossRef] [PubMed]
72. Higuchi, M.; Celino, F.T.; Shimizu-Yamaguchi, S.; Miura, C.; Miura, T. Taurine plays an important role in the protection of spermatogonia from oxidative stress. *Amino Acids* **2012**, *43*, 2359–2369. [CrossRef]
73. Tabassum, H.; Rehman, H.; Banerjee, B.D.; Raisuddin, S.; Parvez, S. Attenuation of tamoxifen-induced hepatotoxicity by taurine in mice. *Clin. Chim. Acta* **2006**, *370*, 129–136. [CrossRef]
74. Miyazaki, T.; Ito, T.; Baseggio Conrado, A.; Murakami, S. Editorial for Special Issue on "Regulation and Effect of Taurine on Metabolism". *Metabolites* **2022**, *12*, 795. [CrossRef]
75. De Carvalho, F.G.; Batitucci, G.; Abud, G.F.; de Freitas, E.C. Taurine and Exercise: Synergistic Effects on Adipose Tissue Metabolism and Inflammatory Process in Obesity. *Adv. Exp. Med. Biol.* **2022**, *1370*, 279–289. [CrossRef] [PubMed]
76. De Carvalho, F.G.; Munoz, V.R.; Brandao, C.F.C.; Simabuco, F.M.; Pavan, I.C.B.; Nakandakari, S.; Pauli, J.R.; De Moura, L.P.; Ropelle, E.R.; Marchini, J.S.; et al. Taurine upregulates insulin signaling and mitochondrial metabolism in vitro but not in adipocytes of obese women. *Nutrition* **2022**, *93*, 111430. [CrossRef]
77. Brons, C.; Spohr, C.; Storgaard, H.; Dyerberg, J.; Vaag, A. Effect of taurine treatment on insulin secretion and action, and on serum lipid levels in overweight men with a genetic predisposition for type II diabetes mellitus. *Eur. J. Clin. Nutr.* **2004**, *58*, 1239–1247. [CrossRef] [PubMed]
78. Nakaya, Y.; Minami, A.; Harada, N.; Sakamoto, S.; Niwa, Y.; Ohnaka, M. Taurine improves insulin sensitivity in the Otsuka Long-Evans Tokushima Fatty rat, a model of spontaneous type 2 diabetes. *Am. J. Clin. Nutr.* **2000**, *71*, 54–58. [CrossRef]
79. Anuradha, C.V.; Balakrishnan, S.D. Taurine attenuates hypertension and improves insulin sensitivity in the fructose-fed rat, an animal model of insulin resistance. *Can. J. Physiol. Pharmacol.* **1999**, *77*, 749–754. [CrossRef]

80. Sarnobat, D.; Moffett, R.C.; Ma, J.; Flatt, P.R.; McClenaghan, N.H.; Tarasov, A.I. Taurine rescues pancreatic beta-cell stress by stimulating alpha-cell transdifferentiation. *Biofactors* **2023**, *49*, 646–662. [CrossRef]
81. Tagawa, R.; Kobayashi, M.; Sakurai, M.; Yoshida, M.; Kaneko, H.; Mizunoe, Y.; Nozaki, Y.; Okita, N.; Sudo, Y.; Higami, Y. Long-Term Dietary Taurine Lowers Plasma Levels of Cholesterol and Bile Acids. *Int. J. Mol. Sci.* **2022**, *23*, 1793. [CrossRef] [PubMed]
82. Guo, J.; -Gao, Y.; Cao, X.; Zhang, J.; Chen, W. Cholesterollowing effect of taurine in HepG2 cell. *Lipids Health Dis.* **2017**, *16*, 56. [CrossRef]
83. Yokogoshi, H.; Mochizuki, H.; Nanami, K.; Hida, Y.; Miyachi, F.; Oda, H. Dietary taurine enhances cholesterol degradation and reduces serum and liver cholesterol concentrations in rats fed a high-cholesterol diet. *J. Nutr.* **1999**, *129*, 1705–1712. [CrossRef] [PubMed]
84. Balkan, J.; Kanbagli, O.; Hatipoglu, A.; Kucuk, M.; Cevikbas, U.; Aykac-Toker, G.; Uysal, M. Improving effect of dietary taurine supplementation on the oxidative stress and lipid levels in the plasma, liver and aorta of rabbits fed on a high-cholesterol diet. *Biosci. Biotechnol. Biochem.* **2002**, *66*, 1755–1758. [CrossRef]
85. Zhang, M.; Bi, L.F.; Fang, J.H.; Su, X.L.; Da, G.L.; Kuwamori, T.; Kagamimori, S. Beneficial effects of taurine on serum lipids in overweight or obese non-diabetic subjects. *Amino Acids* **2004**, *26*, 267–271. [CrossRef] [PubMed]
86. Pansani, M.C.; Azevedo, P.S.; Rafacho, B.P.; Minicucci, M.F.; Chiuso-Minicucci, F.; Zorzella-Pezavento, S.G.; Marchini, J.S.; Padovan, G.J.; Fernandes, A.A.; Matsubara, B.B.; et al. Atrophic cardiac remodeling induced by taurine deficiency in Wistar rats. *PLoS ONE* **2012**, *7*, e41439. [CrossRef]
87. Mozaffari, M.S.; Tan, B.H.; Lucia, M.A.; Schaffer, S.W. Effect of drug-induced taurine depletion on cardiac contractility and metabolism. *Biochem. Pharmacol.* **1986**, *35*, 985–989. [CrossRef]
88. Lake, N. Loss of cardiac myofibrils: Mechanism of contractile deficits induced by taurine deficiency. *Am. J. Physiol.* **1993**, *264*, H1323–H1326. [CrossRef]
89. Satoh, H.; Nakatani, T.; Tanaka, T.; Haga, S. Cardiac functions and taurine's actions at different extracellular calcium concentrations in forced swimming stress-loaded rats. *Biol. Trace Elem. Res.* **2002**, *87*, 171–182. [CrossRef]
90. Franconi, F.; Martini, F.; Stendardi, I.; Matucci, R.; Zilletti, L.; Giotti, A. Effect of taurine on calcium levels and contractility in guinea-pig ventricular strips. *Biochem. Pharmacol.* **1982**, *31*, 3181–3185. [CrossRef]
91. Schaffer, S.W.; Seyed-Mozaffari, M.; Kramer, J.; Tan, B.H. Effect of taurine depletion and treatment on cardiac contractility and metabolism. *Prog. Clin. Biol. Res.* **1985**, *179*, 167–175.
92. Kaplan, J.L.; Stern, J.A.; Fascetti, A.J.; Larsen, J.A.; Skolnik, H.; Peddle, G.D.; Kienle, R.D.; Waxman, A.; Cocchiaro, M.; Gunther-Harrington, C.T.; et al. Taurine deficiency and dilated cardiomyopathy in golden retrievers fed commercial diets. *PLoS ONE* **2018**, *13*, e0209112. [CrossRef]
93. Samadi, M.; Haghi-Aminjan, H.; Sattari, M.; Hooshangi Shayesteh, M.R.; Bameri, B.; Armandeh, M.; Naddafi, M.; Eghbal, M.A.; Abdollahi, M. The role of taurine on chemotherapy-induced cardiotoxicity: A systematic review of non-clinical study. *Life Sci.* **2021**, *265*, 118813. [CrossRef]
94. Ahmadian, M.; Dabidi Roshan, V.; Ashourpore, E. Taurine Supplementation Improves Functional Capacity, Myocardial Oxygen Consumption, and Electrical Activity in Heart Failure. *J. Diet. Suppl.* **2017**, *14*, 422–432. [CrossRef] [PubMed]
95. Ahmadian, M.; Roshan, V.D.; Aslani, E.; Stannard, S.R. Taurine supplementation has anti-atherogenic and anti-inflammatory effects before and after incremental exercise in heart failure. *Ther. Adv. Cardiovasc. Dis.* **2017**, *11*, 185–194. [CrossRef] [PubMed]
96. Azuma, J.; Sawamura, A.; Awata, N.; Ohta, H.; Hamaguchi, T.; Harada, H.; Takihara, K.; Hasegawa, H.; Yamagami, T.; Ishiyama, T.; et al. Therapeutic effect of taurine in congestive heart failure: A double-blind crossover trial. *Clin. Cardiol.* **1985**, *8*, 276–282. [CrossRef]
97. Beyranvand, M.R.; Khalafi, M.K.; Roshan, V.D.; Choobineh, S.; Parsa, S.A.; Piranfar, M.A. Effect of taurine supplementation on exercise capacity of patients with heart failure. *J. Cardiol.* **2011**, *57*, 333–337. [CrossRef] [PubMed]
98. Azuma, J.; Sawamura, A.; Awata, N. Usefulness of taurine in chronic congestive heart failure and its prospective application. *Jpn. Circ. J.* **1992**, *56*, 95–99. [CrossRef] [PubMed]
99. Yamauchi-Takihara, K.; Azuma, J.; Kishimoto, S.; Onishi, S.; Sperelakis, N. Taurine prevention of calcium paradox-related damage in cardiac muscle. Its regulatory action on intracellular cation contents. *Biochem. Pharmacol.* **1988**, *37*, 2651–2658. [CrossRef]
100. Henry, E.F.; MacCormack, T.J. Taurine protects cardiac contractility in killifish, Fundulus heteroclitus, by enhancing sarcoplasmic reticular Ca^{2+} cycling. *J. Comp. Physiol. B* **2018**, *188*, 89–99. [CrossRef]
101. Gates, M.A.; Morash, A.J.; Lamarre, S.G.; MacCormack, T.J. Intracellular taurine deficiency impairs cardiac contractility in rainbow trout (*Oncorhynchus mykiss*) without affecting aerobic performance. *J. Comp. Physiol. B* **2022**, *192*, 49–60. [CrossRef]
102. Satoh, H.; Sperelakis, N. Taurine inhibition of fast Na^+ current in embryonic chick ventricular myocytes. *Eur. J. Pharmacol.* **1992**, *218*, 83–89. [CrossRef]
103. Oz, E.; Erbas, D.; Gelir, E.; Aricioglu, A. Taurine and calcium interaction in protection of myocardium exposed to ischemic reperfusion injury. *Gen. Pharmacol.* **1999**, *33*, 137–141. [CrossRef]
104. Wong, A.P.; Niedzwiecki, A.; Rath, M. Myocardial energetics and the role of micronutrients in heart failure: A critical review. *Am. J. Cardiovasc. Dis.* **2016**, *6*, 81–92. [PubMed]

105. Dragan, S.; Buleu, F.; Christodorescu, R.; Cobzariu, F.; Iurciuc, S.; Velimirovici, D.; Xiao, J.; Luca, C.T. Benefits of multiple micronutrient supplementation in heart failure: A comprehensive review. *Crit. Rev. Food Sci. Nutr.* **2019**, *59*, 965–981. [CrossRef] [PubMed]
106. Razzaghi, A.; Choobineh, S.; Gaeini, A.; Soori, R. Interaction of exercise training with taurine attenuates infarct size and cardiac dysfunction via Akt-Foxo3a-Caspase-8 signaling pathway. *Amino Acids* **2023**, *55*, 869–880. [CrossRef] [PubMed]
107. Li, C.; Zhou, Y.; Niu, Y.; He, W.; Wang, X.; Zhang, X.; Wu, Y.; Zhang, W.; Zhao, L.; Zheng, H.; et al. Deficiency of Pdk1 drives heart failure by impairing taurine homeostasis through Slc6a6. *FASEB J.* **2023**, *37*, e23134. [CrossRef]
108. Li, S.; Wang, D.; Zhang, M.; Zhang, C.; Piao, F. Taurine Ameliorates Apoptosis via AKT Pathway in the Kidney of Diabetic Rats. *Adv. Exp. Med. Biol.* **2022**, *1370*, 227–233. [CrossRef]
109. Li, M.; Gao, Y.; Wang, Z.; Wu, B.; Zhang, J.; Xu, Y.; Han, X.; Phouthapane, V.; Miao, J. Taurine inhibits Streptococcus uberis-induced NADPH oxidase-dependent neutrophil extracellular traps via TAK1/MAPK signaling pathways. *Front. Immunol.* **2022**, *13*, 927215. [CrossRef]
110. Liu, C.; He, P.; Guo, Y.; Tian, Q.; Wang, J.; Wang, G.; Zhang, Z.; Li, M. Taurine attenuates neuronal ferroptosis by regulating GABA(B)/AKT/GSK3beta/beta-catenin pathway after subarachnoid hemorrhage. *Free Radic. Biol. Med.* **2022**, *193*, 795–807. [CrossRef]
111. Das, J.; Vasan, V.; Sil, P.C. Taurine exerts hypoglycemic effect in alloxan-induced diabetic rats, improves insulin-mediated glucose transport signaling pathway in heart and ameliorates cardiac oxidative stress and apoptosis. *Toxicol. Appl. Pharmacol.* **2012**, *258*, 296–308. [CrossRef]
112. Wei, C.; Ding, X.; Liu, C.; Pei, Y.; Zhong, Y.; Sun, W. Mechanism of taurine in alleviating myocardial oxidative stress in rats after burn through p38 MAPK signaling pathway. *Minerva Med.* **2019**, *110*, 472–475. [CrossRef] [PubMed]
113. Azuma, M.; Takahashi, K.; Fukuda, T.; Ohyabu, Y.; Yamamoto, I.; Kim, S.; Iwao, H.; Schaffer, S.W.; Azuma, J. Taurine attenuates hypertrophy induced by angiotensin II in cultured neonatal rat cardiac myocytes. *Eur. J. Pharmacol.* **2000**, *403*, 181–188. [CrossRef]
114. Takatani, T.; Takahashi, K.; Uozumi, Y.; Matsuda, T.; Ito, T.; Schaffer, S.W.; Fujio, Y.; Azuma, J. Taurine prevents the ischemia-induced apoptosis in cultured neonatal rat cardiomyocytes through Akt/caspase-9 pathway. *Biochem. Biophys. Res. Commun.* **2004**, *316*, 484–489. [CrossRef] [PubMed]
115. Sedaghat, M.; Choobineh, S.; Ravasi, A.A. Taurine with combined aerobic and resistance exercise training alleviates myocardium apoptosis in STZ-induced diabetes rats via Akt signaling pathway. *Life Sci.* **2020**, *258*, 118225. [CrossRef] [PubMed]
116. Ghosh, J.; Das, J.; Manna, P.; Sil, P.C. Taurine prevents arsenic-induced cardiac oxidative stress and apoptotic damage: Role of NF-kappa B, p38 and JNK MAPK pathway. *Toxicol. Appl. Pharmacol.* **2009**, *240*, 73–87. [CrossRef]
117. Yousuf, M.; Shamsi, A.; Mohammad, T.; Azum, N.; Alfaifi, S.Y.M.; Asiri, A.M.; Mohamed Elasbali, A.; Islam, A.; Hassan, M.I.; Haque, Q.M.R. Inhibiting Cyclin-Dependent Kinase 6 by Taurine: Implications in Anticancer Therapeutics. *ACS Omega* **2022**, *7*, 25844–25852. [CrossRef] [PubMed]
118. Feng, X.; Hu, W.; Hong, Y.; Ruan, L.; Hu, Y.; Liu, D. Taurine Ameliorates Iron Overload-Induced Hepatocyte Injury via the Bcl-2/VDAC1-Mediated Mitochondrial Apoptosis Pathway. *Oxid. Med. Cell. Longev.* **2022**, *2022*, 4135752. [CrossRef]
119. Zhao, D.; Zhang, X.; Feng, Y.; Bian, Y.; Fu, Z.; Wu, Y.; Ma, Y.; Li, C.; Wang, J.; Dai, J.; et al. Taurine Alleviates LPS-Induced Acute Lung Injury by Suppressing TLR-4/NF-kappaB Pathway. *Adv. Exp. Med. Biol.* **2022**, *1370*, 63–72. [CrossRef] [PubMed]
120. Wu, G.; San, J.; Pang, H.; Du, Y.; Li, W.; Zhou, X.; Yang, X.; Hu, J.; Yang, J. Taurine attenuates AFB1-induced liver injury by alleviating oxidative stress and regulating mitochondria-mediated apoptosis. *Toxicon* **2022**, *215*, 17–27. [CrossRef]
121. Kp, A.D.; Shimoga Janakirama, A.R.; Martin, A. SIRT1 activation by Taurine: In vitro evaluation, molecular docking and molecular dynamics simulation studies. *J. Nutr. Biochem.* **2022**, *102*, 108948. [CrossRef] [PubMed]
122. Mozaffari, M.S.; Patel, C.; Abdelsayed, R.; Schaffer, S.W. Accelerated NaCl-induced hypertension in taurine-deficient rat: Role of renal function. *Kidney Int.* **2006**, *70*, 329–337. [CrossRef] [PubMed]
123. Li, W.; Yang, J.; Lyu, Q.; Wu, G.; Lin, S.; Yang, Q.; Hu, J. Taurine attenuates isoproterenol-induced H9c2 cardiomyocytes hypertrophy by improving antioxidative ability and inhibiting calpain-1-mediated apoptosis. *Mol. Cell. Biochem.* **2020**, *469*, 119–132. [CrossRef]
124. Gentile, S.; Bologna, E.; Terracina, D.; Angelico, M. Taurine-induced diuresis and natriuresis in cirrhotic patients with ascites. *Life Sci.* **1994**, *54*, 1585–1593. [CrossRef]
125. Dlouha, H.; McBroom, M.J. Atrial natriuretic factor in taurine-treated normal and cardiomyopathic hamsters. *Proc. Soc. Exp. Biol. Med.* **1986**, *181*, 411–415. [CrossRef]
126. Guizoni, D.M.; Vettorazzi, J.F.; Carneiro, E.M.; Davel, A.P. Modulation of endothelium-derived nitric oxide production and activity by taurine and taurine-conjugated bile acids. *Nitric Oxide* **2020**, *94*, 48–53. [CrossRef] [PubMed]
127. Dharmashankar, K.; Widlansky, M.E. Vascular endothelial function and hypertension: Insights and directions. *Curr. Hypertens. Rep.* **2010**, *12*, 448–455. [CrossRef] [PubMed]
128. Su, J.B. Vascular endothelial dysfunction and pharmacological treatment. *World J. Cardiol.* **2015**, *7*, 719–741. [CrossRef] [PubMed]
129. Gambardella, J.; Khondkar, W.; Morelli, M.B.; Wang, X.; Santulli, G.; Trimarco, V. Arginine and Endothelial Function. *Biomedicines* **2020**, *8*, 277. [CrossRef]
130. Fennessy, F.M.; Moneley, D.S.; Wang, J.H.; Kelly, C.J.; Bouchier-Hayes, D.J. Taurine and vitamin C modify monocyte and endothelial dysfunction in young smokers. *Circulation* **2003**, *107*, 410–415. [CrossRef]

131. El Idrissi, A.; Okeke, E.; Yan, X.; Sidime, F.; Neuwirth, L.S. Taurine regulation of blood pressure and vasoactivity. *Adv. Exp. Med. Biol.* **2013**, *775*, 407–425. [CrossRef]
132. Yildiz, O.; Ulusoy, K.G. Effects of taurine on vascular tone. *Amino Acids* **2022**, *54*, 1527–1540. [CrossRef] [PubMed]
133. Hagiwara, K.; Kuroki, G.; Yuan, P.X.; Suzuki, T.; Murakami, M.; Hano, T.; Sasano, H.; Yanagisawa, T. The effect of taurine on the salt-dependent blood pressure increase in the voltage-dependent calcium channel beta 3-subunit-deficient mouse. *J. Cardiovasc. Pharmacol.* **2003**, *41* (Suppl. S1), S127–S131. [PubMed]
134. Meldrum, M.J.; Tu, R.; Patterson, T.; Dawson, R., Jr.; Petty, T. The effect of taurine on blood pressure, and urinary sodium, potassium and calcium excretion. *Adv. Exp. Med. Biol.* **1994**, *359*, 207–215. [CrossRef] [PubMed]
135. Sun, B.; Maruta, H.; Ma, Y.; Yamashita, H. Taurine Stimulates AMP-Activated Protein Kinase and Modulates the Skeletal Muscle Functions in Rats via the Induction of Intracellular Calcium Influx. *Int. J. Mol. Sci.* **2023**, *24*, 4125. [CrossRef] [PubMed]
136. Ra, S.G.; Choi, Y.; Akazawa, N.; Kawanaka, K.; Ohmori, H.; Maeda, S. Effects of Taurine Supplementation on Vascular Endothelial Function at Rest and After Resistance Exercise. *Adv. Exp. Med. Biol.* **2019**, *1155*, 407–414. [CrossRef]
137. Katakawa, M.; Fukuda, N.; Tsunemi, A.; Mori, M.; Maruyama, T.; Matsumoto, T.; Abe, M.; Yamori, Y. Taurine and magnesium supplementation enhances the function of endothelial progenitor cells through antioxidation in healthy men and spontaneously hypertensive rats. *Hypertens. Res.* **2016**, *39*, 848–856. [CrossRef]
138. Guizoni, D.M.; Freitas, I.N.; Victorio, J.A.; Possebom, I.R.; Araujo, T.R.; Carneiro, E.M.; Davel, A.P. Taurine treatment reverses protein malnutrition-induced endothelial dysfunction of the pancreatic vasculature: The role of hydrogen sulfide. *Metabolism* **2021**, *116*, 154701. [CrossRef]
139. Casey, R.G.; Gang, C.; Joyce, M.; Bouchier-Hayes, D.J. Taurine attenuates acute hyperglycaemia-induced endothelial cell apoptosis, leucocyte-endothelial cell interactions and cardiac dysfunction. *J. Vasc. Res.* **2007**, *44*, 31–39. [CrossRef]
140. Moloney, M.A.; Casey, R.G.; O'Donnell, D.H.; Fitzgerald, P.; Thompson, C.; Bouchier-Hayes, D.J. Two weeks taurine supplementation reverses endothelial dysfunction in young male type 1 diabetics. *Diabetes Vasc. Dis. Res.* **2010**, *7*, 300–310. [CrossRef]
141. Ferreira Abud, G.; Giolo De Carvalho, F.; Batitucci, G.; Travieso, S.G.; Bueno Junior, C.R.; Barbosa Junior, F.; Marchini, J.S.; de Freitas, E.C. Taurine as a possible antiaging therapy: A controlled clinical trial on taurine antioxidant activity in women ages 55 to 70. *Nutrition* **2022**, *101*, 111706. [CrossRef]
142. Jong, C.J.; Azuma, J.; Schaffer, S. Mechanism underlying the antioxidant activity of taurine: Prevention of mitochondrial oxidant production. *Amino Acids* **2012**, *42*, 2223–2232. [CrossRef]
143. Kang, Y.J.; Choi, M.J. Liver Antioxidant Enzyme Activities Increase After Taurine in Ovariectomized Rats. *Adv. Exp. Med. Biol.* **2017**, *975 Pt 2*, 1071–1080. [CrossRef]
144. Sun, Q.; Wang, B.; Li, Y.; Sun, F.; Li, P.; Xia, W.; Zhou, X.; Li, Q.; Wang, X.; Chen, J.; et al. Taurine Supplementation Lowers Blood Pressure and Improves Vascular Function in Prehypertension: Randomized, Double-Blind, Placebo-Controlled Study. *Hypertension* **2016**, *67*, 541–549. [CrossRef] [PubMed]
145. Maia, A.R.; Batistas, T.M.; Victorio, J.A.; Clerici, S.P.; Delbin, M.A.; Carneiro, E.M.; Davel, A.P. Taurine upplementation reduces blood pressure and prevents endothelial dysfunction and oxidative stress in post-weaning protein-restricted rats. *PLoS ONE* **2014**, *9*, e105851. [CrossRef]
146. Trachtman, H.; Del Pizzo, R.; Rao, P.; Rujikarn, N.; Sturman, J.A. Taurine lowers blood pressure in the spontaneously hypertensive rat by a catecholamine independent mechanism. *Am. J. Hypertens.* **1989**, *2*, 909–912. [CrossRef] [PubMed]
147. Scabora, J.E.; de Lima, M.C.; Lopes, A.; de Lima, I.P.; Mesquita, F.F.; Torres, D.B.; Boer, P.A.; Gontijo, J.A. Impact of taurine supplementation on blood pressure in gestational protein-restricted offspring: Effect on the medial solitary tract nucleus cell numbers, angiotensin receptors, and renal sodium handling. *J. Renin-Angiotensin-Aldosterone Syst.* **2015**, *16*, 47–58. [CrossRef] [PubMed]
148. Abebe, W.; Mozaffari, M.S. Effects of chronic taurine treatment on reactivity of the rat aorta. *Amino Acids* **2000**, *19*, 615–623. [CrossRef]
149. Sener, G.; Ozer Sehirli, A.; Ipci, Y.; Cetinel, S.; Cikler, E.; Gedik, N.; Alican, I. Taurine treatment protects against chronic nicotine-induced oxidative changes. *Fundam. Clin. Pharmacol.* **2005**, *19*, 155–164. [CrossRef]
150. Liang, W.; Yang, Q.; Wu, G.; Lin, S.; Yang, J.; Feng, Y.; Hu, J. Effects of Taurine and L-Arginine on the Apoptosis of Vascular Smooth Muscle Cells in Insulin Resistance Hypertensive Rats. *Adv. Exp. Med. Biol.* **2017**, *975 Pt 2*, 813–819. [CrossRef]
151. Forzano, I.; Avvisato, R.; Varzideh, F.; Jankauskas, S.S.; Cioppa, A.; Mone, P.; Salemme, L.; Kansakar, U.; Tesorio, T.; Trimarco, V.; et al. L-Arginine in diabetes: Clinical and preclinical evidence. *Cardiovasc. Diabetol.* **2023**, *22*, 89. [CrossRef]
152. Trimarco, V.; Izzo, R.; Lombardi, A.; Coppola, A.; Fiorentino, G.; Santulli, G. Beneficial effects of L-Arginine in patients hospitalized for COVID-19: New insights from a randomized clinical trial. *Pharmacol. Res.* **2023**, *191*, 106702. [CrossRef] [PubMed]
153. Gambardella, J.; Fiordelisi, A.; Spigno, L.; Boldrini, L.; Lungonelli, G.; Di Vaia, E.; Santulli, G.; Sorriento, D.; Cerasuolo, F.A.; Trimarco, V.; et al. Effects of Chronic Supplementation of L-Arginine on Physical Fitness in Water Polo Players. *Oxid. Med. Cell. Longev.* **2021**, *2021*, 6684568. [CrossRef]
154. Moludi, J.; Qaisar, S.A.; Kadhim, M.M.; Ahmadi, Y.; Davari, M. Protective and therapeutic effectiveness of taurine supplementation plus low calorie diet on metabolic parameters and endothelial markers in patients with diabetes mellitus: A randomized, clinical trial. *Nutr. Metab.* **2022**, *19*, 49. [CrossRef] [PubMed]
155. Waldron, M.; Patterson, S.D.; Tallent, J.; Jeffries, O. The Effects of Oral Taurine on Resting Blood Pressure in Humans: A Meta-Analysis. *Curr. Hypertens. Rep.* **2018**, *20*, 81. [CrossRef] [PubMed]

156. Gutierrez-Hellin, J.; Varillas-Delgado, D. Energy Drinks and Sports Performance, Cardiovascular Risk, and Genetic Associations; Future Prospects. *Nutrients* **2021**, *13*, 715. [CrossRef]
157. Ozan, M.; Buzdagli, Y.; Eyipinar, C.D.; Baygutalp, N.K.; Yuce, N.; Oget, F.; Kan, E.; Baygutalp, F. Does Single or Combined Caffeine and Taurine Supplementation Improve Athletic and Cognitive Performance without Affecting Fatigue Level in Elite Boxers? A Double-Blind, Placebo-Controlled Study. *Nutrients* **2022**, *14*, 4399. [CrossRef]
158. Kurtz, J.A.; VanDusseldorp, T.A.; Doyle, J.A.; Otis, J.S. Taurine in sports and exercise. *J. Int. Soc. Sports Nutr.* **2021**, *18*, 39. [CrossRef] [PubMed]
159. Pollard, C.M.; McStay, C.L.; Meng, X. Public Concern about the Sale of High-Caffeine Drinks to Children 12 Years or Younger: An Australian Regulatory Perspective. *Biomed Res. Int.* **2015**, *2015*, 707149. [CrossRef]
160. Dawodu, A.; Cleaver, K. Behavioural correlates of energy drink consumption among adolescents: A review of the literature. *J. Child Health Care* **2017**, *21*, 446–462. [CrossRef]
161. Kaur, A.; Yousuf, H.; Ramgobin-Marshall, D.; Jain, R.; Jain, R. Energy drink consumption: A rising public health issue. *Rev. Cardiovasc. Med.* **2022**, *23*, 83. [CrossRef]
162. Erdmann, J.; Wicinski, M.; Wodkiewicz, E.; Nowaczewska, M.; Slupski, M.; Otto, S.W.; Kubiak, K.; Huk-Wieliczuk, E.; Malinowski, B. Effects of Energy Drink Consumption on Physical Performance and Potential Danger of Inordinate Usage. *Nutrients* **2021**, *13*, 2506. [CrossRef] [PubMed]
163. Nuss, T.; Morley, B.; Scully, M.; Wakefield, M. Energy drink consumption among Australian adolescents associated with a cluster of unhealthy dietary behaviours and short sleep duration. *Nutr. J.* **2021**, *20*, 64. [CrossRef] [PubMed]
164. Kriebs, A. Taurine levels modulate aging. *Nat. Aging* **2023**, *3*, 758–759. [CrossRef]
165. Ferreira, J. Systemic taurine decline drives aging. *Lab Anim.* **2023**, *52*, 175. [CrossRef]
166. Izquierdo, J.M. Taurine as a possible therapy for immunosenescence and inflammaging. *Cell. Mol. Immunol.* **2023**, *online ahead of print*. [CrossRef]
167. Barbiera, A.; Sorrentino, S.; Fard, D.; Lepore, E.; Sica, G.; Dobrowolny, G.; Tamagnone, L.; Scicchitano, B.M. Taurine Administration Counteracts Aging-Associated Impingement of Skeletal Muscle Regeneration by Reducing Inflammation and Oxidative Stress. *Antioxidants* **2022**, *11*, 1016. [CrossRef] [PubMed]
168. Singh, P.; Gollapalli, K.; Mangiola, S.; Schranner, D.; Yusuf, M.A.; Chamoli, M.; Shi, S.L.; Lopes Bastos, B.; Nair, T.; Riermeier, A.; et al. Taurine deficiency as a driver of aging. *Science* **2023**, *380*, eabn9257. [CrossRef] [PubMed]
169. Vidal Valero, M. Taurine supplement makes animals live longer—What it means for people is unclear. *Nature* **2023**, *online ahead of print*. [CrossRef]
170. McGaunn, J.; Baur, J.A. Taurine linked with healthy aging. *Science* **2023**, *380*, 1010–1011. [CrossRef] [PubMed]
171. Qian, W.; Li, M.; Yu, L.; Tian, F.; Zhao, J.; Zhai, Q. Effects of Taurine on Gut Microbiota Homeostasis: An Evaluation Based on Two Models of Gut Dysbiosis. *Biomedicines* **2023**, *11*, 1048. [CrossRef] [PubMed]
172. Graham, F. Daily briefing: Taurine makes animals live longer—But don't binge on Red Bulls yet. *Nature* **2023**, *online ahead of print*. [CrossRef]
173. Jun, H.; Choi, M.J. Relationship Between Taurine Intake and Cardiometabolic Risk Markers in Korean Elderly. *Adv. Exp. Med. Biol.* **2019**, *1155*, 301–311. [CrossRef] [PubMed]
174. Lopez-Otin, C.; Blasco, M.A.; Partridge, L.; Serrano, M.; Kroemer, G. Hallmarks of aging: An expanding universe. *Cell* **2023**, *186*, 243–278. [CrossRef] [PubMed]
175. McHugh, D.; Gil, J. Senescence and aging: Causes, consequences, and therapeutic avenues. *J. Cell Biol.* **2018**, *217*, 65–77. [CrossRef] [PubMed]
176. Watanabe, S.; Kawamoto, S.; Ohtani, N.; Hara, E. Impact of senescence-associated secretory phenotype and its potential as a therapeutic target for senescence-associated diseases. *Cancer Sci.* **2017**, *108*, 563–569. [CrossRef]
177. Kumari, R.; Jat, P. Mechanisms of Cellular Senescence: Cell Cycle Arrest and Senescence Associated Secretory Phenotype. *Front. Cell Dev. Biol.* **2021**, *9*, 645593. [CrossRef]
178. Coppe, J.P.; Desprez, P.Y.; Krtolica, A.; Campisi, J. The senescence-associated secretory phenotype: The dark side of tumor suppression. *Annu. Rev. Pathol.* **2010**, *5*, 99–118. [CrossRef]
179. Mohamad Kamal, N.S.; Safuan, S.; Shamsuddin, S.; Foroozandeh, P. Aging of the cells: Insight into cellular senescence and detection Methods. *Eur. J. Cell Biol.* **2020**, *99*, 151108. [CrossRef]
180. Kowald, A.; Passos, J.F.; Kirkwood, T.B.L. On the evolution of cellular senescence. *Aging Cell* **2020**, *19*, e13270. [CrossRef]
181. Yi, S.; Lin, K.; Jiang, T.; Shao, W.; Huang, C.; Jiang, B.; Li, Q.; Lin, D. NMR-based metabonomic analysis of HUVEC cells during replicative senescence. *Aging* **2020**, *12*, 3626–3646. [CrossRef]
182. Ji, H.; Zhao, G.; Luo, J.; Zhao, X.; Zhang, M. Taurine postponed the replicative senescence of rat bone marrow-derived multipotent stromal cells in vitro. *Mol. Cell. Biochem.* **2012**, *366*, 259–267. [CrossRef]
183. Ito, T.; Yoshikawa, N.; Inui, T.; Miyazaki, N.; Schaffer, S.W.; Azuma, J. Tissue depletion of taurine accelerates skeletal muscle senescence and leads to early death in mice. *PLoS ONE* **2014**, *9*, e107409. [CrossRef]
184. Ito, T.; Yamamoto, N.; Nakajima, S.; Schaffer, S.W. Beta-Catenin and SMAD3 Are Associated with Skeletal Muscle Aging in the Taurine Transpoeter Knockout Mouse. *Adv. Exp. Med. Biol.* **2017**, *975 Pt 1*, 497–502. [CrossRef]
185. Kaushik, S.; Cuervo, A.M. Proteostasis and aging. *Nat. Med.* **2015**, *21*, 1406–1415. [CrossRef]

186. Hetz, C.; Zhang, K.; Kaufman, R.J. Mechanisms, regulation and functions of the unfolded protein response. *Nat. Rev. Mol. Cell Biol.* **2020**, *21*, 421–438. [CrossRef]
187. Du, G.; Liu, Z.; Yu, Z.; Zhuo, Z.; Zhu, Y.; Zhou, J.; Li, Y.; Chen, H. Taurine represses age-associated gut hyperplasia in Drosophila via counteracting endoplasmic reticulum stress. *Aging Cell* **2021**, *20*, e13319. [CrossRef]
188. Yang, Y.; Zhang, Y.; Liu, X.; Zuo, J.; Wang, K.; Liu, W.; Ge, J. Exogenous taurine attenuates mitochondrial oxidative stress and endoplasmic reticulum stress in rat cardiomyocytes. *Acta Biochim. Biophys. Sin.* **2013**, *45*, 359–367. [CrossRef]
189. Chowdhury, S.; Sinha, K.; Banerjee, S.; Sil, P.C. Taurine protects cisplatin induced cardiotoxicity by modulating inflammatory and endoplasmic reticulum stress responses. *Biofactors* **2016**, *42*, 647–664. [CrossRef]
190. Ren, Q.; Zhang, G.; Dong, C.; Li, Z.; Zhou, D.; Huang, L.; Li, W.; Huang, G.; Yan, J. Parental Folate Deficiency Inhibits Proliferation and Increases Apoptosis of Neural Stem Cells in Rat Offspring: Aggravating Telomere Attrition as a Potential Mechanism. *Nutrients* **2023**, *15*, 2843. [CrossRef]
191. Gao, Z.; Daquinag, A.C.; Fussell, C.; Zhao, Z.; Dai, Y.; Rivera, A.; Snyder, B.E.; Eckel-Mahan, K.L.; Kolonin, M.G. Age-associated telomere attrition in adipocyte progenitors predisposes to metabolic disease. *Nat. Metab.* **2020**, *2*, 1482–1497. [CrossRef]
192. Varzideh, F.; Gambardella, J.; Kansakar, U.; Jankauskas, S.S.; Santulli, G. Molecular Mechanisms Underlying Pluripotency and Self-Renewal of Embryonic Stem Cells. *Int. J. Mol. Sci.* **2023**, *24*, 8386. [CrossRef]
193. Mashyakhy, M.; Alkahtani, A.; Abumelha, A.S.; Sharroufna, R.J.; Alkahtany, M.F.; Jamal, M.; Robaian, A.; Binalrimal, S.; Chohan, H.; Patil, V.R.; et al. Taurine Augments Telomerase Activity and Promotes Chondrogenesis in Dental Pulp Stem Cells. *J. Pers. Med.* **2021**, *11*, 491. [CrossRef]
194. Gokarn, R.; Solon-Biet, S.; Youngson, N.A.; Wahl, D.; Cogger, V.C.; McMahon, A.C.; Cooney, G.J.; Ballard, J.W.O.; Raubenheimer, D.; Morris, M.J.; et al. The Relationship Between Dietary Macronutrients and Hepatic Telomere Length in Aging Mice. *J. Gerontol. A Biol. Sci. Med. Sci.* **2018**, *73*, 446–449. [CrossRef]
195. Xu, H.; Liu, Y.Y.; Li, L.S.; Liu, Y.S. Sirtuins at the Crossroads between Mitochondrial Quality Control and Neurodegenerative Diseases: Structure, Regulation, Modifications, and Modulators. *Aging Dis.* **2023**, *14*, 794–824. [CrossRef]
196. Grabowska, W.; Sikora, E.; Bielak-Zmijewska, A. Sirtuins, a promising target in slowing down the ageing process. *Biogerontology* **2017**, *18*, 447–476. [CrossRef]
197. Chang, H.C.; Guarente, L. SIRT1 and other sirtuins in metabolism. *Trends Endocrinol. Metab.* **2014**, *25*, 138–145. [CrossRef]
198. Houtkooper, R.H.; Pirinen, E.; Auwerx, J. Sirtuins as regulators of metabolism and healthspan. *Nat. Rev. Mol. Cell Biol.* **2012**, *13*, 225–238. [CrossRef]
199. Watroba, M.; Dudek, I.; Skoda, M.; Stangret, A.; Rzodkiewicz, P.; Szukiewicz, D. Sirtuins, epigenetics and longevity. *Ageing Res. Rev.* **2017**, *40*, 11–19. [CrossRef]
200. Chen, C.; Zhou, M.; Ge, Y.; Wang, X. SIRT1 and aging related signaling pathways. *Mech. Ageing Dev.* **2020**, *187*, 111215. [CrossRef]
201. Abd Elwahab, A.H.; Ramadan, B.K.; Schaalan, M.F.; Tolba, A.M. A Novel Role of SIRT1/ FGF-21 in Taurine Protection Against Cafeteria Diet-Induced Steatohepatitis in Rats. *Cell. Physiol. Biochem.* **2017**, *43*, 644–659. [CrossRef] [PubMed]
202. Liu, J.; Ai, Y.; Niu, X.; Shang, F.; Li, Z.; Liu, H.; Li, W.; Ma, W.; Chen, R.; Wei, T.; et al. Taurine protects against cardiac dysfunction induced by pressure overload through SIRT1-p53 activation. *Chem. Biol. Interact.* **2020**, *317*, 108972. [CrossRef]
203. Sun, Q.; Hu, H.; Wang, W.; Jin, H.; Feng, G.; Jia, N. Taurine attenuates amyloid beta 1-42-induced mitochondrial dysfunction by activating of SIRT1 in SK-N-SH cells. *Biochem. Biophys. Res. Commun.* **2014**, *447*, 485–489. [CrossRef]
204. Chou, C.T.; Lin, W.F.; Kong, Z.L.; Chen, S.Y.; Hwang, D.F. Taurine prevented cell cycle arrest and restored neurotrophic gene expression in arsenite-treated SH-SY5Y cells. *Amino Acids* **2013**, *45*, 811–819. [CrossRef]
205. Brunet, A.; Goodell, M.A.; Rando, T.A. Ageing and rejuvenation of tissue stem cells and their niches. *Nat. Rev. Mol. Cell Biol.* **2023**, *24*, 45–62. [CrossRef] [PubMed]
206. Oh, J.; Lee, Y.D.; Wagers, A.J. Stem cell aging: Mechanisms, regulators and therapeutic opportunities. *Nat. Med.* **2014**, *20*, 870–880. [CrossRef] [PubMed]
207. Guo, J.; Huang, X.; Dou, L.; Yan, M.; Shen, T.; Tang, W.; Li, J. Aging and aging-related diseases: From molecular mechanisms to interventions and treatments. *Signal Transduct. Target. Ther.* **2022**, *7*, 391. [CrossRef]
208. Li, X.W.; Gao, H.Y.; Liu, J. The role of taurine in improving neural stem cells proliferation and differentiation. *Nutr. Neurosci.* **2017**, *20*, 409–415. [CrossRef]
209. Han, X.; Chesney, R.W. Knockdown of TauT expression impairs human embryonic kidney 293 cell development. *Adv. Exp. Med. Biol.* **2013**, *776*, 307–320. [CrossRef]
210. Huang, X.; Liu, J.; Wu, W.; Hu, P.; Wang, Q. Taurine enhances mouse cochlear neural stem cell transplantation via the cochlear lateral wall for replacement of degenerated spiral ganglion neurons via sonic hedgehog signaling pathway. *Cell Tissue Res.* **2019**, *378*, 49–57. [CrossRef]
211. Zhou, C.; Zhang, X.; Xu, L.; Wu, T.; Cui, L.; Xu, D. Taurine promotes human mesenchymal stem cells to differentiate into osteoblast through the ERK pathway. *Amino Acids* **2014**, *46*, 1673–1680. [CrossRef] [PubMed]
212. Gutierrez-Castaneda, N.E.; Gonzalez-Corona, J.; Griego, E.; Galvan, E.J.; Ochoa-de la Paz, L.D. Taurine Promotes Differentiation and Maturation of Neural Stem/Progenitor Cells from the Subventricular Zone via Activation of GABA(A) Receptors. *Neurochem. Res.* **2023**, *48*, 2206–2219. [CrossRef]
213. Hernandez-Benitez, R.; Ramos-Mandujano, G.; Pasantes-Morales, H. Taurine stimulates proliferation and promotes neurogenesis of mouse adult cultured neural stem/progenitor cells. *Stem Cell Res.* **2012**, *9*, 24–34. [CrossRef] [PubMed]

214. Yao, X.; Huang, H.; Li, Z.; Liu, X.; Fan, W.; Wang, X.; Sun, X.; Zhu, J.; Zhou, H.; Wei, H. Taurine Promotes the Cartilaginous Differentiation of Human Umbilical Cord-Derived Mesenchymal Stem Cells In Vitro. *Neurochem. Res.* **2017**, *42*, 2344–2353. [CrossRef]
215. Miyazaki, T.; Honda, A.; Ikegami, T.; Matsuzaki, Y. The role of taurine on skeletal muscle cell differentiation. *Adv. Exp. Med. Biol.* **2013**, *776*, 321–328. [CrossRef] [PubMed]
216. Elango, R. Tolerable Upper Intake Level for Individual Amino Acids in Humans: A Narrative Review of Recent Clinical Studies. *Adv. Nutr.* **2023**, *14*, 885–894. [CrossRef] [PubMed]
217. Garcia-Montero, C.; Fraile-Martinez, O.; Gomez-Lahoz, A.M.; Pekarek, L.; Castellanos, A.J.; Noguerales-Fraguas, F.; Coca, S.; Guijarro, L.G.; Garcia-Honduvilla, N.; Asunsolo, A.; et al. Nutritional Components in Western Diet Versus Mediterranean Diet at the Gut Microbiota-Immune System Interplay. Implications for Health and Disease. *Nutrients* **2021**, *13*, 699. [CrossRef] [PubMed]
218. Finicelli, M.; Di Salle, A.; Galderisi, U.; Peluso, G. The Mediterranean Diet: An Update of the Clinical Trials. *Nutrients* **2022**, *14*, 2956. [CrossRef]
219. Rana, S.K.; Sanders, T.A. Taurine concentrations in the diet, plasma, urine and breast milk of vegans compared with omnivores. *Br. J. Nutr.* **1986**, *56*, 17–27. [CrossRef]
220. Elshorbagy, A.; Jerneren, F.; Basta, M.; Basta, C.; Turner, C.; Khaled, M.; Refsum, H. Amino acid changes during transition to a vegan diet supplemented with fish in healthy humans. *Eur. J. Nutr.* **2017**, *56*, 1953–1962. [CrossRef]
221. Caine, J.J.; Geracioti, T.D. Taurine, energy drinks, and neuroendocrine effects. *Clevel. Clin. J. Med.* **2016**, *83*, 895–904. [CrossRef] [PubMed]
222. Stapleton, P.P.; Charles, R.P.; Redmond, H.P.; Bouchier-Hayes, D.J. Taurine and human nutrition. *Clin. Nutr.* **1997**, *16*, 103–108. [CrossRef] [PubMed]
223. Hwang, E.S.; Ki, K.N.; Chung, H.Y. Proximate composition, amino Acid, mineral, and heavy metal content of dried laver. *Prev Nutr. Food Sci.* **2013**, *18*, 139–144. [CrossRef]
224. Purchas, R.W.; Rutherfurd, S.M.; Pearce, P.D.; Vather, R.; Wilkinson, B.H. Concentrations in beef and lamb of taurine, carnosine, coenzyme Q_{10}, and creatine. *Meat Sci.* **2004**, *66*, 629–637. [CrossRef] [PubMed]
225. Zhao, X.; Li, Q.; Meng, Q.; Yue, C.; Xu, C. Identification and expression of cysteine sulfinate decarboxylase, possible regulation of taurine biosynthesis in Crassostrea gigas in response to low salinity. *Sci. Rep.* **2017**, *7*, 5505. [CrossRef]
226. Vidot, H.; Cvejic, E.; Carey, S.; Strasser, S.I.; McCaughan, G.W.; Allman-Farinelli, M.; Shackel, N.A. Randomised clinical trial: Oral taurine supplementation versus placebo reduces muscle cramps in patients with chronic liver disease. *Aliment. Pharmacol. Ther.* **2018**, *48*, 704–712. [CrossRef]
227. Hladun, O.; Papaseit, E.; Martin, S.; Barriocanal, A.M.; Poyatos, L.; Farre, M.; Perez-Mana, C. Interaction of Energy Drinks with Prescription Medication and Drugs of Abuse. *Pharmaceutics* **2021**, *13*, 491. [CrossRef]
228. Rubio, C.; Camara, M.; Giner, R.M.; Gonzalez-Munoz, M.J.; Lopez-Garcia, E.; Morales, F.J.; Moreno-Arribas, M.V.; Portillo, M.P.; Bethencourt, E. Caffeine, D-glucuronolactone and Taurine Content in Energy Drinks: Exposure and Risk Assessment. *Nutrients* **2022**, *14*, 5103. [CrossRef]
229. McBroom, M.J.; Welty, J.D. Comparison of taurine-verapamil interaction in hamsters and rats. *Comp. Biochem. Physiol. C Comp. Pharmacol. Toxicol.* **1985**, *80*, 217–219. [CrossRef]
230. Shao, A.; Hathcock, J.N. Risk assessment for the amino acids taurine, L-glutamine and L-arginine. *Regul. Toxicol. Pharmacol.* **2008**, *50*, 376–399. [CrossRef]

Disclaimer/Publisher's Note: The statements, opinions and data contained in all publications are solely those of the individual author(s) and contributor(s) and not of MDPI and/or the editor(s). MDPI and/or the editor(s) disclaim responsibility for any injury to people or property resulting from any ideas, methods, instructions or products referred to in the content.

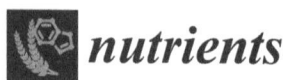

Article

Glucosamine Use Is Associated with a Higher Risk of Cardiovascular Diseases in Patients with Osteoarthritis: Results from a Large Study in 685,778 Subjects

Huan Yu [1], Junhui Wu [1,2], Hongbo Chen [1,2], Mengying Wang [1], Siyue Wang [1], Ruotong Yang [1], Siyan Zhan [1], Xueying Qin [1], Tao Wu [1], Yiqun Wu [1,*] and Yonghua Hu [1,3,*]

[1] Department of Epidemiology and Biostatistics, School of Public Health, Peking University Health Science Center, Beijing 100191, China
[2] School of Nursing, Peking University, No. 38 Xueyuan Road, Beijing 100191, China
[3] Medical Informatics Center, Peking University, Beijing 100191, China
* Correspondence: qywu118@163.com (Y.W.); yhhu@bjmu.edu.cn (Y.H.)

Abstract: Glucosamine is widely used around the world and as a popular dietary supplement and treatment in patients with osteoarthritis in China; however, the real-world cardiovascular risk of glucosamine in long-term use is still unclear. A retrospective, population-based cohort study was performed, based on the Beijing Medical Claim Data for Employees from 1 January 2010 to 31 December 2017. Patients newly diagnosed with osteoarthritis were selected and divided into glucosamine users and non-glucosamine users. The glucosamine users group was further divided into adherent, partially adherent, and non-adherent groups according to the medication adherence. New-onset cardiovascular diseases (CVD) events, coronary heart diseases (CHD), and stroke, were identified during the observational period. COX proportional regression models were used to estimate the risks. Of the 685,778 patients newly diagnosed with osteoarthritis including 240,419 glucosamine users and 445,359 non-users, the mean age was 56.49 (SD: 14.45) years and 59.35% were females. During a median follow-up of 6.13 years, 64,600 new-onset CVD, 26,530 CHD, and 17,832 stroke events occurred. Glucosamine usage was significantly associated with CVD (HR: 1.10; 95% CI: 1.08–1.11) and CHD (HR: 1.12; 95% CI: 1.09–1.15), but not with stroke (HR: 1.03; 95% CI: 0.99–1.06). The highest CVD risk was shown in the adherent group (HR: 1.68; 95% CI: 1.59–1.78), followed by the partially adherent group (HR: 1.26, 95% CI: 1.22–1.30), and the non-adherent group (HR: 1.03; 95% CI: 1.02–1.05), with a significant dose–response relationship (p-trend < 0.001). In this longitudinal study, adherent usage of glucosamine was significantly associated with a higher risk for cardiovascular diseases in patients with osteoarthritis.

Keywords: glucosamine; cardiovascular disease; osteoarthritis; epidemiology

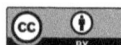

1. Introduction

Glucosamine is a nutritional supplement for joint cartilage, which is widely used for managing the symptoms of osteoarthritis [1,2] and is regularly consumed in approximately one-fifth of adults in the United States, Australia, and the United Kingdom [3–5]. Despite low potential toxicity reported in previous studies, the patients exposed to glucosamine experienced increased fasting blood glucose and reduced insulin sensitivity [6–9]. Biochemical studies have shown that glucosamine is an inhibitor of nitric oxide (NO) synthesis [10], which might affect microvascular remodeling and endothelial function regulation [11,12], and cause glucosamine a potential risk factor of cardiovascular disease. Since patients with osteoarthritis are at a high risk of cardiovascular disease [13–15], it is necessary to know whether glucosamine use in patients with osteoarthritis brings an additional risk for cardiovascular disease (CVD).

Previous randomized control trials focusing on evaluating the efficacy did not find excess cardiovascular risks of glucosamine compared with placebo or celecoxib in patients with osteoarthritis [16–20]. Nevertheless, these studies had a limited sample size and contained a follow-up period of no more than 2 years [16–20]. Recently, large cohort studies in the general population were designed to explore the association of habitual glucosamine use with the risk of CVD [5,21]. However, in these studies, the use of glucosamine was reported by participants without detailed records of the dosage and duration, and the association of glucosamine with cardiovascular events in patients with osteoarthritis is still unclear. Therefore, based on a comprehensive database with medication information from all hospitals, pharmacies, and medical facilities, we aimed to assess the association of glucosamine use with CVD in 685,778 patients with osteoarthritis in a real-world setting in Beijing, China.

2. Materials and Methods

2.1. Data Source

A retrospective cohort study was performed from 1 January 2010 to 31 December, based on the Beijing Medical Claim Data for Employees (BMCDE). The database was described elsewhere [22]. Briefly, it contained all of the medical and pharmacy records for about 20 million residents who enrolled in the urban employee basic medical insurance (UEBMI) program in Beijing. The UEBMI is basic medical insurance covering more than 92% of urban employees, workers, and retirees in China [23–25]. The BMCDE database includes sale information of drugs from all sources in Beijing, including all of the hospitals and retail pharmacies, and part of the data records from the database were manually validated by comparing with the original medical and pharmacy files. Demographic, diseases, and detailed medical information were derived from the database. All of the data were collected for administrative purposes without any personal identifiers. Therefore, this study was exempted from ethics committee review by the Ethics Committee of the Peking University Health Science Center.

2.2. Population

Of the 20.8 million residents enrolled in UEBMI, those who were newly diagnosed with osteoarthritis from 1 January 2010 to 31 December 2012, were selected. Then, the participants who newly started taking glucosamine within one year after diagnosis of osteoarthritis were considered as the exposure group (the distribution of period time from diagnosis of osteoarthritis to starting taking glucosamine is shown in Table S1), and those who never use glucosamine were used as the control group. A two-year wash-out period was used to identify the new patients with osteoarthritis and the new glucosamine users, which meant that the participants diagnosed with osteoarthritis or taking glucosamine within two years before baseline were excluded as old cases or former users. Newly diagnosed osteoarthritis was determined by the International Classification of Diseases (ICD)-10 code (M0–M2). To control potential bias caused by the disease course and to estimate the long-term effect of glucosamine on CVD, those under 18 years or with <1-year follow-up time were excluded in both the glucosamine group and non-glucosamine group. Missing data were defined as missing any of the covariates, and the participants with missing data were excluded.

2.3. Exposure, Outcome, and Covariates

Of 685,778 participants from 774,912 patients newly diagnosed with osteoarthritis, there were 240,419 who newly started taking glucosamine within one year after diagnosis of osteoarthritis, and 445,359 patients never took glucosamine, while 89,134 patients who started taking glucosamine more than one year after the diagnosis of osteoarthritis were excluded from the main analyses (Figure A1). To further compare the differences among the groups with different adherence, the glucosamine group was further classified into adherent, partially adherent, and non-adherent groups. The proportion of the days covered (PDC) was used to quantify the adherence of glucosamine, based on the dosage of prescription recorded in the database and the daily defined dose (DDD) [26,27]. The PDC was calculated as the proportion of days on which a person had an available supply of glucosamine, which represents the adherence to which a person continued to fill glucosamine prescriptions over time. According to PDC, those who used glucosamine were divided into three subgroups, including adherent (PDC $\geq$ 80%), partially adherent (20% $\leq$ PDC < 80%), and non-adherent (PDC < 20%) [26].

The incident CVD, coronary heart disease (CHD), and stroke events of the subjects were observed from the index date to 31 December 2017, which were identified by the primary diagnosis at each inpatient or outpatient encounter during the follow-up. Each participant had only one outcome in this study. The primary outcomes were overall cardiovascular diseases, with an ICD code of I00-I99. The secondary outcomes were CHD and stroke, with an ICD code of I20-I25 or I60-I64, respectively.

Several covariates were adjusted, including age, sex, hypertension, medication, Charlson Comorbidity Index (CCI), and health care utilization index (HCUI) at the baseline [28]. Hypertension was defined as diagnosis with an ICD-10 code of I10-I15 or having antihypertensive prescriptions before the index date. Medications included lipid treatment, antiplatelet treatment (including aspirin, clopidogrel, indobufen, ticagrelor, ticlopidine, prasugrel, and cangrelor), and NSAIDs' therapy (except aspirin and indobufen), which was determined using the pharmacy records before the index date. CCI is a weighted score categorizing and integrating comorbidities of patients based on the ICD diagnosis codes, including 19 comorbidities [29]. The higher scores indicated more comorbidities and poorer health status, and more details about CCI are shown in Table S2. HCUI was calculated as the frequency of hospital visits in the past 12 months before the index date. Moreover, considering the indication bias of adherence, we selected the PDC of antidiabetic drugs as a negative control adjusted in the sensitivity analysis. The PDC of antidiabetic drugs was calculated in the same way as that mentioned before.

2.4. Statistical Analysis

The normal continuous variables were performed by the mean (standard deviation, SD), non-normal continuous variables by the median (interquartile range, IQR), while the categorical variables were represented by the number (percentage). The baseline characteristics were compared between groups using ANOVA, Wilcoxon test, or χ^2 test. The index date was defined as the date of the first diagnosis of osteoarthritis in the non-glucosamine group, or the date when the patients first used glucosamine in the glucosamine group. The follow-up period was determined from the index date to the outcome occurrence or to 31 December 2017, which came first. The incidence rate of cardiovascular events was calculated and presented with 95% confidence intervals per 1000 person-years. The 95% CI of the incidence rate was calculated using the following formula:

$$95\% \text{ CI} = \text{the number of events/cumulative person-years} \\ \pm 1.96 \times \text{sqrt (the number of events)/cumulative person-years} \quad (1)$$

Hazard ratios (HRs) and 95% CIs were reported to estimate the risk of cardiovascular events using the Cox proportional regression model after adjusting for age, sex, hypertension, medication, CCI, and HCUI. Sex (female or male), hypertension, lipid treatment, antiplatelet treatment, and NSAIDs' therapy (yes or no) were analyzed as binary variables, while age, CCI, and HCUI were the continuous variables. Subgroup analysis stratified by age and sex in different adherence groups was then performed after adjusting for the other covariates.

Five sensitivity analyses were performed to prove our results. First, the 1:2 propensity score matching (PSM) within a caliper of 0.03 was conducted between the adherent glucosamine users and non-glucosamine users to reduce potential indication bias. The propensity scores for each participant between the groups were calculated using a logistic regression model including the index year and all of the covariates mentioned before.

The patients were matched according to the propensity score, and the association was then reported in the matched patients. Second, to avoid the indication bias caused by adherence, the PDC of antidiabetic drugs was additionally adjusted as a negative control on the original model, to reduce the potential confounding. Third, patients with lower than 2 years follow-up time were excluded to further explore the long-term effect of glucosamine. Fourth, we included all of the patients newly diagnosed with osteoarthritis whether or not they took glucosamine within one year. Fifth, to validate our results and test potential residual confounding due to the course of the disease, follow-up time was defined separately as the period from the diagnosis of osteoarthritis to the outcomes.

A two-tailed p value less than 0.05 was considered statistically significant. PSM was analyzed by the "MatchIt" package in R 3.6.3 with a caliper of 0.03. Otherwise, the statistical analyses were completed using SAS version 9.4.

3. Results

3.1. Characteristics of Study Population

A total of 685,778 participants with a new diagnosis of osteoarthritis were included in the main analysis. The average age was 56.49 (SD: 14.45) years, 59.35% were female, 21.20% presented with hypertension, 37.29% were undergoing lipid treatment, 27.74% were undergoing antiplatelet treatment, 29.67% were undergoing NSAIDs therapy, the mean of the CCI was 0.67 (SD: 0.91), and the median of HCUI was 21 (IQR: 6, 45). Among them, 240,419 subjects were glucosamine users and 445,359 were non-users, respectively. Table 1 shows the characteristics of study subjects according to their glucosamine-using status. When compared with non-users, the glucosamine users were older, more likely to be females, more likely to have hypertension, more likely to have lipid treatment or antiplatelet treatment, less likely to have NSAIDs therapy, had higher CCI, and had lower HCUI.

Table 1. Characteristics of the study population.

Characteristics	Glucosamine Non-Users (n = 445,359)	Glucosamine Users (n= 240,419)	p Value
Age, years, mean (SD)	55.44 (15.40)	58.43 (12.24)	<0.001
Female, n(%)	247,181 (55.50)	159,826 (66.48)	<0.001
Hypertension, n(%)	89,394 (20.07)	55,974 (23.28)	<0.001
Lipid treatment, n(%)	153,169 (34.39)	102,571 (42.66)	<0.001
Antiplatelet treatment [1], n(%)	113,118 (25.40)	77,084 (32.06)	<0.001
NSAIDs therapy [2], n(%)	140,099 (31.46)	63,387 (26.37)	<0.001
CCI, mean (SD)	0.65 (0.93)	0.71 (0.86)	<0.001
HCUI, median (IQR)	22 (7, 45)	20 (6, 45)	<0.001

NSAIDs, non-steroidal anti-inflammatory drug; CCI, Charlson Comorbidity Index; HCUI, health care utilization index; IQR, interquartile range. [1] Antiplatelet treatment included usage of aspirin, clopidogrel, indobufen, ticagrelor, ticlopidine, prasugrel, and cangrelor. [2] NSAIDs therapy here did not include aspirin and indobufen.

3.2. Incidence of CVD Events

The median follow-up time was 6.13 (IQR: 5.57–6.75) years overall, 6.15 (IQR: 5.61–6.81) for non-users, and 6.01 (IQR: 5.48–6.68) for glucosamine users. There were 64,600 new-onset CVD events, with an overall incidence rate of 15.61 (95% CI: 15.49–15.73) per 1000 person-years. There were 26,530 and 17,832 CHD and stroke events, with incidence rates of 6.25 (95% CI: 6.18–6.33) and 4.18 (95% CI: 4.12–4.24) per 1000 person-years, respectively. Compared with the non-users, the glucosamine users had significantly higher incidence rates of overall CVD events, CHD, but not stroke (Table 2). Among the glucosamine users with different adherence levels, a higher incidence was observed in the group with a higher adherence (Table S3).

Table 2. Incidence of cardiovascular disease events.

	Glucosamine Non-Users		Glucosamine Users		p Value [2]
	Number of Events	Incidence [1] (95% CI)	Number of Events	Incidence [1] (95% CI)	
Overall CVD	40,858	15.08 (14.93, 15.23)	23,742	16.63 (16.42, 16.84)	<0.001
CHD	16,686	6.01 (5.91, 6.10)	9844	6.72 (6.59, 6.85)	<0.001
Stroke	11,742	4.21 (4.13, 4.28)	6090	4.13 (4.03, 4.23)	0.57

CVD, cardiovascular disease; CHD, coronary heart disease; CI, confidence interval. [1] "Incidence" indicates crude incidence without adjusting for any covariates. [2] "p values" were calculated for the difference between incidences of two groups.

3.3. Association of Glucosamine with Cardiovascular Events

The association of glucosamine with cardiovascular events is shown in Figure 1 and model adjustment is shown in Table A1. Glucosamine usage was significantly associated with overall CVD (HR: 1.10, 95% CI: 1.08–1.11), CHD (HR: 1.12, 95% CI: 1.09–1.15) but not stroke (HR: 1.03, 95% CI: 0.99–1.06). The cardiovascular risks for glucosamine use with different adherence levels were further explored. The highest HR was observed in the adherent group for CVD (HR: 1.68, 95% CI: 1.59–1.78), CHD (HR: 1.69, 95% CI: 1.56–1.84), and stroke (HR: 1.53, 95% CI: 1.37–1.70) followed by the partially adherent group, then the non-adherent group, compared to non-users. A significant dose–response relationship was shown for glucosamine with CVD, CHD, and stroke events in all of the subjects (p-trend < 0.001 for each).

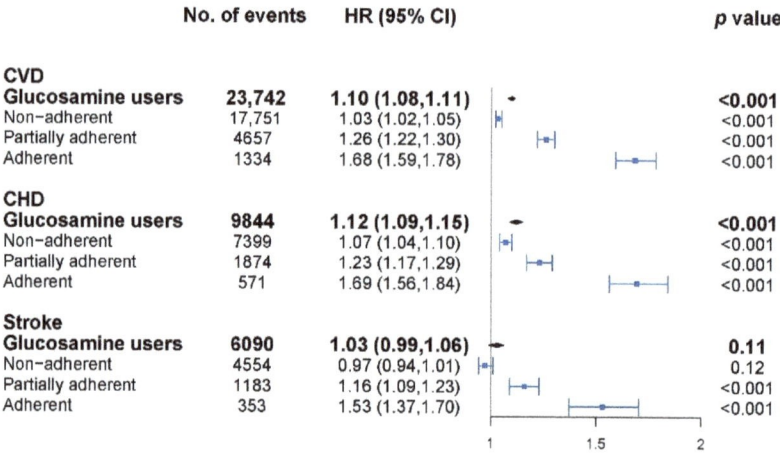

Figure 1. Association of glucosamine users with cardiovascular disease (CVD) at different adherence levels. CVD, cardiovascular disease; CHD, coronary heart disease; HR, hazard ratios; CI, confidence interval. HRs were calculated compared with glucosamine non-users, and were adjusted for age, sex, hypertension, medication, Charlson Comorbidity Index (CCI), and health care utilization index (HCUI). The dots indicate the HRs and the lines between bars represents the 95% confidence intervals.

The subgroup analysis for CVD is shown in Table S4. The similar trends among the glucosamine users with different adherence were found when stratified by sex or age (p for trend < 0.001 for each).

3.4. Sensitivity Analysis

After the 1:2 PSM, 8022 adherent glucosamine users and 16,043 matched glucosamine non-users were included, while one glucosamine user was matched to only one control due to the strict caliper. The baseline characteristics showed no significant difference (Table S5), and the adherent glucosamine use was still significantly associated with CVD,

CHD, and stroke (Table S6). The results were consistent with those in the main analysis when the PDC of antidiabetic drugs was additionally adjusted considering the indication bias (Table S7), or when patients with lower than 2 years follow-up time were excluded (Table S8). Among 774,912 patients newly diagnosed with osteoarthritis whether or not they took glucosamine within one year, the glucosamine use was significantly associated with CVD, CHD, and stroke with a significant trend for each (p for trend < 0.001) (Table S9). Lastly, to avoid potential confounding due to the course of disease, follow-up time was defined separately as the period from the diagnosis of osteoarthritis to the outcomes, and a significant association was also estimated for CVD, CHD, and stroke (Table S10)

4. Discussion

Despite several studies [5,21] that were conducted to evaluate the association of glucosamine with CVD risks in the general population, the association was still unclear in patients with osteoarthritis who were at a higher risk of cardiovascular events. In this retrospective cohort study, based on a comprehensive database with prescription information for nearly 0.7 million patients newly diagnosed with osteoarthritis, we assessed CVD, CHD, and stroke risks between glucosamine users and non-users in patients with osteoarthritis. According to the results, we found that glucosamine was significantly associated with a higher risk for CVD and CHD, especially in patients who had a higher adherence. Although no statistically significant association of glucosamine use with stroke was found, a 53% increase in the risk of stroke was estimated in adherent glucosamine users significantly. Taking glucosamine was already strongly recommended against in patients with osteoarthritis in America [1], and was given a weak recommendation in Europe [2] by Guidelines, due to its limited efficacy. The present study provides additional safety considerations for long-term glucosamine use for the guidelines.

Most importantly, this study provides new references for screening people at high risk of cardiovascular diseases in patients with osteoarthritis. The association of glucosamine usage and CVD risks among patients with osteoarthritis in previous studies was inconsistent. Several randomized clinical trials reported no significant association between glucosamine and CVD risks in patients with osteoarthritis [16–20], but the evidence was insufficient due to the lack of sample size and the short follow-up of no more than 2 years. The randomized clinical trials with a three-year follow-up found that there was no significant difference in the levels of blood pressure, lipids, and glucose between patients with osteoarthritis taking crystalline glucosamine sulfate and those with placebo [30], but these biochemical markers are not synonymous with cardiovascular events. Recently, two cohort studies reported habitual glucosamine users had a lower risk for CVD in general population [5,21]. However, patients with osteoarthritis were at higher risk for cardiovascular events [13–15], which had potentially mechanistic differences from general population. Meanwhile, another cohort study using the same database as the above two studies found that glucosamine use was associated with a lower incidence of type 2 diabetes in patients who initially were free of diabetes, cancer, or cardiovascular disease at baseline. However, again, these participants were rather healthy at baseline [31]. The results of those studies could not be directly extrapolated to those in patients with osteoarthritis, which might cause the main difference from our research. In the present research, the association was estimated by the patient-based design and the adjustment for comorbidities, medications, and health-care utilization. Moreover, a dose–response relationship between glucosamine and cardiovascular events was first found in this study, indicating that glucosamine use and its adherence are important when considering the risk for CVD in patients with osteoarthritis. Previous studies have not analyzed the association of glucosamine with cardiovascular events in terms of medication adherence. In this research, analyzing the different adherence groups separately rather than together helped to ensure the authenticity of the results. Although the relationship should be interpreted with caution due to the difference of characteristics among the groups, we performed multiple adjustments of covariates and subgroup/sensitivity analyses to minimize the differences, and our results were stable in all of the analyses.

Further research is still needed to determine the association. For specific cardiovascular disease, different effects of glucosamine were observed between CHD and stroke, which might indicate different biological and other aspects of different events.

A higher CVD risk in glucosamine users among the patients with osteoarthritis is also biologically plausible. First, previous studies showed that glucosamine may increase fasting blood glucose, accelerate atherosclerosis, and reduce insulin sensitivity [6–9,32–37], which have been widely identified as risk factors for cardiovascular diseases [38–41]. Second, glucosamine could inhibit the synthesis of nitric oxide (NO) [10]. As a protective signaling molecule, NO plays an important role in preventing atherosclerosis [42]. Suppression of NO might accelerate atherosclerosis.

This large population-based cohort study was based on comprehensive medical and pharmacy information for nearly 20 million residents in Beijing, China. During a median observational period of 6.13 years, the long-term CVD risks were assessed in patients using glucosamine with different adherence levels. Due to the comprehensive prescription-recording system, covering all of the pharmacy records from all of the hospitals and pharmacies, the glucosamine-taking frequency can be obtained in detail. Additionally, multiple sensitivity analyses were performed to validate the results. Although the huge number of participants showed a relatively low difference in outcome between groups with low p-values, we still found adherent glucosamine users had a 68% increase in risk for CVD compared with that in non-users. The results provide real-world evidence on the association of glucosamine use with CVD events and insights into screening individuals with a high CVD risk in patients with osteoarthritis based on a medical insurance database.

This study has several limitations. First, the participants in this research were all from Beijing, the capital city of China, who had a relatively high income and convenient medical services. The interpretation of the results should be cautious. Second, the adherence levels of glucosamine users were determined by the prescription dispensation. The dispensation did not necessarily indicate the actual drug consumption. However, any underestimation was likely to have been the same across groups, meaning that our results were conservative. Meanwhile, the dispensations outside the system could not be obtained, but the possibility was low. Third, the severity of osteoarthritis, BMI, physical activity, alcohol, and smoke status, etc. could not be obtained in our database, which was an inherent drawback of insurance database research and caused potential confounding. We could not rule out whether glucosamine users, especially those who used adherently, had more severe osteoarthritis, less physical activity, or a higher BMI, i.e., they were at a higher risk of CVD. However, in the sensitivity analysis of this study, our results were stable after matching covariates including hypertension, CCI, and HCUI, which were closely correlated with osteoarthritis severity, physical activity, and BMI at baseline. The relativity was helpful to reduce the potential confounding. Although some previous studies considered that the PSM was not the best matching method [43], our results still showed a high degree of consistency after matching. Meanwhile, in another sensitivity analysis, we adjusted PDC for antidiabetic drugs to reduce the potential bias due to the patients' health status and severity of osteoarthritis. Moreover, the genetic aspects affecting risk of CVD could not obtained in our database, but we considered them to be a nondifferential misclassification between the groups, which made the results more conservative. Further research is still needed to prove our results with more covariates. Furthermore, the CVD risk of the combination of glucosamine with other medication, such as chondroitin, is still needed to be explored in the future.

5. Conclusions

In this longitudinal study, adherent usage of glucosamine was significantly associated with a higher risk for CVD in patients with osteoarthritis. The results suggested that the risks and benefits of glucosamine need to be revisited. Considering the potential residual confounding, the findings should be interpreted cautiously.

Supplementary Materials: The following supporting information can be downloaded at: https://www.mdpi.com/article/10.3390/nu14183694/s1, Table S1: The distribution of period time from diagnosis of osteoarthritis to starting taking glucosamine; Table S2: The items and weights in Charlson Comorbidity Index (CCI); Table S3: Incidence of cardiovascular disease (CVD) events; Table S4: Association of glucosamine users with cardiovascular disease (CVD) in subgroups; Table S5: Characteristics of the study population after 1:2 propensity score matching; Table S6: Incidence of CVD events after 1:2 propensity score matching; Table S7: Association of glucosamine users with CVD adjusting for adherence of antidiabetic drugs; Table S8: Association of glucosamine users with CVD excluding patients with <2 years follow-up period; Table S9: Association of glucosamine users with CVD including all patients newly diagnosed with osteoarthritis; Table S10: Association of glucosamine users with CVD from the diagnosis of osteoarthritis to the outcomes.

Author Contributions: Conceptualization, H.Y., Y.W., and Y.H.; methodology, H.Y., J.W., H.C., and Y.W.; software, H.Y., M.W., S.W., and R.Y.; validation, S.Z., X.Q., T.W., Y.W., and Y.H.; formal analysis, H.Y., J.W., and Y.W.; investigation, X.Q., T.W., Y.W., and Y.H.; resources, Y.H.; data curation, Y.W. and Y.H.; writing—original draft preparation, H.Y.; writing—review and editing, S.Z., Y.W., and Y.H.; visualization, H.Y. and Y.W.; supervision, Y.H.; project administration, Y.H.; funding acquisition, X.Q., T.W., Y.W., and Y.H. All authors have read and agreed to the published version of the manuscript.

Funding: This research was funded by the National Natural Science Foundation of China, grant numbers 81872695, and 81972158.

Institutional Review Board Statement: This study was considered exempted from Institutional Review Board approval because this study was for administrative purposes and do not have any identifying personal information, such as full name and citizen's ID number.

Informed Consent Statement: Not applicable.

Data Availability Statement: Not applicable.

Conflicts of Interest: The authors declare no conflict of interest.

Appendix A

Table A1. Model adjustment of association between glucosamine use with cardiovascular disease (CVD).

Adjusted Covariates	HR (95% CI) for Glucosamine Use
None	1.11 (1.09, 1.13)
+Age	1.06 (1.04, 1.07)
+Sex	1.09 (1.08, 1.11)
+Hypertension	1.10 (1.08, 1.11)
+Lipid treatment	1.07 (1.05, 1.09)
+Antiplatelet treatment	1.06 (1.05, 1.08)
+NSAIDs therapy	1.06 (1.05, 1.08)
+CCI	1.09 (1.07, 1.10)
+HCUI (full model)	1.10 (1.08, 1.11)

NSAIDs, non-steroidal anti-inflammatory drug; CCI, Charlson Comorbidity Index; HCUI, health care utilization index; HR, hazard ratio; CI, confidence interval.

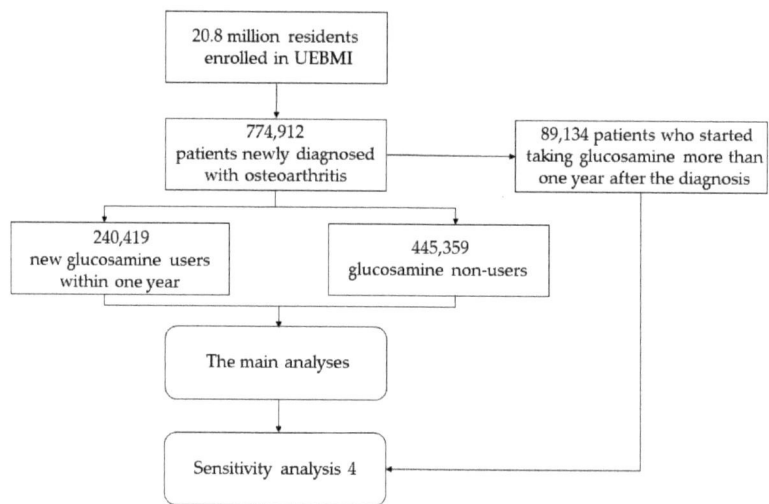

Figure A1. Flow chart of the study. UEBMI, urban employee basic medical insurance.

References

1. Kolasinski, S.L.; Neogi, T.; Hochberg, M.C.; Oatis, C.; Guyatt, G.; Block, J.; Callahan, L.; Copenhaver, C.; Dodge, C.; Felson, D.; et al. 2019 American College of Rheumatology/Arthritis Foundation Guideline for the Management of Osteoarthritis of the Hand, Hip, and Knee. *Arthritis Rheumatol.* **2020**, *72*, 220–233. [CrossRef]
2. Bruyère, O.; Honvo, G.; Veronese, N.; Arden, N.K.; Branco, J.; Curtis, E.M.; Al-Daghri, N.M.; Herrero-Beaumont, G.; Martel-Pelletier, J.; Pelletier, J.P.; et al. An updated algorithm recommendation for the management of knee osteoarthritis from the European Society for Clinical and Economic Aspects of Osteoporosis, Osteoarthritis and Musculoskeletal Diseases (ESCEO). *Semin. Arthritis Rheum.* **2019**, *49*, 337–350. [CrossRef]
3. Barnes, P.M.; Bloom, B.; Nahin, R.L. Complementary and alternative medicine use among adults and children: United States, 2007. *Natl. Health Stat. Rep.* **2008**, *10*, 1–23.
4. Sibbritt, D.; Adams, J.; Lui, C.W.; Broom, A.; Wardle, J. Who uses glucosamine and why? A study of 266,848 Australians aged 45 years and older. *PLoS ONE* **2012**, *7*, e41540. [CrossRef] [PubMed]
5. Ma, H.; Li, X.; Sun, D.; Zhou, T.; Ley, S.H.; Gustat, J.; Heianza, Y.; Qi, L. Association of habitual glucosamine use with risk of cardiovascular disease: Prospective study in UK Biobank. *BMJ* **2019**, *365*, l1628. [CrossRef] [PubMed]
6. Pham, T.; Cornea, A.; Blick, K.E.; Jenkins, A.; Scofield, R.H. Oral glucosamine in doses used to treat osteoarthritis worsens insulin resistance. *Am. J. Med. Sci.* **2007**, *333*, 333–339. [CrossRef]
7. Almada, A.; Harvey, P.; Platt, K. Effect of chronic oral glucosamine sulfate upon fasting insulin resistance index (FIRI) in non-diabetic individuals. *Faseb J.* **2000**, *14*, A750.
8. Monauni, T.; Zenti, M.G.; Cretti, A.; Daniels, M.C.; Targher, G.; Caruso, B.; Caputo, M.; McClain, D.; Del Prato, S.; Giaccari, A.; et al. Effects of glucosamine infusion on insulin secretion and insulin action in humans. *Diabetes* **2000**, *49*, 926–935. [CrossRef]
9. Biggee, B.A.; Blinn, C.M.; Nuite, M.; Silbert, J.E.; McAlindon, T.E. Effects of oral glucosamine sulphate on serum glucose and insulin during an oral glucose tolerance test of subjects with osteoarthritis. *Ann. Rheum. Dis.* **2007**, *66*, 260–262. [CrossRef]
10. Meininger, C.J.; Kelly, K.A.; Li, H.; Haynes, T.E.; Wu, G. Glucosamine inhibits inducible nitric oxide synthesis. *Biochem. Biophys. Res. Commun.* **2000**, *279*, 234–239. [CrossRef]
11. Numaguchi, K.; Egashira, K.; Takemoto, M.; Kadokami, T.; Shimokawa, H.; Sueishi, K.; Takeshita, A. Chronic inhibition of nitric oxide synthesis causes coronary microvascular remodeling in rats. *Hypertension* **1995**, *26*, 957–962. [CrossRef] [PubMed]
12. Toda, N. Age-related changes in endothelial function and blood flow regulation. *Pharmacol. Ther.* **2012**, *133*, 159–176. [CrossRef] [PubMed]
13. Kendzerska, T.; Jüni, P.; King, L.K.; Croxford, R.; Stanaitis, I.; Hawker, G.A. The longitudinal relationship between hand, hip and knee osteoarthritis and cardiovascular events: A population-based cohort study. *Osteoarthr. Cartil.* **2017**, *25*, 1771–1780. [CrossRef] [PubMed]
14. Schieir, O.; Tosevski, C.; Glazier, R.H.; Hogg-Johnson, S.; Badley, E.M. Incident myocardial infarction associated with major types of arthritis in the general population: A systematic review and meta-analysis. *Ann. Rheum. Dis.* **2017**, *76*, 1396–1404. [CrossRef]
15. Atiquzzaman, M.; Karim, M.E.; Kopec, J.; Wong, H.; Anis, A.H. Role of Nonsteroidal Antiinflammatory Drugs in the Association between Osteoarthritis and Cardiovascular Diseases: A Longitudinal Study. *Arthritis Rheumatol.* **2019**, *71*, 1835–1843. [CrossRef] [PubMed]

16. Clegg, D.O.; Reda, D.J.; Harris, C.L.; Klein, M.A.; O'Dell, J.R.; Hooper, M.M.; Bradley, J.D.; Bingham, C.O.; Weisman, M.H.; Jackson, C.G.; et al. Glucosamine, chondroitin sulfate, and the two in combination for painful knee osteoarthritis. *N. Engl. J. Med.* **2006**, *354*, 795–808. [CrossRef] [PubMed]
17. Hochberg, M.C.; Martel-Pelletier, J.; Monfort, J.; Möller, I.; Castillo, J.R.; Arden, N.; Berenbaum, F.; Blanco, F.J.; Conaghan, P.G.; Doménech, G.; et al. Combined chondroitin sulfate and glucosamine for painful knee osteoarthritis: A multicentre, randomised, double-blind, non-inferiority trial versus celecoxib. *Ann. Rheum. Dis.* **2016**, *75*, 37–44. [CrossRef]
18. Roman-Blas, J.A.; Castañeda, S.; Sánchez-Pernaute, O.; Largo, R.; Herrero-Beaumont, G. Combined Treatment with Chondroitin Sulfate and Glucosamine Sulfate Shows no Superiority over Placebo for Reduction of Joint Pain and Functional Impairment in Patients with Knee Osteoarthritis: A Six-Month Multicenter, Randomized, Double-Blind, Placebo-Controlled Clinical Trial. *Arthritis Rheumatol.* **2017**, *69*, 77–85. [CrossRef]
19. McAlindon, T.E.; LaValley, M.P.; Gulin, J.P.; Felson, D.T. Glucosamine and chondroitin for treatment of osteoarthritis: A systematic quality assessment and meta-analysis. *JAMA* **2000**, *283*, 1469–1475. [CrossRef]
20. Sawitzke, A.D.; Shi, H.; Finco, M.F.; Dunlop, D.D.; Harris, C.L.; Singer, N.G.; Bradley, J.D.; Silver, D.; Jackson, C.G.; Lane, N.E.; et al. Clinical efficacy and safety of glucosamine, chondroitin sulphate, their combination, celecoxib or placebo taken to treat osteoarthritis of the knee: 2-year results from GAIT. *Ann. Rheum. Dis.* **2010**, *69*, 1459–1464. [CrossRef]
21. Li, Z.H.; Gao, X.; Chung, V.C.; Zhong, W.F.; Fu, Q.; Lv, Y.B.; Wang, Z.H.; Shen, D.; Zhang, X.R.; Zhang, P.D.; et al. Associations of regular glucosamine use with all-cause and cause-specific mortality: A large prospective cohort study. *Ann. Rheum. Dis.* **2020**, *79*, 829–836. [CrossRef] [PubMed]
22. Wu, Y.; Yang, C.; Xi, H.; Zhang, Y.; Zhou, Z.; Hu, Y. Prescription of antibacterial agents for acute upper respiratory tract infections in Beijing, 2010–2012. *Eur. J. Clin. Pharmacol.* **2016**, *72*, 359–364. [CrossRef] [PubMed]
23. Tian, Y.; Liu, H.; Wu, Y.; Si, Y.; Song, J.; Cao, Y.; Li, M.; Wu, Y.; Wang, X.; Chen, L.; et al. Association between ambient fine particulate pollution and hospital admissions for cause specific cardiovascular disease: Time series study in 184 major Chinese cities. *BMJ* **2019**, *367*, l6572. [CrossRef] [PubMed]
24. Tian, Y.; Liu, H.; Si, Y.; Cao, Y.; Song, J.; Li, M.; Wu, Y.; Wang, X.; Xiang, X.; Juan, J.; et al. Association between temperature variability and daily hospital admissions for cause-specific cardiovascular disease in urban China: A national time-series study. *PLoS Med.* **2019**, *16*, e1002738. [CrossRef]
25. Yip, W.C.; Hsiao, W.C.; Chen, W.; Hu, S.; Ma, J.; Maynard, A. Early appraisal of China's huge and complex health-care reforms. *Lancet* **2012**, *379*, 833–842. [CrossRef]
26. Benner, J.S.; Glynn, R.J.; Mogun, H.; Neumann, P.J.; Weinstein, M.C.; Avorn, J. Long-term persistence in use of statin therapy in elderly patients. *JAMA* **2002**, *288*, 455–461. [CrossRef] [PubMed]
27. WHO Collaborating Centre for Drug Statistics Methodology. ATC/DDD Index 2022. Available online: https://www.whocc.no/atc_ddd_index/ (accessed on 14 June 2022).
28. Xie, J.; Strauss, V.Y.; Martinez-Laguna, D.; Carbonell-Abella, C.; Diez-Perez, A.; Nogues, X.; Collins, G.S.; Khalid, S.; Delmestri, A.; Turkiewicz, A.; et al. Association of Tramadol vs Codeine Prescription Dispensation with Mortality and Other Adverse Clinical Outcomes. *JAMA* **2021**, *326*, 1504–1515. [CrossRef] [PubMed]
29. Charlson, M.E.; Carrozzino, D.; Guidi, J.; Patierno, C. Charlson Comorbidity Index: A Critical Review of Clinimetric Properties. *Psychother. Psychosom.* **2022**, *91*, 8–35. [CrossRef]
30. Palma Dos Reis, R.; Giacovelli, G.; Girolami, F.; André, R.; Bonazzi, A.; Rovati, L.C. Crystalline glucosamine sulfate in the treatment of osteoarthritis: Evidence of long-term cardiovascular safety from clinical trials. *Open Rheumatol. J.* **2011**, *5*, 69–77. [CrossRef]
31. Ma, H.; Li, X.; Zhou, T.; Sun, D.; Liang, Z.; Li, Y.; Heianza, Y.; Qi, L. Glucosamine Use, Inflammation, and Genetic Susceptibility, and Incidence of Type 2 Diabetes: A Prospective Study in UK Biobank. *Diabetes Care* **2020**, *43*, 719–725. [CrossRef]
32. Traxinger, R.R.; Marshall, S. Coordinated regulation of glutamine:fructose-6-phosphate amidotransferase activity by insulin, glucose, and glutamine. Role of hexosamine biosynthesis in enzyme regulation. *J. Biol. Chem.* **1991**, *266*, 10148–10154. [CrossRef]
33. Marshall, S.; Bacote, V.; Traxinger, R.R. Discovery of a metabolic pathway mediating glucose-induced desensitization of the glucose transport system. Role of hexosamine biosynthesis in the induction of insulin resistance. *J. Biol. Chem.* **1991**, *266*, 4706–4712. [CrossRef]
34. Baron, A.D.; Zhu, J.S.; Zhu, J.H.; Weldon, H.; Maianu, L.; Garvey, W.T. Glucosamine induces insulin resistance in vivo by affecting GLUT 4 translocation in skeletal muscle. Implications for glucose toxicity. *J. Clin. Investig.* **1995**, *96*, 2792–2801. [CrossRef] [PubMed]
35. Kim, Y.B.; Zhu, J.S.; Zierath, J.R.; Shen, H.Q.; Baron, A.D.; Kahn, B.B. Glucosamine infusion in rats rapidly impairs insulin stimulation of phosphoinositide 3-kinase but does not alter activation of Akt/protein kinase B in skeletal muscle. *Diabetes* **1999**, *48*, 310–320. [CrossRef] [PubMed]
36. Patti, M.E.; Virkamäki, A.; Landaker, E.J.; Kahn, C.R.; Yki-Järvinen, H. Activation of the hexosamine pathway by glucosamine in vivo induces insulin resistance of early postreceptor insulin signaling events in skeletal muscle. *Diabetes* **1999**, *48*, 1562–1571. [CrossRef]
37. Werstuck, G.H.; Khan, M.I.; Femia, G.; Kim, A.J.; Tedesco, V.; Trigatti, B.; Shi, Y. Glucosamine-induced endoplasmic reticulum dysfunction is associated with accelerated atherosclerosis in a hyperglycemic mouse model. *Diabetes* **2006**, *55*, 93–101. [CrossRef]

38. Haffner, S.M. Pre-diabetes, insulin resistance, inflammation and CVD risk. *Diabetes Res. Clin. Pract.* **2003**, *61* (Suppl. 1), S9–S18. [CrossRef]
39. Caccamo, G.; Bonura, F.; Bonura, F.; Vitale, G.; Novo, G.; Evola, S.; Evola, G.; Grisanti, M.R.; Novo, S. Insulin resistance and acute coronary syndrome. *Atherosclerosis* **2010**, *211*, 672–675. [CrossRef]
40. Effoe, V.S.; Wagenknecht, L.E.; Echouffo Tcheugui, J.B.; Chen, H.; Joseph, J.J.; Kalyani, R.R.; Bell, R.A.; Wu, W.H.; Casanova, R.; Bertoni, A.G. Sex Differences in the Association between Insulin Resistance and Incident Coronary Heart Disease and Stroke Among Blacks without Diabetes Mellitus: The Jackson Heart Study. *J. Am. Heart Assoc.* **2017**, *6*, e004229. [CrossRef]
41. Kernan, W.N.; Inzucchi, S.E.; Viscoli, C.M.; Brass, L.M.; Bravata, D.M.; Horwitz, R.I. Insulin resistance and risk for stroke. *Neurology* **2002**, *59*, 809–815. [CrossRef]
42. Balarini, C.M.; Leal, M.A.; Gomes, I.B.; Pereira, T.M.; Gava, A.L.; Meyrelles, S.S.; Vasquez, E.C. Sildenafil restores endothelial function in the apolipoprotein E knockout mouse. *J. Transl. Med.* **2013**, *11*, 3. [CrossRef] [PubMed]
43. King, G.; Nielsen, R.J.P.A. Why Propensity Scores Should Not Be Used for Matching. *Political Anal.* **2019**, *27*, 1–20. [CrossRef]

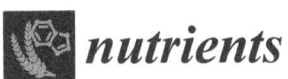

Article

Effects of L-Arginine Plus Vitamin C Supplementation on Physical Performance, Endothelial Function, and Persistent Fatigue in Adults with Long COVID: A Single-Blind Randomized Controlled Trial

Matteo Tosato [1], Riccardo Calvani [1,*], Anna Picca [1,2], Francesca Ciciarello [1], Vincenzo Galluzzo [1], Hélio José Coelho-Júnior [1,3], Angela Di Giorgio [1], Clara Di Mario [4], Jacopo Gervasoni [1], Elisa Gremese [1,3,4], Paolo Maria Leone [1], Antonio Nesci [1], Anna Maria Paglionico [1], Angelo Santoliquido [1,5], Luca Santoro [1], Lavinia Santucci [6], Barbara Tolusso [4], Andrea Urbani [1,7], Federico Marini [8], Emanuele Marzetti [1,3] and Francesco Landi [1,3] on behalf of the Gemelli against COVID-19 Post-Acute Care Team

1. Fondazione Policlinico Universitario A. Gemelli IRCCS, 00168 Rome, Italy
2. Department of Medicine and Surgery, LUM University, 70010 Casamassima, Italy
3. Department of Geriatrics and Orthopedics, Università Cattolica del Sacro Cuore, 00168 Rome, Italy
4. Immunology Core Facility, Gemelli Science Technological Park (GSTeP), Fondazione Policlinico Universitario A. Gemelli IRCCS, 00168 Rome, Italy
5. Department of Cardiovascular Sciences, Università Cattolica del Sacro Cuore, 00168 Rome, Italy
6. Metabolomics Research Core Facility, Gemelli Science and Technology Park (GSTeP), Fondazione Policlinico Universitario A. Gemelli IRCCS, 00168 Rome, Italy
7. Department of Biochemistry and Clinical Biochemistry, Università Cattolica del Sacro Cuore, 00168 Rome, Italy
8. Department of Chemistry, Sapienza University of Rome, 00185 Rome, Italy
* Correspondence: riccardo.calvani@policlinicogemelli.it; Tel.: +39-(06)-3015-5559

Citation: Tosato, M.; Calvani, R.; Picca, A.; Ciciarello, F.; Galluzzo, V.; Coelho-Júnior, H.J.; Di Giorgio, A.; Di Mario, C.; Gervasoni, J.; Gremese, E.; et al. Effects of L-Arginine Plus Vitamin C Supplementation on Physical Performance, Endothelial Function, and Persistent Fatigue in Adults with Long COVID: A Single-Blind Randomized Controlled Trial. *Nutrients* 2022, *14*, 4984. https://doi.org/10.3390/nu14234984

Academic Editors: Bruno Trimarco and Gaetano Santulli

Received: 13 September 2022
Accepted: 20 November 2022
Published: 23 November 2022

Publisher's Note: MDPI stays neutral with regard to jurisdictional claims in published maps and institutional affiliations.

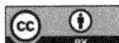

Copyright: © 2022 by the authors. Licensee MDPI, Basel, Switzerland. This article is an open access article distributed under the terms and conditions of the Creative Commons Attribution (CC BY) license (https://creativecommons.org/licenses/by/4.0/).

Abstract: Long COVID, a condition characterized by symptom and/or sign persistence following an acute COVID-19 episode, is associated with reduced physical performance and endothelial dysfunction. Supplementation of L-arginine may improve endothelial and muscle function by stimulating nitric oxide synthesis. A single-blind randomized, placebo-controlled trial was conducted in adults aged between 20 and 60 years with persistent fatigue attending a post-acute COVID-19 outpatient clinic. Participants were randomized 1:1 to receive twice-daily orally either a combination of 1.66 g L-arginine plus 500 mg liposomal vitamin C or a placebo for 28 days. The primary outcome was the distance walked on the 6 min walk test. Secondary outcomes were handgrip strength, flow-mediated dilation, and fatigue persistence. Fifty participants were randomized to receive either L-arginine plus vitamin C or a placebo. Forty-six participants (median (interquartile range) age 51 (14), 30 [65%] women), 23 per group, received the intervention to which they were allocated and completed the study. At 28 days, L-arginine plus vitamin C increased the 6 min walk distance (+30 (40.5) m; placebo: +0 (75) m, $p = 0.001$) and induced a greater improvement in handgrip strength (+3.4 (7.5) kg) compared with the placebo (+1 (6.6) kg, $p = 0.03$). The flow-mediated dilation was greater in the active group than in the placebo (14.3% (7.3) vs. 9.4% (5.8), $p = 0.03$). At 28 days, fatigue was reported by two participants in the active group (8.7%) and 21 in the placebo group (80.1%; $p < 0.0001$). L-arginine plus vitamin C supplementation improved walking performance, muscle strength, endothelial function, and fatigue in adults with long COVID. This supplement may, therefore, be considered to restore physical performance and relieve persistent symptoms in this patient population.

Keywords: post-acute COVID-19 syndrome; SARS-CoV-2; 6 min walk test; handgrip strength; flow-mediated dilation; nitric oxide; nutraceuticals; oral supplement; persistent symptoms

1. Introduction

A large share of COVID-19 survivors reports long-lasting clinical sequelae weeks or months after symptom onset: a condition known as post-acute COVID-19 syndrome or long COVID [1,2]. Long COVID encompasses a constellation of respiratory, cardiovascular, gastrointestinal, and neurological signs and symptoms, such as dyspnea, fatigue, dysrhythmias, heartburn, and memory and attention difficulties ("brain fog"), with a substantial impact on quality of life [3,4]. Long COVID is also associated with reduced physical function, which may hamper the complete resumption of pre-infection daily activities [5,6]. Several processes are currently being investigated for their involvement in the pathophysiology of long COVID, including viral persistence, chronic inflammation, autoimmunity, perturbation in metabolic and redox homeostasis, and endothelial dysfunction [7,8]. The heterogeneity of clinical manifestations of long COVID has hampered the devising of specific treatments for the condition, such that its management is mostly based on symptomatic treatments and healthy lifestyle recommendations.

Several nutritional supplements and bioactive foods are being investigated to counteract long COVID [9]. L-arginine is a key regulator of immune, respiratory, and endothelial function [10,11]. Its pleiotropic properties are regulated by two main metabolizing enzymes, nitric oxide (NO) synthase and arginase [12]. The flux of L-arginine towards NO synthesis is associated with beneficial effects on immune and vascular health, while its catabolism to ornithine by arginase has been associated with an abnormal immune response and endothelial dysfunction [13,14]. Accumulating evidence indicates that L-arginine metabolism is altered in patients with COVID-19 [10,11]. During acute COVID-19, the upregulation of arginase activity reduces the circulating levels of L-arginine and shifts its metabolism away from NO production to induce immune and endothelial dysfunction, inflammation, and thrombosis, which ultimately lead to vascular occlusion and multiorgan failure [11]. Indeed, lower plasma levels of L-arginine and higher arginase activity have been found both in patients with COVID-19 and in children with the multisystem inflammatory syndrome (MIS-C) compared with healthy controls [15]. A decrease in plasma L-arginine levels has also been described in acute COVID-19 and is associated with the expansion of myeloid-derived suppressor cells and impaired T-cell proliferation, two cardinal inflammatory features of severe disease [16,17].

Based on these observations, strategies to restore circulating levels of L-arginine and increase NO bioavailability have been proposed to counteract immune, respiratory, and vascular complications of COVID-19 [11,18]. Vitamin C may support the beneficial effects of L-arginine on endothelial function by increasing intracellular tetrahydrobiopterin, a co-factor needed for the oxidation of L-arginine to NO, in endothelial cells [12,19]. In vitro, L-arginine supplementation restores the proliferative capacity of T-cells obtained from patients with acute respiratory distress syndrome during COVID-19 [17]. Furthermore, oral L-arginine supplementation has been shown to reduce the need for respiratory support and the length of hospital stay in patients with severe COVID-19 [20]. Finally, oral supplementation with L-arginine plus vitamin C reduced the burden of persisting symptoms and ameliorated perceived exertion in a large cohort of patients with long COVID [21].

Previous studies have shown that L-arginine supplementation improves respiratory function and exercise tolerance in patients with pulmonary diseases [22] and in those with congestive heart failure [23] as well as in heart transplant recipients [24]. In addition, supplementation with L-arginine may increase aerobic and anaerobic performance in healthy adults, especially in untrained individuals [25,26]. However, other studies found no effects of L-arginine supplementation on human performance [27,28].

To further explore the potential benefits of L-arginine supplementation on COVID-19 outcomes, we conducted a single-blind randomized controlled trial to assess the effects of a 28-day oral supplementation with L-arginine plus vitamin C on physical performance, muscle strength, endothelial function, fatigue persistence, and systemic L-arginine bioavailability in adults with long COVID.

2. Materials and Methods

2.1. Study Design and Participants

This was a single-center, single-blind, placebo-controlled randomized clinical trial that was conducted at the post-acute COVID-19 outpatient clinic of the Fondazione Policlinico A. Gemelli IRCCS (Rome, Italy) [29] from 1 July 2021 to 30 April 30, 2022. The study protocol was approved by the institutional ethics committee (prot. no. 0013008/20). Written informed consent was collected from all participants prior to enrolment. The trial was conducted in accordance with the guidelines of the International Council for Harmonization of Technical Requirements for Pharmaceuticals for Human Use Good Clinical Practice and the principles of the Declaration of Helsinki. The trial was registered on ClinicalTrials.gov (NCT04947488).

Eligible participants were men and women aged between 20 and 60 years who met the following criteria: (a) previous confirmed SARS-CoV-2 infection, certified by a positive RT–PCR molecular swab test; (b) a negative COVID-19 swab test at least four weeks prior to the start of trial operations; (c) long COVID diagnosis according to the World Health Organization criteria [30]; and (d) persistent fatigue, operationalized as the response "most or all the time" to item seven of the Center for Epidemiological Studies Depression Scale ("I felt that everything I did was an effort") [31]. The main exclusion criteria were intolerance to either supplement ingredient (i.e., L-arginine and vitamin C), conditions and/or therapies that may interfere with trial outcomes and procedures (e.g., pregnancy or breastfeeding, chronic pulmonary disease, diabetes, use of antihypertensive drugs, steroids, or non-steroidal anti-inflammatory drugs, immunosuppressants, nitrates), and engagement in other intervention trials for long COVID.

Eligible participants were randomized using a random number generator in a 1:1 ratio to receive a twice-daily oral supplementation with either a combination of 1.66 g L-arginine plus 500 mg liposomal vitamin C (Bioarginina® C, Farmaceutici Damor, Naples, Italy) or a placebo for 28 days. Vials containing the active supplement or the placebo were supplied by Farmaceutici Damor and were made to be indistinguishable in appearance.

The primary endpoint was the change from baseline to day 28 in the distance walked on the 6 min walk test. The secondary endpoints were changes from baseline to day 28 in handgrip strength and flow-mediated dilation, and fatigue persistence through day 28. Serum L-arginine levels were measured before the intervention and at 28 days. Participants were asked to refrain from exercising and consuming any vasoactive products (e.g., tobacco, caffeinated drinks) for at least 12 h prior to the assessment of physical performance, muscle strength, endothelial function, and blood draw. The last consumption of the supplements occurred the evening before the tests. Outcome assessors were unaware of the group assignment. Adverse events were recorded and compared between the intervention groups.

2.2. Anthropometric and Clinical Data

Body height and weight were measured through a standard stadiometer and an analog medical scale, respectively. Body mass index (BMI, kg/m^2) was calculated as the ratio between the weight and the square of height. The severity of the acute COVID-19 episode was categorized as follows: (a) no hospitalization, (b) hospitalization, and (c) intensive care unit (ICU) admission. The time from COVID-19 diagnosis to the study inclusion was calculated based on self-report.

2.3. Measurement of Serum L-Arginine Concentration

Blood samples were collected at the baseline and after 28 days of intervention. Blood was drawn after overnight fasting using standard collection tubes (BD Vacutainer®; Becton, Dickinson and Co., Franklin Lakes, NJ, USA). Samples were left at room temperature for 30 min and were then centrifuged at $1000\times g$ for 10 min at 4 °C. Serum aliquots were stored at −80 °C until analysis. Serum samples from 20 age- and sex-matched blood donors without evidence of previous SARS-CoV-2 infection were collected and used as a "healthy" reference. Serum L-arginine levels were determined using an in-house validated liquid chromatography with tandem mass spectrometry method [32]. The chromatographic separation was performed with an ACQUITY UPLC I-Class System (Waters, Milford, MA, USA) using a HILIC column. Analyte detection was accomplished with a triple quadrupole Xevo-TQs Micro (Waters) equipped with an electrospray ion source operating in positive ion mode. A multiple reaction monitoring experiment was optimized for the detection and quantification of L-arginine.

2.4. Primary Outcome

The primary outcome measure was the distance walked on the 6 min walk test [33]. The test is a valid and easy-to-perform measure of exercise capacity in people with chronic lung disease and is increasingly being used to assess the sequelae of COVID-19 [34]. All participants completed the test at baseline and after 28 days of intervention. The test was performed on a 20 m-long indoor hallway, with markers placed at each end of the track, as previously described [35]. The total distance walked in 6 min was recorded in meters.

2.5. Secondary Outcomes

All secondary outcome measures were collected at baseline and after 28 days of intervention.

Muscle strength was assessed by handgrip strength testing [36] using a hydraulic hand-held dynamometer (North Coast Medical, Inc., Morgan Hill, CA, USA) according to international standard protocols, as detailed elsewhere [37]. Briefly, the participant was requested to sit on a standard chair, with the elbow near the trunk and bent at 90°, the hand in a neutral position, with the thumb pointing upwards. The measure was obtained after participants performed one familiarization trial with both hands. The highest reading (reported in kg) out of three trials was used for the analysis. Handgrip strength values at the baseline and post-intervention were compared with age- and sex-specific reference values [37].

The endothelial function was assessed non-invasively by measuring the brachial artery dilation following a transient period of forearm ischemia (flow-mediated dilation test) [38]. Flow-mediated dilation was measured by Doppler ultrasonography, using an iU22 2D ultrasound system (Philips Electronics, Amsterdam, The Netherlands) according to standard protocols [38,39], as described elsewhere [40]. In brief, the diameter of the brachial artery was measured at baseline and after the abrupt release of a blood pressure cuff that arrested the forearm circulation (by applying a pressure of 250 mmHg for 5 min). Flow-mediated dilation, which is mainly mediated by NO, was expressed as the percent increase in the arterial diameter following cuff release compared with the baseline diameter.

The persistence of fatigue was operationalized as the response "most or all the time" to item seven of the Center for Epidemiological Studies Depression Scale (CES-D, "I felt that everything I did was an effort") [31]. This operationalization of fatigue is commonly used in studies on physical frailty [41]. Furthermore, item seven of the CES-D was shown to be more related to fatigue than to depression [42].

2.6. Statistical Analysis

For the estimation of the sample size, we used reference values for the 6 min walk test in healthy adults published by Chetta et al. [43]. A sample size of 42 participants, 21 per intervention arm, was estimated to provide 80% power to detect a between-group difference of at least 35 m on the 6 min walk test, considering a standard deviation of 50 m and an alpha level of 5%. The recruitment target was increased to 50 participants (25 per group) to account for a 20% dropout rate. The 35 m cut-point was chosen as it corresponds to the minimal clinically important difference for the test [44].

The normal distribution of data were assessed via the Shapiro–Wilk test. Anthropometric, clinical, and functional characteristics of the study participants were reported as the median (interquartile range, IQR) for continuous variables and as absolute values (percentages) for categorical variables. Changes from baseline for continuous variables were expressed as deltas (values at 28 days minus the values at baseline), and differences between the intervention groups were evaluated using the Student's *t*-test for normally distributed variables or the Mann–Whitney U test for skewed variables. Mean differences and effect size values (Cohen's d for Student's *t*-test and rank biserial correlation for Mann–Whitney U test) were reported. Chi-squared or Fisher tests were used to assess differences between groups in categorical variables. Analyses of intervention effects were based on the intention-to-treat principle. All tests were two-sided with a statistical significance set at $p < 0.05$. All analyses were performed using Jamovi freeware version 2.0.0.0 (The Jamovi project, 2021; retrieved from https://www.jamovi.org; accessed on 19 July 2021).

Multivariate classification models, based on partial least squares discriminant analysis (PLS–DA) [45], were built and validated by double cross-validation [46] to gain a more comprehensive appraisal of the effects of interventions on the variables of interest. The potential influence of confounding factors (i.e., age and sex) was also evaluated. Multivariate analyses were performed using in-house routines running under the MATLAB R2015b environment (The MathWorks, Natick, MA, USA) and are detailed in Supplementary Material.

3. Results

Out of 94 candidate participants screened, 50 (53.2%) met the inclusion criteria and agreed to be randomized to receive either the L-arginine plus vitamin C (n = 25) or placebo (n = 25) intervention. Two participants in each group withdrew their consent before receiving the allocated intervention and were not included in the analysis (Figure 1).

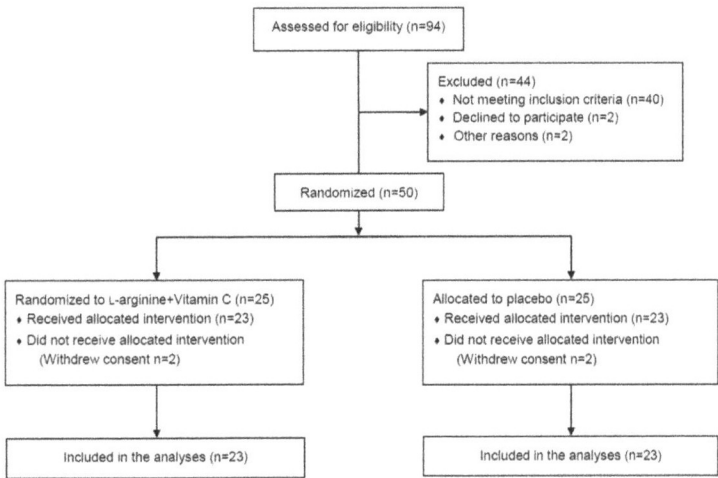

Figure 1. CONSORT diagram of participant flow through the study.

The anthropometric, clinical, and functional characteristics of the study participants at baseline were comparable between the intervention groups (Table 1).

Participants had a median (IQR) age of 50.5 (14.0) years and were predominantly women (65.2%). Approximately half of the participants needed hospitalization during the acute COVID-19 episode, and four (8.7%) were admitted to ICU. The median (IQR) time that elapsed from COVID-19 diagnosis to inclusion in the study was 254.0 (136.5) days. The median (IQR) distance walked on the 6 min walk test was 520 (90) m, while the handgrip strength was 22.6 (14.4) kg. Flow-mediated dilation at baseline was 9.8%. The median (IQR) serum L-arginine concentration was 170.6 (88.0) μM, with no differences between the intervention groups. However, serum L-arginine values were lower than those observed in the sample without evidence of previous SARS-CoV-2 infection (median

(IQR) 222.1 (23.1) µM; $p = 0.04$). At 28 days, serum L-arginine concentrations increased more in the participants who received L-arginine plus vitamin C supplementation (+60.2 (85.8) µM) than in the placebo group (+11.0 (90.8) µM; $p = 0.02$; mean difference 62.4 µM, 95% confidence interval (CI): 11.1–113.7 µM; effect size = 0.72) (Figure 2). After 28 days of L-arginine plus vitamin C supplementation, serum L-arginine levels in the active group (222.8 (88.6) µM) were comparable to those of the controls with no previous SARS-CoV-2 infection ($p = 0.8$).

Table 1. Baseline characteristics of study participants.

Characteristic	L-Arginine + Vitamin C ($n = 23$)	Placebo ($n = 23$)	Total ($n = 46$)
Age, years	50.0 (16.5)	51.0 (11.0)	50.5 (14.0)
Women, n (%)	15 (65.2)	15 (65.2)	30 (65.2)
BMI, kg/m^2	24.8 (5.9)	25.5 (6.5)	25.0 (6.5)
Severity of acute COVID-19, n (%)			
No hospitalization	8 (34.8)	12 (52.2)	20 (43.5)
Hospitalization	13 (56.5)	9 (39.1)	22 (47.8)
ICU admission	2 (8.7)	2 (8.7)	4 (8.7)
Time from COVID-19 diagnosis, days	240.0 (118.5)	269.0 (127.0)	254.0 (136.5)
6 min walk test distance, m	520.0 (49.5)	540.0 (120.0)	520.0 (90.0)
Handgrip, kg	22.5 (16.0)	22.6 (12.3)	22.6 (14.4)
Flow-mediated dilation, %	10.5 (5.2)	8.9 (5.8)	9.8 (6.0)
Serum L-arginine, µM	167.2 (76.8)	175.0 (93.1)	170.6 (88.0)

Abbreviations: BMI, body mass index; ICU, intensive care unit. Data are expressed as median (interquartile range) for continuous variables and number (percent) for categorical variables.

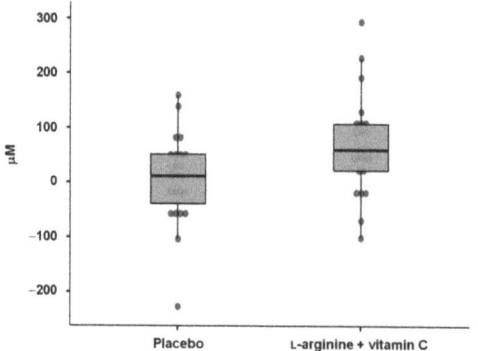

Figure 2. Changes from baseline to day 28 in serum L-arginine levels in the two intervention groups.

L-arginine plus vitamin C supplementation was safe and well tolerated, and no adverse events were recorded.

Efficacy Endpoints

L-arginine plus vitamin C significantly increased the distance walked on the 6 min walk test (median (IQR) change from baseline: +30.0 (40.5) m) compared with the placebo (+0.0 (75.0) m; $p = 0.001$; mean difference = 50 m, 95% CI: 20.0–80.0 m; effect size = 0.56) (Figure 3).

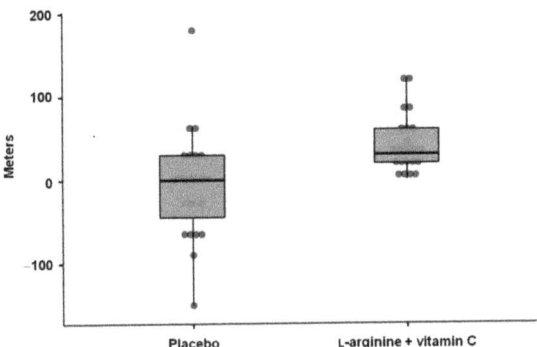

Figure 3. Changes from baseline to day 28 in the 6 min walk test distance in the two intervention groups.

At 28 days, L-arginine plus vitamin C supplementation induced greater improvements in handgrip strength (+3.4 (7.5) kg) compared with the placebo (+1.0 (6.6) kg, $p = 0.03$; mean difference = 3.4 kg, 95% CI: 0.5–9.4 kg; effect size = 0.37) (Figure 4A). At baseline, around 60% of the study participants had a handgrip strength below the 25th percentile of age- and sex-specific reference values [37]. After 28 days of intervention, more participants who received L-arginine plus vitamin C than those in the placebo group (57% vs. 30%) were above the first quartile of handgrip strength reference values [37], although the difference between the groups did not reach the statistical significance ($p = 0.07$).

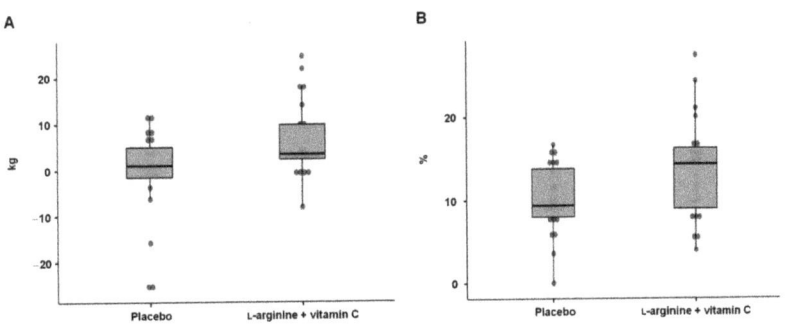

Figure 4. Changes from baseline to day 28 in (**A**) handgrip strength and (**B**) flow-mediated dilation in the two intervention groups.

Flow-mediated dilation was greater in participants who received L-arginine plus vitamin C compared with the placebo (14.3% (7.3) vs. 9.4% (5.8), $p = 0.03$; mean difference = 3.4%; 95% CI: 0.4–6.5; effect size = 0.66) (Figure 4B).

Finally, on day 28, fatigue was reported by two participants (8.7%) in the L-arginine plus vitamin C supplementation group and 21 (80.1%) in the placebo group ($p < 0.0001$).

As described in Supplementary Material S1, the multivariate classification showed a high degree of correlation among the four variables of interest (i.e., 6 min walk distance, handgrip strength, flow-mediated dilation, and serum L-arginine concentration). The average classification accuracy of the participants in the two intervention arms was 77.7 ± 1.9% ($p < 0.001$). Participant classification was unaffected by age. Treatment effects were more evident in women than men. This may be due to the low number of male participants, most of whom were, however, correctly classified in the full model.

4. Discussion

In the present clinical trial, we showed that the L-arginine plus vitamin C supplementation improved walking performance, muscle strength, and endothelial function, reduced fatigue and restored serum L-arginine concentrations in adults with long COVID. These findings support the view that increasing NO bioavailability through the synergistic effects of L-arginine and vitamin C ameliorates post-acute COVID-19 sequelae [19].

The 6 min walking distance is a useful metrics of exercise capacity after COVID-19, as it correlates with the severity of acute disease and with pulmonary function/structure impairment in the post-acute phase [34,47]. In our study, participants allocated in the L-arginine plus vitamin C group showed clinically meaningful improvements [44] from baseline in the distance walked on the 6 min test compared with those who received a placebo. This finding aligns with previous evidence on the beneficial effects of L-arginine supplementation on pulmonary function and exercise capacity of patients with chronic lung diseases [22]. A short-term oral administration of L-arginine significantly decreased the mean pulmonary arterial pressure and vascular resistance and improved peak oxygen consumption and dead-space ventilation in patients with precapillary pulmonary hypertension [48]. A 12-week L-arginine supplementation combined with a home-based walking program increased the 6 min walking distance, peak aerobic capacity, and quality of life in clinically stable patients with pulmonary arterial hypertension [49]. Moreover, oral L-arginine supplementation boosted NO synthesis, improved endothelial function, and increased exercise tolerance in patients with congestive heart failure [50] and in heart transplant recipients [24].

A recent systematic review and meta-analysis on the effects of L-arginine supplementation on athletic performance indicated that either acute or chronic L-arginine supplementation could enhance both aerobic and anaerobic performance [25]. Based on these findings, the authors concluded that L-arginine supplementation with 1.5–2 g daily from four to seven weeks and 10–12 g daily for eight weeks could be recommended to improve aerobic and anaerobic performance, respectively [25]. Interestingly, untrained or moderately trained individuals seem to obtain greater gains in exercise performance after L-arginine supplementation than those who are highly trained [26]. While no conclusive evidence exists on the beneficial effects of L-arginine supplementation on human performance, our findings indicate that a short course of L-arginine plus vitamin C supplementation may positively impact the exercise capacity of adults with long COVID.

Handgrip strength is a valid indicator of general health and a powerful predictor of disability, morbidity, and mortality across all life stages [51–54]. During an acute COVID-19 episode, low handgrip strength has been associated with an increased risk of hospitalization and poor outcomes [55–57]. In adults who survived severe COVID-19, handgrip strength values after six months of hospital discharge were significantly lower than the healthy controls [58]. Moreover, in a cohort of 541 individuals who recovered from COVID-19, low handgrip strength values were associated with a higher number of persistent symptoms, including fatigue and dyspnea [59]. In our study, approximately 60% of participants had low handgrip strength at baseline. Those who received L-arginine plus vitamin C experienced a greater increase in handgrip strength than the participants in the placebo group after 28 days of intervention. Remarkably, at day 28, more than half of the participants randomized to L-arginine plus vitamin C had handgrip strength values above the 25th percentile of age- and sex-specific reference values [37], compared with 30% in the placebo group. Indeed, L-arginine supplementation (either alone or in combination with other amino acids and derivatives) is among the nutritional strategies proposed to preserve muscle mass and function/strength and manage sarcopenia in older adults [60,61].

Flow-mediated dilation is a non-invasive measure of endothelial function and vascular health [62]. Recent studies showed that patients with acute COVID-19 and convalescent survivors had reduced flow-mediated dilation values, which supports the central role of endothelial dysfunction throughout the disease course [40,63–65]. In the present investigation, L-arginine plus vitamin C supplementation induced a greater flow-mediated dilation than the placebo. Since flow-mediated dilation is, at least partly, mediated by NO bioavailability [66], our findings provide the first evidence that the combination of L-arginine plus vitamin C may be effective at improving endothelial function in post-acute COVID-19 through increasing NO synthesis. This view is in line with the results of a meta-analysis of randomized clinical trials showing that short-term oral L-arginine supplementation improves endothelial function in both healthy individuals and those with cardiovascular disease [67].

Fatigue is one of the most prevalent and burdensome symptoms in people with long COVID [2,68]. Of note, after 28 days of L-arginine plus vitamin C supplementation, only two participants reported fatigue compared with 21 who had received a placebo. This finding is in keeping with recent evidence from a large Italian multicenter clinical study of patients with long COVID, which reported an amelioration of fatigue and perceived exertion following 30 days of supplementation with L-arginine plus vitamin C [21]. Hence, the synergistic effects of L-arginine and vitamin C on NO synthesis may play a favorable role not only on the endothelial function, but also on immune response regulation, two major determinants of fatigue in long COVID and chronic fatigue syndromes [69–71].

Some limitations should be taken into account in the interpretation of the study results. The sample size was adequately powered for the primary outcome. However, owing to the small number of participants and the single-center nature of the study, our results should be considered preliminary. Further trials with larger populations, conducted in multiple centers, and using different study methodologies (e.g., longer intervention, crossover design) are warranted to confirm these promising findings. The levels of physical activity as well as dietary habits of study participants may have influenced the intervention effects. However, participants were requested to refrain from exercising and limit the ingestion of foods rich in arginine or with vasoactive properties for at least 12 h before study visits. Multivariate analyses suggested that the effects of L-arginine plus vitamin C supplementation were more evident in women. However, the study was not powered to evaluate sex-specific differences in the response to treatments. Because a data safety monitoring board was not appointed, we opted for a single-blind approach to maximize participant safety. As mentioned earlier, to preserve the trial integrity, all outcome measures were assessed by investigators who were blind to the participant group assignment. Although well-established physical performance and muscle strength measures were used, it is possible that more sophisticated aerobic and anaerobic tests might provide additional information on the effects of L-arginine plus vitamin C supplementation in adults with long COVID. Finally, while the evaluation of serum L-arginine levels provided relevant information on the effectiveness of the proposed intervention, we cannot exclude the possibility that a more comprehensive evaluation of L-arginine metabolism (e.g., measurement of citrulline, ornithine, and methyl-arginine compounds) may provide further insights into the mechanisms by which the beneficial effects of L-arginine and vitamin C supplementation on the outcomes of interest are conveyed.

5. Conclusions

L-arginine plus vitamin C supplementation improved exercise capacity, muscle strength, endothelial function, and fatigue in adults with long COVID. The combination of L-arginine plus vitamin C may therefore be proposed as a remedy to restore physical performance and relieve persistent symptoms in people with long COVID.

Supplementary Materials: The following supporting information can be downloaded at: https://www.mdpi.com/article/10.3390/nu14234984/s1, Multivariate Classification by Partial Least Squares Discriminant Analysis.

Author Contributions: Conceptualization, M.T., R.C. and F.L.; methodology, A.P., H.J.C.-J., C.D.M., J.G., E.G., L.S. (Lavinia Santucci) and B.T.; validation, A.S., L.S. (Luca Santoro), A.U. and E.M.; formal analysis, M.T., R.C., H.J.C.-J. and F.M.; investigation, F.C., V.G., A.D.G., P.M.L., A.N. and A.M.P.; resources, E.G., A.S., A.U. and F.L.; writing—original draft preparation, R.C.; writing—review and editing, M.T. and E.M.; supervision, A.U. and F.L. All authors have read and agreed to the published version of the manuscript.

Funding: This research received no external funding.

Institutional Review Board Statement: The study was conducted in accordance with the Declaration of Helsinki and was approved by the ethics committee of Università Cattolica del Sacro Cuore di Roma/Fondazione Policlinico Universitario A. Gemelli IRCCS (prot. no. 0013008/20).

Informed Consent Statement: Informed consent was obtained from all subjects involved in the study.

Data Availability Statement: The data presented in this study are available from the corresponding author upon reasonable request pending approval by the Gemelli Against COVID Scientific Committee.

Acknowledgments: The study was supported by the Italian Ministry of Health—Ricerca Corrente 2022. The authors thank all of the investigators of the Gemelli Against COVID-19 Post-Acute Care Team (Steering committee: Landi Francesco, Gremese Elisa. Coordination: Bernabei Roberto, Fantoni Massimo, Antonio Gasbarrini. Field investigators: Gastroenterology team: Settanni Carlo Romano, Porcari Serena. Geriatric team: Benvenuto Francesca, Bramato Giulia, Brandi Vincenzo, Carfì Angelo, Ciciarello Francesca, Lo Monaco Maria Rita, Martone Anna Maria, Marzetti Emanuele, Napolitano Carmen, Galluzzo Vincenzo, Pagano Francesco, Pais Cristina, Rocchi Sara, Rota Elisabetta, Salerno Andrea, Tosato Matteo, Tritto Marcello, Calvani Riccardo, Zazzara Maria Beatrice, Catalano Lucio, Picca Anna, Savera Giulia. Infectious disease team: Cauda Roberto, Murri Rita, Cingolani Antonella, Ventura Giulio, Taddei Eleonora, Moschese Davide, Ciccullo Arturo, Fantoni Massimo. Internal Medicine team: Stella Leonardo, Addolorato Giovanni, Franceschi Francesco, Mingrone Gertrude, Zocco Maria Assunta. Microbiology team: Sanguinetti Maurizio, Cattani Paola, Marchetti Simona, Posteraro Brunella, Sali Michela. Neurology team: Bizzarro Alessandra, Alessandra Lauria. Ophthalmology team: Rizzo Stanislao, Savastano Maria Cristina, Gambini Gloria, Cozzupoli Grazia Maria, Culiersi Carola. Otolaryngology team: Passali Giulio Cesare, Paludetti Gaetano, Galli Jacopo, Crudo Fabrizio, Di Cintio Giovanni, Longobardi Ylenia, Tricarico Laura, Santantonio Mariaconsiglia, Di Cesare Tiziana, Guarino Mariateresa, Corbò Marco, Settimi Stefano, Mele Dario, Brigato Francesca. Pediatric team: Buonsenso Danilo, Valentini Piero, Sinatti Dario, De Rose Gabriella. Pneumology team: Richeldi Luca, Lombardi Francesco, Calabrese Angelo, Varone Francesco, Leone Paolo Maria, Siciliano Matteo, Corbo Giuseppe Maria, Montemurro Giuliano, Calvello Mariarosaria, Intini Enrica, Simonetti Jacopo, Pasciuto Giuliana, Adiletta Veronica, Sofia Carmelo, Licata Maria Angela. Psychiatry team: Sani Gabriele, Delfina Janiri, Simonetti Alessio, Modica Marco, Montanari Silvia, Catinari Antonello, Terenzi Beatrice. Radiology team: Natale Luigi, Larici Anna Rita, Marano Riccardo, Pirronti Tommaso, Infante Amato. Rheumatology team: Paglionico Annamaria, Petricca Luca, Tolusso Barbara, Alivernini Stefano, Di Mario Clara. Vascular disease team: Santoliquido Angelo, Santoro Luca, Nesci Antonio, Di Giorgio Angela, D'Alessandro Alessia.

Conflicts of Interest: The authors declare no conflict of interest. The L-arginine plus vitamin C supplement and placebo were donated by Farmaceutici Damor, Naples, Italy. The supplier had no role in the design of the study; in the collection, analyses, or interpretation of the data; in the writing of the manuscript; or in the decision to publish the results.

References

1. Nalbandian, A.; Sehgal, K.; Gupta, A.; Madhavan, M.V.; McGroder, C.; Stevens, J.S.; Cook, J.R.; Nordvig, A.S.; Shalev, D.; Sehrawat, T.S.; et al. Post-acute COVID-19 syndrome. *Nat. Med.* **2021**, *27*, 601–615. [CrossRef] [PubMed]
2. Tosato, M.; Carfì, A.; Martis, I.; Pais, C.; Ciciarello, F.; Rota, E.; Tritto, M.; Salerno, A.; Zazzara, M.B.; Martone, A.M.; et al. Prevalence and Predictors of Persistence of COVID-19 Symptoms in Older Adults: A Single-Center Study. *J. Am. Med. Dir. Assoc.* **2021**, *22*, 1840–1844. [CrossRef]
3. Groff, D.; Sun, A.; Ssentongo, A.E.; Ba, D.M.; Parsons, N.; Poudel, G.R.; Lekoubou, A.; Oh, J.S.; Ericson, J.E.; Ssentongo, P.; et al. Short-term and Long-term Rates of Postacute Sequelae of SARS-CoV-2 Infection: A Systematic Review. *JAMA Netw. Open* **2021**, *4*, e2128568. [CrossRef]

4. Subramanian, A.; Nirantharakumar, K.; Hughes, S.; Myles, P.; Williams, T.; Gokhale, K.M.; Taverner, T.; Chandan, J.S.; Brown, K.; Simms-Williams, N.; et al. Symptoms and risk factors for long COVID in non-hospitalized adults. *Nat. Med.* **2022**, *28*, 1706–1714. [CrossRef] [PubMed]
5. Belli, S.; Balbi, B.; Prince, I.; Cattaneo, D.; Masocco, F.; Zaccaria, S.; Bertalli, L.; Cattini, F.; Lomazzo, A.; Dal Negro, F.; et al. Low physical functioning and impaired performance of activities of daily life in COVID-19 patients who survived hospitalisation. *Eur. Respir. J.* **2020**, *56*, 2002096. [CrossRef] [PubMed]
6. Davis, H.E.; Assaf, G.S.; McCorkell, L.; Wei, H.; Low, R.J.; Re'em, Y.; Redfield, S.; Austin, J.P.; Akrami, A. Characterizing long COVID in an international cohort: 7 months of symptoms and their impact. *EClinicalMedicine* **2021**, *38*, 101019. [CrossRef] [PubMed]
7. Mehandru, S.; Merad, M. Pathological sequelae of long-haul COVID. *Nat. Immunol.* **2022**, *23*, 194–202. [CrossRef]
8. Merad, M.; Blish, C.A.; Sallusto, F.; Iwasaki, A. The immunology and immunopathology of COVID-19. *Science* **2022**, *375*, 1122–1127. [CrossRef]
9. Tosato, M.; Ciciarello, F.; Zazzara, M.B.; Pais, C.; Savera, G.; Picca, A.; Galluzzo, V.; Coelho-Júnior, H.J.; Calvani, R.; Marzetti, E.; et al. Nutraceuticals and Dietary Supplements for Older Adults with Long COVID-19. *Clin. Geriatr. Med.* **2022**, *38*, 565–591. [CrossRef]
10. Adebayo, A.; Varzideh, F.; Wilson, S.; Gambardella, J.; Eacobacci, M.; Jankauskas, S.S.; Donkor, K.; Kansakar, U.; Trimarco, V.; Mone, P.; et al. l-Arginine and COVID-19: An Update. *Nutrients* **2021**, *13*, 3951. [CrossRef]
11. Durante, W. Targeting Arginine in COVID-19-Induced Immunopathology and Vasculopathy. *Metabolites* **2022**, *12*, 240. [CrossRef] [PubMed]
12. Lundberg, J.O.; Weitzberg, E. Nitric oxide signaling in health and disease. *Cell* **2022**, *185*, 2853–2878. [CrossRef]
13. Martí i Líndez, A.A.; Reith, W. Arginine-dependent immune responses. *Cell. Mol. Life Sci.* **2021**, *78*, 5303–5324. [CrossRef]
14. Pernow, J.; Jung, C. Arginase as a potential target in the treatment of cardiovascular disease: Reversal of arginine steal? *Cardiovasc. Res.* **2013**, *98*, 334–343. [CrossRef]
15. Rees, C.A.; Rostad, C.A.; Mantus, G.; Anderson, E.J.; Chahroudi, A.; Jaggi, P.; Wrammert, J.; Ochoa, J.B.; Ochoa, A.; Basu, R.K.; et al. Altered amino acid profile in patients with SARS-CoV-2 infection. *Proc. Natl. Acad. Sci. USA* **2021**, *118*, e2101708118. [CrossRef] [PubMed]
16. Sacchi, A.; Grassi, G.; Notari, S.; Gili, S.; Bordoni, V.; Tartaglia, E.; Casetti, R.; Cimini, E.; Mariotti, D.; Garotto, G.; et al. Expansion of Myeloid Derived Suppressor Cells Contributes to Platelet Activation by L-Arginine Deprivation during SARS-CoV-2 Infection. *Cells* **2021**, *10*, 2111. [CrossRef] [PubMed]
17. Reizine, F.; Lesouhaitier, M.; Gregoire, M.; Pinceaux, K.; Gacouin, A.; Maamar, A.; Painvin, B.; Camus, C.; Le Tulzo, Y.; Tattevin, P.; et al. SARS-CoV-2-Induced ARDS Associates with MDSC Expansion, Lymphocyte Dysfunction, and Arginine Shortage. *J. Clin. Immunol.* **2021**, *41*, 515–525. [CrossRef]
18. Gambardella, J.; Khondkar, W.; Morelli, M.B.; Wang, X.; Santulli, G.; Trimarco, V. Arginine and Endothelial Function. *Biomedicines* **2020**, *8*, 277. [CrossRef]
19. Morelli, M.B.; Gambardella, J.; Castellanos, V.; Trimarco, V.; Santulli, G. Vitamin C and Cardiovascular Disease: An Update. *Antioxidants* **2020**, *9*, 1227. [CrossRef]
20. Fiorentino, G.; Coppola, A.; Izzo, R.; Annunziata, A.; Bernardo, M.; Lombardi, A.; Trimarco, V.; Santulli, G.; Trimarco, B. Effects of adding L-arginine orally to standard therapy in patients with COVID-19: A randomized, double-blind, placebo-controlled, parallel-group trial. Results of the first interim analysis. *EClinicalMedicine* **2021**, *40*, 101125. [CrossRef]
21. Izzo, R.; Trimarco, V.; Mone, P.; Aloè, T.; Capra Marzani, M.; Diana, A.; Fazio, G.; Mallardo, M.; Maniscalco, M.; Marazzi, G.; et al. Combining L-Arginine with vitamin C improves long-COVID symptoms: The LINCOLN Survey. *Pharmacol. Res.* **2022**, *183*, 106360. [CrossRef] [PubMed]
22. Scott, J.A.; Maarsingh, H.; Holguin, F.; Grasemann, H. Arginine Therapy for Lung Diseases. *Front. Pharmacol.* **2021**, *12*, 627503. [CrossRef] [PubMed]
23. Doutreleau, S.; Mettauer, B.; Piquard, F.; Rouyer, O.; Schaefer, A.; Lonsdorfer, J.; Geny, B. Chronic L-arginine supplementation enhances endurance exercise tolerance in heart failure patients. *Int. J. Sports Med.* **2006**, *27*, 567–572. [CrossRef] [PubMed]
24. Doutreleau, S.; Rouyer, O.; Di Marco, P.; Lonsdorfer, E.; Richard, R.; Piquard, F.; Geny, B. L-arginine supplementation improves exercise capacity after a heart transplant. *Am. J. Clin. Nutr.* **2010**, *91*, 1261–1267. [CrossRef]
25. Viribay, A.; Burgos, J.; Fernández-Landa, J.; Seco-Calvo, J.; Mielgo-Ayuso, J. Effects of Arginine Supplementation on Athletic Performance Based on Energy Metabolism: A Systematic Review and Meta-Analysis. *Nutrients* **2020**, *12*, 1300. [CrossRef]
26. Bescós, R.; Sureda, A.; Tur, J.A.; Pons, A. The effect of nitric-oxide-related supplements on human performance. *Sports Med.* **2012**, *42*, 99–117. [CrossRef]
27. Abel, T.; Knechtle, B.; Perret, C.; Eser, P.; Von Arx, P.; Knecht, H. Influence of chronic supplementation of arginine aspartate in endurance athletes on performance and substrate metabolism — a randomized, double-blind, placebo-controlled study. *Int. J. Sports Med.* **2005**, *26*, 344–349. [CrossRef]
28. Alvares, T.S.; Conte-Junior, C.A.; Silva, J.T.; Paschoalin, V.M.F. L-arginine does not improve biochemical and hormonal response in trained runners after 4 weeks of supplementation. *Nutr. Res.* **2014**, *34*, 31–39. [CrossRef]

29. Landi, F.; Gremese, E.; Bernabei, R.; Fantoni, M.; Gasbarrini, A.; Settanni, C.R.; Benvenuto, F.; Bramato, G.; Carfi, A.; Ciciarello, F.; et al. Post-COVID-19 global health strategies: The need for an interdisciplinary approach. *Aging Clin. Exp. Res.* **2020**, *32*, 1613–1620. [CrossRef]
30. A Clinical Case Definition of Post COVID-19 Condition by a Delphi Consensus, 6 October 2021. Available online: https://www.who.int/publications/i/item/WHO-2019-nCoV-Post_COVID-19_condition-Clinical_case_definition-2021.1 (accessed on 8 September 2022).
31. Radloff, L.S. The CES-D Scale: A Self-Report Depression Scale for Research in the General Population. *Appl. Psychol. Meas.* **1977**, *1*, 385–401. [CrossRef]
32. Santucci, L.; Lomuscio, S.; Canu, F.; Primiano, A.; Persichilli, S.; Urbani, A.; Gervasoni, J. A rapid method for determination of underivatized arginine-related metabolites in human plasma using LC-MS/MS. In Proceedings of the 54° National Conference of Società Italiana di Biochimica Clinica e Biologia Molecolare Clinica (SIBioC), Genoa, Italy, 5–7 October 2022; Volume 46. Available online: https://bc.sibioc.it/bc/numero/bcnum/206 (accessed on 18 November 2022).
33. Guyatt, G.H.; Sullivan, M.J.; Thompson, P.J.; Fallen, E.L.; Pugsley, S.O.; Taylor, D.W.; Berman, L.B. The 6-minute walk: A new measure of exercise capacity in patients with chronic heart failure. *Can. Med. Assoc. J.* **1985**, *132*, 919–921. [PubMed]
34. Ferioli, M.; Prediletto, I.; Bensai, S.; Betti, S.; Daniele, F.; Scioscio, V.D.; Modolon, C.; Rimondi, M.R.; Nava, S.; Fasano, L. The role of 6MWT in Covid-19 follow up. *Eur. Respir. J.* **2021**, *58*, OA4046. [CrossRef]
35. Galluzzo, V.; Ciciarello, F.; Tosato, M.; Zazzara, M.B.; Pais, C.; Savera, G.; Calvani, R.; Picca, A.; Marzetti, E.; Landi, F. Association between vitamin D status and physical performance in COVID-19 survivors: Results from the Gemelli against COVID-19 post-acute care project. *Mech. Ageing Dev.* **2022**, *205*, 111684. [CrossRef] [PubMed]
36. Patrizio, E.; Calvani, R.; Marzetti, E.; Cesari, M. Physical Functional Assessment in Older Adults. *J. Frailty Aging* **2021**, *10*, 141–149. [CrossRef] [PubMed]
37. Landi, F.; Calvani, R.; Martone, A.M.; Salini, S.; Zazzara, M.B.; Candeloro, M.; Coelho-Junior, H.J.; Tosato, M.; Picca, A.; Marzetti, E. Normative values of muscle strength across ages in a "real world" population: Results from the longevity check-up 7+ project. *J. Cachexia Sarcopenia Muscle* **2020**, *11*, 1562–1569. [CrossRef]
38. Deanfield, J.; Donald, A.; Ferri, C.; Giannattasio, C.; Halcox, J.; Halligan, S.; Lerman, A.; Mancia, G.; Oliver, J.J.; Pessina, A.C.; et al. Endothelial function and dysfunction. Part I: Methodological issues for assessment in the different vascular beds: A statement by the Working Group on Endothelin and Endothelial Factors of the European Society of Hypertension. *J. Hypertens.* **2005**, *23*, 7–17. [CrossRef]
39. Corretti, M.C.; Anderson, T.J.; Benjamin, E.J.; Celermajer, D.; Charbonneau, F.; Creager, M.A.; Deanfield, J.; Drexler, H.; Gerhard-Herman, M.; Herrington, D.; et al. Guidelines for the ultrasound assessment of endothelial-dependent flow-mediated vasodilation of the brachial artery: A report of the international brachial artery reactivity task force. *J. Am. Coll. Cardiol.* **2002**, *39*, 257–265. [CrossRef]
40. Santoro, L.; Falsetti, L.; Zaccone, V.; Nesci, A.; Tosato, M.; Giupponi, B.; Savastano, M.C.; Moroncini, G.; Gasbarrini, A.; Landi, F.; et al. Impaired Endothelial Function in Convalescent Phase of COVID-19: A 3 Month Follow Up Observational Prospective Study. *J. Clin. Med.* **2022**, *11*, 1774. [CrossRef]
41. Fried, L.P.; Tangen, C.M.; Walston, J.; Newman, A.B.; Hirsch, C.; Gottdiener, J.; Seeman, T.; Tracy, R.; Kop, W.J.; Burke, G.; et al. Frailty in older adults: Evidence for a phenotype. *J. Gerontol. A Biol. Sci. Med. Sci.* **2001**, *56*, M146–M156. [CrossRef]
42. Michielsen, H.J.; De Vries, J.; Van Heck, G.L. Psychometric qualities of a brief self-rated fatigue measure: The Fatigue Assessment Scale. *J. Psychosom. Res.* **2003**, *54*, 345–352. [CrossRef]
43. Chetta, A.; Zanini, A.; Pisi, G.; Aiello, M.; Tzani, P.; Neri, M.; Olivieri, D. Reference values for the 6-min walk test in healthy subjects 20-50 years old. *Respir. Med.* **2006**, *100*, 1573–1578. [CrossRef] [PubMed]
44. Bohannon, R.W.; Crouch, R. Minimal clinically important difference for change in 6-minute walk test distance of adults with pathology: A systematic review. *J. Eval. Clin. Pract.* **2017**, *23*, 377–381. [CrossRef] [PubMed]
45. Ståhle, L.; Wold, S. Partial least squares analysis with cross-validation for the two-class problem: A Monte Carlo study. *J. Chemom.* **1987**, *1*, 185–196. [CrossRef]
46. Szymańska, E.; Saccenti, E.; Smilde, A.K.; Westerhuis, J.A. Double-check: Validation of diagnostic statistics for PLS-DA models in metabolomics studies. *Metabolomics* **2012**, *8*, 3–16. [CrossRef]
47. Huang, L.; Yao, Q.; Gu, X.; Wang, Q.; Ren, L.; Wang, Y.; Hu, P.; Guo, L.; Liu, M.; Xu, J.; et al. 1-year outcomes in hospital survivors with COVID-19: A longitudinal cohort study. *Lancet* **2021**, *398*, 747–758. [CrossRef]
48. Nagaya, N.; Uematsu, M.; Oya, H.; Sato, N.; Sakamaki, F.; Kyotani, S.; Ueno, K.; Nakanishi, N.; Yamagishi, M.; Miyatake, K. Short-term oral administration of L-arginine improves hemodynamics and exercise capacity in patients with precapillary pulmonary hypertension. *Am. J. Respir. Crit. Care Med.* **2001**, *163*, 887–891. [CrossRef]
49. Brown, M.B.; Kempf, A.; Collins, C.M.; Long, G.M.; Owens, M.; Gupta, S.; Hellman, Y.; Wong, V.; Farber, M.; Lahm, T. A prescribed walking regimen plus arginine supplementation improves function and quality of life for patients with pulmonary arterial hypertension: A pilot study. *Pulm. Circ.* **2018**, *8*, 2045893217743966. [CrossRef]
50. Bednarz, B.; Jaxa-Chamiec, T.; Gebalska, J.; Herbaczyńska-Cedro, K.; Ceremuzyński, L.; Herbaczynska-Cedro, K.; Ceremuzynski, L. L-arginine supplementation prolongs exercise capacity in congestive heart failure. *Kardiol. Pol.* **2004**, *60*, 348–353.
51. Sayer, A.A.; Kirkwood, T.B.L. Grip strength and mortality: A biomarker of ageing? *Lancet* **2015**, *386*, 226–227. [CrossRef]

52. Gale, C.R.; Martyn, C.N.; Cooper, C.; Sayer, A.A. Grip strength, body composition, and mortality. *Int. J. Epidemiol.* **2007**, *36*, 228–235. [CrossRef]
53. Rantanen, T.; Harris, T.; Leveille, S.G.; Visser, M.; Foley, D.; Masaki, K.; Guralnik, J.M. Muscle strength and body mass index as long-term predictors of mortality in initially healthy men. *J. Gerontol. A Biol. Sci. Med. Sci.* **2000**, *55*, M168–M173. [CrossRef] [PubMed]
54. Ortega, F.B.; Silventoinen, K.; Tynelius, P.; Rasmussen, F. Muscular strength in male adolescents and premature death: Cohort study of one million participants. *BMJ* **2012**, *345*, e7279. [CrossRef] [PubMed]
55. Cheval, B.; Sieber, S.; Maltagliati, S.; Millet, G.P.; Formánek, T.; Chalabaev, A.; Cullati, S.; Boisgontier, M.P. Muscle strength is associated with COVID-19 hospitalization in adults 50 years of age or older. *J. Cachexia Sarcopenia Muscle* **2021**, *12*, 1136–1143. [CrossRef] [PubMed]
56. Kara, Ö.; Kara, M.; Akın, M.E.; Özçakar, L. Grip strength as a predictor of disease severity in hospitalized COVID-19 patients. *Heart Lung* **2021**, *50*, 743–747. [CrossRef]
57. Pucci, G.; D'Abbondanza, M.; Curcio, R.; Alcidi, R.; Campanella, T.; Chiatti, L.; Gandolfo, V.; Veca, V.; Casarola, G.; Leone, M.C.; et al. Handgrip strength is associated with adverse outcomes in patients hospitalized for COVID-19-associated pneumonia. *Intern. Emerg. Med.* **2022**. Online ahead of print. [CrossRef]
58. Sirayder, U.; Inal-Ince, D.; Kepenek-Varol, B.; Acik, C. Long-Term Characteristics of Severe COVID-19: Respiratory Function, Functional Capacity, and Quality of Life. *Int. J. Environ. Res. Public Health* **2022**, *19*, 6304. [CrossRef]
59. Martone, A.M.; Tosato, M.; Ciciarello, F.; Galluzzo, V.; Zazzara, M.B.; Pais, C.; Savera, G.; Calvani, R.; Marzetti, E.; Robles, M.C.; et al. Sarcopenia as potential biological substrate of long COVID-19 syndrome: Prevalence, clinical features, and risk factors. *J. Cachexia Sarcopenia Muscle* **2022**, *13*, 1974–1982. [CrossRef]
60. Calvani, R.; Miccheli, A.; Landi, F.; Bossola, M.; Cesari, M.; Leeuwenburgh, C.; Sieber, C.C.; Bernabei, R.; Marzetti, E. Current nutritional recommendations and novel dietary strategies to manage sarcopenia. *J. Frailty Aging* **2013**, *2*, 38–53. [CrossRef]
61. Hickson, M. Nutritional interventions in sarcopenia: A critical review. *Proc. Nutr. Soc.* **2015**, *74*, 378–386. [CrossRef]
62. Thijssen, D.H.J.; Black, M.A.; Pyke, K.E.; Padilla, J.; Atkinson, G.; Harris, R.A.; Parker, B.; Widlansky, M.E.; Tschakovsky, M.E.; Green, D.J. Assessment of flow-mediated dilation in humans: A methodological and physiological guideline. *Am. J. Physiol. Heart Circ. Physiol.* **2011**, *300*, H2–H12. [CrossRef]
63. Oikonomou, E.; Souvaliotis, N.; Lampsas, S.; Siasos, G.; Poulakou, G.; Theofilis, P.; Papaioannou, T.G.; Haidich, A.B.; Tsaousi, G.; Ntousopoulos, V.; et al. Endothelial dysfunction in acute and long standing COVID-19: A prospective cohort study. *Vascul. Pharmacol.* **2022**, *144*, 106975. [CrossRef] [PubMed]
64. Gao, Y.P.; Zhou, W.; Huang, P.N.; Liu, H.Y.; Bi, X.J.; Zhu, Y.; Sun, J.; Tang, Q.Y.; Li, L.; Zhang, J.; et al. Persistent Endothelial Dysfunction in Coronavirus Disease-2019 Survivors Late After Recovery. *Front. Med.* **2022**, *9*, 809033. [CrossRef]
65. Sardu, C.; Gambardella, J.; Morelli, M.B.; Wang, X.; Marfella, R.; Santulli, G. Hypertension, Thrombosis, Kidney Failure, and Diabetes: Is COVID-19 an Endothelial Disease? A Comprehensive Evaluation of Clinical and Basic Evidence. *J. Clin. Med.* **2020**, *9*, 1417. [CrossRef] [PubMed]
66. Green, D.J.; Dawson, E.A.; Groenewoud, H.M.M.; Jones, H.; Thijssen, D.H.J. Is flow-mediated dilation nitric oxide mediated?: A meta-analysis. *Hypertension* **2014**, *63*, 376–382. [CrossRef] [PubMed]
67. Bai, Y.; Sun, L.; Yang, T.; Sun, K.; Chen, J.; Hui, R. Increase in fasting vascular endothelial function after short-term oral L-arginine is effective when baseline flow-mediated dilation is low: A meta-analysis of randomized controlled trials. *Am. J. Clin. Nutr.* **2009**, *89*, 77–84. [CrossRef]
68. Carfì, A.; Bernabei, R.; Landi, F. Persistent Symptoms in Patients After Acute COVID-19. *JAMA* **2020**, *324*, 603–605. [CrossRef]
69. Komaroff, A.L. Inflammation correlates with symptoms in chronic fatigue syndrome. *Proc. Natl. Acad. Sci. USA* **2017**, *114*, 8914–8916. [CrossRef]
70. Haffke, M.; Freitag, H.; Rudolf, G.; Seifert, M.; Doehner, W.; Scherbakov, N.; Hanitsch, L.; Wittke, K.; Bauer, S.; Konietschke, F.; et al. Endothelial dysfunction and altered endothelial biomarkers in patients with post-COVID-19 syndrome and chronic fatigue syndrome (ME/CFS). *J. Transl. Med.* **2022**, *20*, 138. [CrossRef]
71. Zazzara, M.B.; Bellieni, A.; Calvani, R.; Coelho-Junior, H.J.; Picca, A.; Marzetti, E. Inflammaging at the Time of COVID-19. *Clin. Geriatr. Med.* **2022**, *38*, 473–481. [CrossRef]

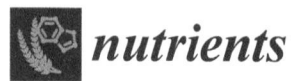

Article

Effect of Dietary Coenzyme Q10 Plus NADH Supplementation on Fatigue Perception and Health-Related Quality of Life in Individuals with Myalgic Encephalomyelitis/Chronic Fatigue Syndrome: A Prospective, Randomized, Double-Blind, Placebo-Controlled Trial

Jesús Castro-Marrero [1,*,†], Maria Jose Segundo [2,†], Marcos Lacasa [3], Alba Martinez-Martinez [4], Ramon Sanmartin Sentañes [1] and Jose Alegre-Martin [1]

[1] ME/CFS Research Unit, Division of Rheumatology, Vall d'Hebron Hospital Research Institute, Universitat Autònoma de Barcelona, 08035 Barcelona, Spain; rsanmartin@vhebron.net (R.S.S.); jalegre@vhebron.net (J.A.-M.)
[2] Clinical Research Department, Vitae Health Innovation, Montmeló, 08160 Barcelona, Spain; msegundo@vitae.es
[3] Department of Education, Generalitat de Catalunya, Sabadell, 08202 Barcelona, Spain; marcos.lacasa@gmail.com
[4] Medical Oncology Clinical Trials Office, Vall d'Hebron Institute of Oncology, Vall d´Hebron University Hospital, Universitat Autònoma de Barcelona, 08035 Barcelona, Spain; albamartinez@vhio.net
* Correspondence: jesus.castro@vhir.org; Tel.: +34-93-489-3000 (ext. 3753)
† These authors have contributed equally to this work.

Abstract: Myalgic encephalomyelitis/chronic fatigue syndrome (ME/CFS) is a complex, multisystem, and profoundly debilitating neuroimmune disease, probably of post-viral multifactorial etiology. Unfortunately, no accurate diagnostic or laboratory tests have been established, nor are any universally effective approved drugs currently available for its treatment. This study aimed to examine whether oral coenzyme Q10 and NADH (reduced form of nicotinamide adenine dinucleotide) co-supplementation could improve perceived fatigue, unrefreshing sleep, and health-related quality of life in ME/CFS patients. A 12-week prospective, randomized, double-blind, placebo-controlled trial was conducted in 207 patients with ME/CFS, who were randomly allocated to one of two groups to receive either 200 mg of CoQ10 and 20 mg of NADH ($n = 104$) or matching placebo ($n = 103$) once daily. Endpoints were simultaneously evaluated at baseline, and then reassessed at 4- and 8-week treatment visits and four weeks after treatment cessation, using validated patient-reported outcome measures. A significant reduction in cognitive fatigue perception and overall FIS-40 score ($p < 0.001$ and $p = 0.022$, respectively) and an improvement in HRQoL (health-related quality of life) (SF-36) ($p < 0.05$) from baseline were observed within the experimental group over time. Statistically significant differences were also shown for sleep duration at 4 weeks and habitual sleep efficiency at 8 weeks in follow-up visits from baseline within the experimental group ($p = 0.018$ and $p = 0.038$, respectively). Overall, these findings support the use of CoQ10 plus NADH supplementation as a potentially safe therapeutic option for reducing perceived cognitive fatigue and improving the health-related quality of life in ME/CFS patients. Future interventions are needed to corroborate these clinical benefits and also explore the underlying pathomechanisms of CoQ10 and NADH administration in ME/CFS.

Keywords: chronic fatigue syndrome; coenzyme Q10; myalgic encephalomyelitis; mitochondria; nonrestorative sleep; NADH; quality of life

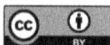

1. Introduction

Myalgic encephalomyelitis, commonly referred to as chronic fatigue syndrome (ME/CFS), is a serious, complex, and chronic multisystem illness of unknown etiology, often triggered by a persistent viral infection (for this reason, it is also known as post-viral fatigue syndrome). It is characterized by unexplained and persistent post-exertional fatigue, which is unrelieved by rest and made worse by physical and mental effort, along with other core symptoms such as the disruption of cognitive, immunometabolic, autonomic, and neuroendocrine pathways [1]. It affects as many as 17 to 24 million people worldwide, and its prevalence is expected to more than double by 2030 [2]. The clinical presentation and symptom frequency and severity may vary between patients, but in general, the illness reduces overall quality of life and social, occupational, and personal activity; indeed, some patients are even bedridden or housebound [3]. Diagnosis of ME/CFS is based on patients' core symptoms according to a consensus of four case criteria developed over the past 25 years, which have been applied both in research and in clinical practice: the 1994 CDC/Fukuda definition [4], the 2003 Canadian Consensus Criteria (also known as CCC) [5], the 2011 International Consensus Criteria (ICC) [6], and, most recently, the 2015 IOM Expert Criteria for Systemic Exertion Intolerance Disease (SEID) [7]. In the clinical diagnosis of ME/CFS, it is important to evaluate the disabling fatigue perception, sleep problems, and health-related quality of life using validated questionnaires such as the fatigue impact scale (FIS-40) [8], Pittsburg sleep quality index (PSQI) [9], and Short Form Health Survey (SF-36) [10]. Unfortunately, at present, there are no commercially available diagnostic tests, no specific lab biomarkers, and no targeted FDA-approved drugs for ME/CFS [11].

Coenzyme Q10 (CoQ10) and the reduced form of nicotinamide adenine dinucleotide (NADH) are key components of the electron transport chain responsible for mitochondrial ATP production, which decreases free radical generation, and, in their reduced forms, they act as powerful antioxidants. CoQ10 and NADH levels and redox status have been shown to be disturbed in ME/CFS. Strong evidence has emerged that mitochondrial dysfunction, disturbed immunometabolism, and increased oxidative stress play a pivotal role in the pathogenesis of numerous illnesses, providing a robust scientific rationale for testing potential "nutraceuticals" that target these processes [12].

As chronic fatigue is a key diagnostic symptom for ME/CFS, it has been suggested that energy metabolism may be disrupted in a subset of patients with ME/CFS. Mitochondrial dysfunction has been considered as a possible underlying pathomechanism of the illness, based on the structural and functional changes reported vis-a-vis healthy controls [12]. Long-chain polyunsaturated fatty acid, prostaglandin and amino acid metabolism, and inefficient ATP biosynthesis have been suggested as consequences of ME/CFS due to perturbed mitochondrial bioenergetic metabolism [13]. Due to the potential role of the mitochondria in ME/CFS, mitochondrial-targeting nutraceutical interventions have been used to assist in improving patient outcomes such as fatigue and their health-related quality of life [14], including CoQ10, NADH, and n-Acetyl-L-carnitine as part of their treatment regime [15–18]. These treatments are administered either alone or in combination with a cocktail of other nutraceutical and/or pharmaceutical-based products.

Over the last decade, a growing body of data has supported the potential clinical use of dietary CoQ10 supplementation in health and chronic illnesses [13,19–25].

Previously, in a proof-of-concept study, our group found a trend towards improvement over time in fatigue perception, response to physical exercise, and biochemical parameters of oxidative stress and mitochondrial metabolism (ATP content, lipid peroxidation, citrate synthase activity, levels of CoQ10 and NADH) in peripheral blood mononuclear cells after CoQ10 plus NADH administration [26–28]. There is evidence of improved mitochondrial respiration following prolonged CoQ10 supplementation [29,30], via mechanisms involving the upregulation of enzymes that regulate fatty acid transport into organelles and also the stimulation of mitochondrial biogenesis [31,32]. Among individuals suffering from a wide range of illnesses, researchers have also reported reductions in reactive oxygen and nitrogen species levels (ROS/RNS), protein carboxylation, DNA damage, protein nitration, and lipid peroxidation following CoQ10 supplementation [33,34]. Other in vivo evidence of reduced levels of oxidative and nitrosative stress following CoQ10 supplementation includes downregulation of iNOS enzyme and NF-kB [35,36]. Coenzyme Q10 has been shown to reduce markers of systemic inflammation in several metabolic, autoimmune, and neurological disorders [37,38]. As for NADH, it is known to facilitate the generation of intracellular ATP [39], and in several studies, it has shown a higher response rate during the first trimester of treatment compared to control subjects [40]. In another proof-of-concept cohort study, our group showed that NADH managed to improve anxiety/depression symptoms and maximum heart rate in ME/CFS following a two-day consecutive challenge test (2-day CPET), findings that may imply an improvement in the oxygen supply to the skeletal muscle and to the brain in individuals with ME/CFS [41].

Data on the potential therapeutic effects of CoQ10 and NADH co-supplementation on fatigue, pain, and sleep impairments in individuals with ME/CFS are scarce. The current study was conducted to evaluate the clinical effects of CoQ10 plus NADH supplementation on fatigue perception, nonrestorative sleep problems, and HRQoL in people with ME/CFS, due to a previous pilot study in which no significant differences were found for chronic pain and sleep quality in ME/CFS.

2. Materials and Methods

2.1. Participants

A 12-week, single-center, randomized, double-blind, placebo-controlled trial was conducted in 242 Caucasian ME/CFS patients consecutively recruited from a single outpatient tertiary referral center (ME/CFS Clinical Unit, Vall d'Hebron University Hospital, Barcelona, Spain) from January 2018 to December 2019. Figure 1 shows a flowchart of the participants prior to analysis. Patients were eligible for the study if they were female, aged 18 years or older, had a confirmed diagnosis of ME/CFS according to the 1994 CDC/Fukuda case definition [4], and provided signed written informed consent. Exclusion criteria included any active medical condition that explained the chronic fatigue (untreated hypothyroidism, sleep apnea, narcolepsy, medication side effects, and iron deficiency anemia), previous diagnosis not unequivocally resolved (chronic hepatitis, malignancy), past or current neuropsychiatric disorders (major depressive disorder with psychotic or melancholic features, bipolar disorder, schizophrenia, delusional disorder, dementias, anorexia nervosa, bulimia nervosa), and participation in another clinical trial of the same or different nature within 30 days prior to study inclusion; inability (in the opinion of the investigator) to follow the instructions or to complete the treatment satisfactorily; failure to provide signed informed consent; consumption of certain drugs/supplements that might influence outcome measures in the last 90 days or whose withdrawal might be a relevant problem, anticoagulant treatment, pregnancy or breast-feeding, smoking, alcohol intake or substance abuse, obesity (BMI > 30 kg/m^2), and hypersensitivity to CoQ10 or NADH. Patients with missing data from the follow-up visits to baseline were considered to have dropped out.

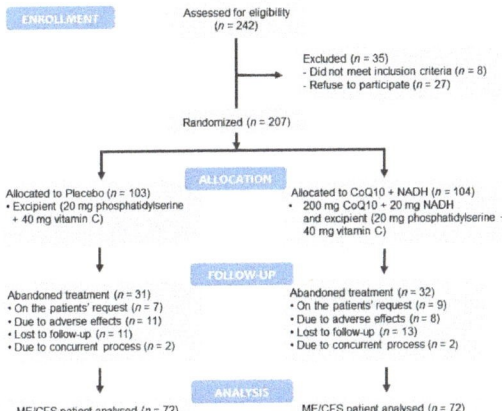

Figure 1. Consolidated Standards of Reporting Trials (CONSORT) flow diagram illustrating the steps of screening, enrollment, assignment, and follow-up of the study participants.

2.2. Intervention

Of the 242 eligible ME/CFS participants screened, 35 were excluded (eight who did not meet the inclusion criteria, and 27 who refused to participate). The remaining 207 participants were allocated to treatment by an independent investigator not otherwise involved in the intervention, using the result of a list of random numbers generated by a computer program. The participants were randomly assigned in a double-blind fashion in a 1:1 ratio to receive either 200 mg of CoQ10 plus 20 mg of NADH ($n = 72$) or a matching placebo ($n = 72$), in four capsules daily for eight weeks; all participants also received their standard therapy for the disease. The CoQ10 was used in combination with NADH, in light of reports that they may have synergistic antioxidant effects and that NADH may enhance CoQ10 absorption [26,27].

Safety information obtained at all study visits included data on adverse events, data from clinical laboratory tests, vital signs, along with the results of the general physical examination. Adverse events, including serious ones, were reviewed throughout the trial by the independent medical monitor, the steering committee, and the independent data and safety monitoring board. Provision was made for investigator-initiated temporary or permanent dose reductions or suspensions due to adverse effects.

During the study, 19 subjects dropped out due to adverse effects: eight in the active group (five epigastralgias, and three dizziness), and 11 in the placebo group (four epigastralgias, five dizziness, one diarrhea, and one muscle spasm). Twenty-four patients were lost to follow-up (13 in the experimental group and 11 in the placebo group). Four discontinued the study due to the presence of a concurrent process (one case of hypotensive treatment in each group, one case of anemia in the experimental group, and one case of foot trauma in the placebo group). Finally, 16 patients withdrew at their own request (nine cases in the experimental group and seven within in the placebo group). The remaining 144 cases of ME/CFS (70%, 72 patients in each treatment group) completed all the study protocol procedures and were included in the overall analysis of outcome measures (see Figure 1).

2.3. Product Tested

Patients randomized to the CoQ10 plus NADH experimental group received four enteric-coated tablets daily consisting of active ingredients (50 mg of CoQ10 and 5 mg of NADH) and excipients (20 mg of phosphatidylserine and 40 mg of vitamin C). Patients randomized to placebo received supplementation comprising four enteric-coated tablets daily containing only excipients. Both experimental and placebo tablets were identical in size, color, opacity, shape, presentation, and packaging. All tablets were manufactured and donated by Vitae Health Innovation, S.L. (Montmeló, Barcelona, Spain). The study pharmacist recorded all treatments supplied on the medication-dispensing forms along with the original script.

2.4. Study Design and Procedures

This unicenter, randomized, double-blind, placebo-controlled cohort study design was conducted to evaluate the clinical benefits of oral CoQ10 plus NADH administration on fatigue perception, unrefreshing sleep problems, and HRQoL in ME/CFS. Clinical visits throughout the study are detailed in Figure 2, which also describes the trial design in both groups. After a verbal description of the study, all participants gave written consent prior to commencement and received no compensation for their participation. Patients were evaluated at baseline, and then at four and eight weeks of treatment, and finally four weeks after the end of treatment by the site investigator. Changes in symptoms were assessed through validated self-reported questionnaires completed by participants under the supervision of two trained investigators (J.C.-M. and J.A.-M.). Compliance was checked through medication logs. Use of concomitant medications was tracked at all follow-up visits. The study protocol was reviewed and approved by the local institutional review board at the participating site (Clinical Research Ethics Committee, Vall d'Hebron University Hospital, Barcelona, Spain; protocol code: VITAE-2015, approved on 24 April 2015). The study protocol was conducted in accordance with the guidelines of the Declaration of Helsinki, and with the current Spanish regulations on clinical research and the standards of good clinical practice of the European Union. It also followed the Consolidated Standards of Reporting Trials (CONSORT) guidelines. The current clinical trial was registered on https://clinicaltrials.gov as NCT03186027 (accessed on 29 June 2017).

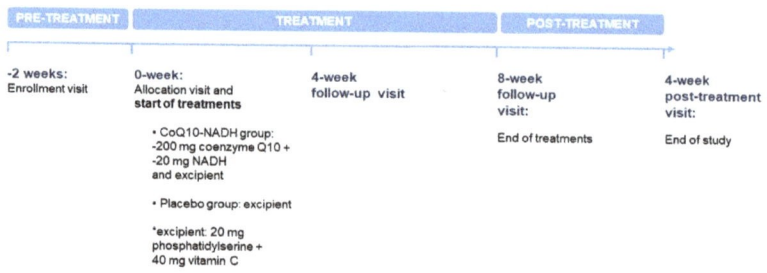

Figure 2. Summary of the study schedule at each visit during the clinical trial.

2.5. Primary Endpoint

The prospectively defined main outcome measure was the change in self-reported fatigue scores assessed using the validated Fatigue Impact Scale (FIS-40) from baseline to the final study visit held three months later. The study was powered to detect a 3-point difference between active treatment group and placebo. The FIS-40 comprises 40 items divided into three domains that describe how perceived fatigue impacts upon cognitive (10 items), physical (10 items), and psychosocial functioning (20 items) over the previous four weeks. Each item is scored from 0 (no fatigue) to 4 (severe fatigue). The total FIS-40 score is calculated by adding together responses from the 40 questions (score range 0–160). Higher scores indicate more functional limitations due to severe fatigue [8].

2.6. Secondary Endpoints

The secondary outcome measures included changes in sleep disturbances and health-related quality of life through validated self-reported PSQI and HRQoL questionnaires, respectively.

2.6.1. Pittsburgh Sleep Quality Index

Sleep disturbances were assessed through the self-administered 19-item Pittsburgh Sleep Quality Index (PSQI) questionnaire. Scores are obtained on each of seven domains of sleep quality: subjective sleep quality, sleep latency, sleep duration, habitual sleep efficiency, sleep perturbations, use of sleeping medication, and daytime dysfunction. Each component is scored from 0 to 3 (0 = no sleep problems and 3 = severe sleep problems). The global PSQI score ranges from 0 to 21 points, with scores of ≥ 5 indicating poorer sleep quality [9].

2.6.2. The 36-Item Short Form Health Survey

The 36-item Short Form Health Survey (SF-36) was used to assess health-related quality of life. The SF-36 is a broadly-based self-reported survey of health-related physical and mental functioning status in ME/CFS and other chronic conditions. It assesses functioning on eight subscales including domains of physical functioning, physical role, bodily pain, general health, social functioning, vitality, emotional role, and mental health, and two additional general subscales covering the physical and mental health domains, rated on a scale from 0 to 100. Lower scores indicate a more negative impact of an individual's health on functioning [10].

2.7. Power and Sample Size Estimation

The sample size was estimated based on data from a previous clinical trial of CoQ10 and NADH supplementation in people with ME/CFS [28]. Allowing for an estimated early drop-out rate of 20%, and accepting an alpha risk of 5% and a beta risk of 20% (two-sided test), a total of 121 subjects in each group was considered necessary to find statistically significant differences between groups, expected to be 10% in the placebo group and 25% in the experimental group (https://www.imim.es/ofertadeserveis/software-public/granmo/, accessed on 12 June 2018).

2.8. Monitoring of Compliance and Adverse Events

All participants were asked to return any remaining study product after the intervention. Adherence was measured by calculating all remaining tablets. Participants who did not take the supplement on more than two non-consecutive days or consecutive days were considered non-compliant ($n = 0$). All adverse events following administration of study product intake were monitored until the end of the study. No serious adverse events or suspected adverse reactions (e.g., events resulting in death, immediately life-threatening events, medically significant events for any reason, events requiring or prolonging hospitalization or resulting in persistent or significant disability/incapacity) were reported during or after the end of the study.

2.9. Statistical Analysis

A descriptive statistical analysis was carried out for all study variables. Results are shown as means ± standard deviation (SD). A Kolmogorov–Smirnov test was used to determine the distribution and normality of data for both groups. Continuous variables were defined by the number of valid cases and expressed as mean ± SD. Categorical variables were described using absolute and relative frequencies of each category over the total of valid values. Differences in comparison analysis between the two groups were assessed using Student's t-test (paired data t-test using the value of the patient as a control) for continuous variables and the Chi-square test for categorical variables. For all comparisons, a two-sided level of statistical significance of 0.05 was considered. All analyses were performed on the data set using all available information with intention-to-treat (ITT) criteria. An analysis of covariance (one-way ANCOVA) was performed using the changes in overall FIS-40 score from baseline to the last follow-up visit of the study as the primary outcome measure, and entering the overall FIS-40, PSQI, and HRQoL scores at baseline as continuous predictors and the enrolling investigator and treatment assigned as categorical predictors. The statistical analysis observed the ICH-E9 guidelines as well as all the rules of good clinical practice. All data were analyzed using the SAS program, version 9.4 (Statistical Analysis System Institute Inc., Cary, NC, USA).

3. Results

3.1. Participants' Characteristics at Baseline

Table 1 shows the demographic and clinical characteristics of the study participants. No statistically significant differences were found in terms of demographic and clinical parameters between the study groups at baseline. No statistically significant differences were observed in the standard drug therapy used within the participants' treatment groups. The following are the most frequent concomitant drugs (more than 90%) that subjects were taking during the study: anticonvulsants (gabapentin), tricyclic antidepressants (duloxetine), anxiolytics/hypnotics (benzodiazepines on demand), NSAIDs (ibuprofen on demand), and opioids (tramadol).

Table 1. Baseline demographic and clinical characteristics of study participants who completed the final assessment.

Variables	CoQ10 + NADH (n = 72)	Placebo (n = 72)	p-Values
Age (years)	45.38 ± 7.81	46.79 ± 6.48	0.238
BMI (kg/m^2)	24.07 ± 4.36	24.88 ± 4.85	0.296
Systolic BP (mmHg)	124.44 ± 10.50	125.32 ± 11.85	0.639
Diastolic BP (mmHg)	75.63 ± 9.33	75.54 ± 8.21	0.954
HR (bpm)	78.96 ± 9.42	77.51 ± 10.78	0.393
Symptom onset (years)	36.94 ± 8.98	36.65 ± 7.95	0.836
Illness duration (months)	97.21 ± 69.40	106.56 ± 74.55	0.437
Concomitant drugs			
Anticonvulsants	27 (37.5)	27 (37.5)	1.000
Tricyclic antidepressants	34 (47.2)	38 (52.8)	0.505
Anxiolytics/hypnotics	14 (19.4)	18 (25.0)	0.422
NSAIDs	48 (66.7)	49 (68.1)	0.858
Opioids	15 (20.8)	24 (33.3)	0.091

Data are expressed as means ± standard deviation (SD) for continuous variables and compared by Student's t-test, and as numbers of participants with percentages (%) for categorical variables and compared by Chi-squared test. Abbreviations: BMI, body mass index; BP, blood pressure; HR, heart rate; NSAIDs, non-steroidal anti-inflammatory drugs.

3.2. Changes in Fatigue Perception among Participants

Table 2 shows participants' scores for fatigue perception over the course of the clinical study. Perception of cognitive fatigue (as indicated by the change in the cognitive domain from FIS-40) improved significantly at the 4- and 8-week visits from baseline within the active group ($p = 0.005$ and $p = 0.010$, respectively). The psychosocial domain showed a nominal improvement in the active group at the 4-week visit, though without reaching statistical significance ($p = 0.053$).

Table 2. Fatigue severity (FIS-40 questionnaire) scores of the participants completing the final assessment.

FIS-40 Domains	CoQ10 + NADH (n = 72)	Placebo (n = 72)	p-Values [1]
Physical functioning			
Baseline	35.31 ± 4.61	34.82 ± 5.85	0.580
4 weeks	34.51 ± 5.39	34.14 ± 6.57	0.708
8 weeks	34.74 ± 5.21	34.42 ± 5.52	0.721
4 weeks post-treatment	35.71 ± 5.26	36.64 ± 5.43	0.554
Cognitive			
Baseline	34.26 ± 5.26	32.97 ± 7.12	0.217
4 weeks	33.14 ± 5.94 **	31.83 ± 7.07	0.232
8 weeks	33.13 ± 6.28 **	32.40 ± 7.00	0.515
4 weeks post-treatment	33.44 ± 6.90	32.97 ± 6.83	0.680
Psychosocial			
Baseline	64.78 ± 11.69	62.31 ± 13.71	0.246
4 weeks	63.44 ± 12.42	61.19 ± 14.29	0.315
8 weeks	63.94 ± 12.69	61.83 ± 14.42	0.352
4 weeks post-treatment	64.79 ± 13.53	62.97 ± 14.91	0.444
Total FIS-40 scores (0–160)			
Baseline	134.35 ± 19.80	130.10 ± 25.35	0.264
4 weeks	131.10 ± 22.15 *	127.17 ± 25.89	0.329
8 weeks	131.81 ± 22.73	128.65 ± 25.60	0.435
4 weeks post-treatment	133.40 ± 24.33	130.58 ± 25.59	0.499

Data are given as means ± SD and compared by paired Student's t-test for within-group comparison analysis and by Student's t-test for independent data for between-group comparison analysis. Significance level was set at * $p < 0.05$ and ** $p < 0.01$. Statistically significant differences were found in the overall FIS-40 score at 4 weeks from baseline ($p = 0.022$) in the experimental group. Abbreviations: FIS-40, 40-item fatigue impact scale. Lower FIS-40 scores indicate an improvement in fatigue perception among participants. [1] p-values for between-group comparison analysis.

In the CoQ10 + NADH group, the total FIS-40 score significantly decreased at the 4-week visit from baseline ($p = 0.022$). However, this improvement was not significant at the follow-up visits from baseline (8 weeks and 4 weeks post-treatment; $p = 0.089$ and $p = 0.071$, respectively). FIS-40 domain scores evolved in parallel between groups over the course of the study.

3.3. Changes in Sleep Quality and Health-Related Quality of Life after CoQ10 Plus NADH Supplementation in the Study Population

3.3.1. Pittsburgh Sleep Quality Index

Table 3 displays participants' sleep quality scores assessed using the PSQI questionnaire. In the between-group comparison analysis, statistically significant differences were displayed for sleep duration at 4-week follow-up visit from baseline in the experimental group ($p = 0.018$). Moreover, in the within-experimental group comparison analysis, we found statistically significant differences for the PSQI domains from baseline over time (all p-values < 0.05).

Table 3. Sleep quality (assessed with the PSQI questionnaire) in participants completing the final assessment.

PSQI Domains	CoQ10 + NADH (n = 72)	Placebo (n = 72)	p-Values [1]
Subjective sleep quality			
Baseline	1.71 ± 1.14	2.01 ± 1.08	0.101
4 weeks	1.67 ± 1.15	2.01 ± 1.08	0.064
8 weeks	1.69 ± 1.23	2.03 ± 1.13	0.091
4 weeks post-treatment	1.94 ± 1.06 *	2.10 ± 1.04	0.383
Sleep latency			
Baseline	2.29 ± 0.88	2.10 ± 1.04	0.226
4 weeks	2.25 ± 0.92	2.10 ± 1.04	0.350
8 weeks	2.40 ± 0.88	2.17 ± 1.05	0.145
4 weeks post-treatment	2.33 ± 0.87	2.07 ± 1.15	0.124
Sleep duration			
Baseline	1.31 ± 1.02	1.71 ± 0.98	0.017
4 weeks	1.28 ± 1.00	1.67 ± 0.96	0.018
8 weeks	1.51 ± 1.03 *	1.75 ± 0.98	0.160
4 weeks post-treatment	1.43 ± 0.96	1.67 ± 1.02	0.155
Habitual sleep efficiency			
Baseline	1.81 ± 1.25	2.03 ± 1.15	0.269
4 weeks	1.68 ± 1.25	1.94 ± 1.19	0.196
8 weeks	1.90 ± 1.13 *	1.97 ± 1.20	0.720
4 weeks post-treatment	1.94 ± 1.11	1.93 ± 1.23	0.943
Sleep disturbances			
Baseline	2.35 ± 0.70	2.35 ± 0.63	1.000
4 weeks	2.31 ± 0.76	2.35 ± 0.63	0.721
8 weeks	2.31 ± 0.64	2.33 ± 0.75	0.811
4 weeks post-treatment	2.36 ± 0.61	2.32 ± 0.65	0.691
Sleeping medication use			
Baseline	1.93 ± 1.23	1.75 ± 1.36	0.404
4 weeks	1.90 ± 1.25	1.75 ± 1.36	0.483
8 weeks	1.96 ± 1.22	1.88 ± 1.36	0.699
4 weeks post-treatment	1.99 ± 1.14	1.81 ± 1.34	0.385
Daytime dysfunction			
Baseline	2.15 ± 0.85	2.15 ± 0.88	1.000
4 weeks	2.13 ± 0.87	2.15 ± 0.88	0.849
8 weeks	2.18 ± 0.79	2.19 ± 0.91	0.922
4 weeks post-treatment	2.22 ± 0.74	2.22 ± 084	1.000
Global PSQI score			
Baseline	14.71 ± 3.47	15.07 ± 3.48	0.533
4 weeks	14.44 ± 3.86	15.03 ± 3.47	0.341
8 weeks	15.03 ± 3.44	15.35 ± 3.70	0.592
4 weeks post-treatment	15.26 ± 3.09	15.18 ± 3.71	0.883

Data are given as means ± SD and compared by paired Student's t-test for within-group comparison analysis and by Student's t-test for independent data in between-group comparison analysis. Significance level was set at * $p < 0.05$. No statistically significant differences were displayed in any PSQI items between groups. Abbreviations: PSQI, Pittsburgh sleep quality index. Lower PSQI scores indicate an improvement in the perception of sleep quality among participants. [1] p-values for between-group comparison analysis.

3.3.2. The Short Form 36-Item Health Survey

Table 4 shows participants' scores on the SF-36 questionnaire. Physical role functioning, general health perception, vitality, social role functioning, emotional role functioning, and mental health status domains did not show any differences in the between-group comparison analysis.

Table 4. Health-related quality of life (SF-36 questionnaire) in participants completing the final assessment.

SF-36 Domains	CoQ10 + NADH (n = 72)	Placebo (n = 72)	p-Values [1]
Physical functioning			
Baseline	25.28 ± 15.72	28.47 ± 18.49	0.266
4 weeks	27.50 ± 17.78 *	30.26 ± 19.70	0.378
8 weeks	29.58 ± 18.98 **	30.35 ± 20.02	0.814
4 weeks post-treatment	28.89 ± 20.70	32.64 ± 21.18	0.284
Physical role functioning			
Baseline	3.47 ± 15.31	3.82 ± 15.51	0.892
4 weeks	4.86 ± 17.12	6.31 ± 21.28	0.654
8 weeks	5.56 ± 17.91	6.60 ± 19.68	0.740
4 weeks post-treatment	6.94 ± 22.29	2.43 ± 10.41	0.121
Bodily pain			
Baseline	15.42 ± 13.68	17.44 ± 14.04	0.381
4 weeks	18.49 ± 15.80 *	18.17 ± 15.50	0.902
8 weeks	18.24 ± 14.61	17.44 ± 17.58	0.769
4 weeks post-treatment	17.58 ± 16.07	18.60 ± 14.07	0.687
General health perception			
Baseline	24.08 ± 15.70	18.36 ± 12.55	0.017
4 weeks	21.79 ± 15.10	18.65 ± 13.53	0.191
8 weeks	21.72 ± 16.44	19.08 ± 13.39	0.292
4 weeks post-treatment	21.93 ± 17.27	17.08 ± 12.35	0.054
Vitality			
Baseline	17.64 ± 17.98	16.32 ± 16.27	0.645
4 weeks	17.08 ± 16.80	16.33 ± 15.95	0.783
8 weeks	16.39 ± 16.43	18.33 ± 19.70	0.521
4 weeks post-treatment	15.28 ± 18.04	13.82 ± 13.93 *	0.588
Social role functioning			
Baseline	30.21 ± 24.35	30.38 ± 23.44	0.965
4 weeks	28.82 ± 24.34	32.32 ± 23.95	0.386
8 weeks	28.13 ± 24.08	32.12 ± 23.72	0.317
4 weeks post-treatment	28.47 ± 23.00	29.69 ± 22.64	0.749
Emotional role functioning			
Baseline	36.11 ± 47.39	36.57 ± 43.75	0.951
4 weeks	36.57 ± 46.19	37.06 ± 43.87	0.948
8 weeks	32.87 ± 43.87	34.26 ± 42.23	0.846
4 weeks post-treatment	29.63 ± 43.89	28.24 ± 39.42	0.842
Mental health status			
Baseline	46.50 ± 21.87	45.67 ± 19.91	0.811
4 weeks	43.89 ± 21.26	47.13 ± 21.80	0.368
8 weeks	45.06 ± 22.43	47.44 ± 19.03	0.491
4 weeks post-treatment	44.72 ± 22.92	44.17 ± 21.37	0.880

Data are given as means ± SD and compared by paired Student's t-test for within-group comparison analysis and by Student's t-test for independent data for between-group comparison analysis. Significance level was set at * $p < 0.05$, and ** $p < 0.01$. No statistically significant differences were found in any SF-36 items in between-group comparison over time. Abbreviations: SF-36, 36-item short form health survey. Higher SF-36 scores indicate better health-related quality of life among participants. [1] p-values for between-group comparison analysis.

The physical functioning showed better scores in the CoQ10 plus NADH group; statistically significant improvements were observed at both visits from baseline during treatment (4-week and 8-week visits; $p = 0.036$ and $p = 0.001$, respectively). The bodily pain domain improved at the 4-week visit from baseline ($p = 0.043$). In the placebo group, a reduction in vitality was observed 4 weeks after treatment discontinuation ($p = 0.042$).

3.4. Clinical Safety and Tolerability Evaluation

With regard to safety data, few adverse effects have been associated with CoQ10 and NADH supplementation [18,39] in other populations. In our study of ME/CFS patients, no relevant treatment-related adverse events were recorded. Our findings demonstrate that oral CoQ10 plus NADH supplementation for eight weeks was safe and potentially well-tolerated by the participants.

4. Discussion

The use of nutritional interventions as antioxidant supplements in order to reduce increased oxidative stress in ME/CFS patients remains a controversial issue [14]. CoQ10 and NADH are two possible candidates for use in the treatment of ME/CFS, and perhaps in other illnesses involving chronic fatigue in which oxidative stress plays a significant role, for at least three main reasons. First, CoQ10 and NADH are bioenergetic cofactors with the potential to boost mitochondrial function. Second, CoQ10 and NADH are powerful free radical scavengers that can mitigate the lipid peroxidation and DNA damage caused by oxidative stress; third, they have powerful antioxidant properties [17].

To the best of our knowledge, this is the first RCT to investigate the beneficial effects of oral CoQ10 plus NADH supplementation on perceived fatigue, nonrestorative problems, and HRQoL in a substantial number of people with ME/CFS. Our results showed that the combination of CoQ10 plus NADH had a positive effect on the perception of fatigue, sleep quality, and HRQoL in ME/CFS. This was highlighted in the improvement in scores observed in the intragroup analysis, although no differences were found in the intergroup analysis.

Coenzyme Q10 and NADH deficiencies have also been described in individuals with ME/CFS and fibromyalgia [26,42], and it has suggested that serum NADH levels are directly correlated with serum CoQ10 concentrations in these patients. CoQ10, also known as ubiquinone, is a fat-soluble, vitamin-like benzoquinone compound that is endogenously synthesized from tyrosine in the human body. It is an essential component in the metabolism of all cells, and a CoQ10 deficiency is linked to the pathogenesis of a range of chronic disorders. It is a strong antioxidant agent that confers resistance to the mitochondrial damage induced by oxidative and nitrosative stress, and it also serves as an anti-inflammatory agent, affecting ATP synthesis and nitric oxide preservation [14]. Chronically activated immune responses and nitrosative and oxidative stress in ME/CFS patients induce disorders such as brain hypoperfusion/hypometabolism, neuroinflammation, DNA damage, mitochondrial dysfunction, secondary autoimmune responses directed against disrupted proteins and lipid membrane components, and dysfunctional intracellular signaling pathways [15].

The administration of NADH alone [43] and in combination with CoQ10 [27,28] has been shown to reduce fatigue in people with ME/CFS. However, although those studies reported beneficial effects, none of them reported the baseline dietary intake characteristics, and this may have influenced the results.

Alongside chronic fatigue, the most hallmark symptoms of ME/CFS are intolerance to physical/mental exercise (post-exertional malaise), alterations in concentration/memory, nonrestorative sleep, orthostatic intolerance, and generalized chronic pain [1]. Given the natural course towards chronicity in ME/CFS, we consider the results obtained in our study to be important. We confirm that CoQ10 plus NADH supplementation has a positive effect on the perception of cognitive fatigue, with significant improvements at 4- and 8-week visits ($p < 0.001$) compared to baseline. Likewise, our dietary nutraceutical combination may have influenced the overall FIS-40 domain score—reducing it at the 4-week visit from baseline ($p = 0.022$), although the difference was not significant at the end of treatment visit (8-weeks vs. baseline, $p = 0.08$)—and also the psychological domain, which showed a marked improvement at the 4-week visit (though also without reaching significance vs. baseline, $p = 0.05$) within the experimental group. In previous research carried out by our group and others, with nutraceutical interventions to assess mitochondrial dysfunction in ME/CFS, fatigue was the primary endpoint in eight out of nine studies [28,43–49]. Of these studies, five found significant differences in fatigue levels following an intervention [28,46–49]; however, other authors reported no significant changes in fatigue levels in ME/CFS [44,45].

The discrepancies between these studies may be due to the heterogeneity of the ME/CFS population (i.e., sociodemographic and clinical characteristics of the patients, diagnostic criteria used, presence of different comorbid health conditions, and pharmacological and non-pharmacological treatments administered), the small sample size, and the short study duration, among other factors.

In experiments on rodents, CoQ10 treatment improved cognitive deficits by modulating mitochondrial functions and was effective in protecting against cognitive impairments and neurodegeneration in experimental animal models [50,51]. Fukuda et al. [44] suggested that ubiquinol-10 supplementation may improve cognitive impairments by modulating energy reserves in ME/CFS, and Dumont et al. [52] reported that CoQ10 administration improved cognitive performance in a transgenic mouse model of Alzheimer's disease.

Clinical trials have shown that oral replacement supplements of CoQ10 plus/or NADH significantly reduce fatigue perception and other symptoms associated with chronic diseases. Several studies in people with fibromyalgia [42] have reported improvements in chronic pain, fatigue, and HRQoL, and studies in other neuroimmune conditions such as remitting–relapsing multiple sclerosis have demonstrated the effectiveness of CoQ10 administration in reducing in vivo inflammation and oxidative stress, and in improving fatigue and anxiety/depression symptoms [52,53]. Based on these findings, new potential therapeutic strategies are now urgently needed [54].

Our intragroup comparison analysis found that ME/CFS patients supplemented with CoQ10 plus NADH showed significant increases in the physical function domain of the SF-36 at both follow-up visits. This result is of interest, because our review of the scientific literature revealed improvements in health-related quality of life after CoQ10 administration in other related chronic conditions such as fibromyalgia and Gulf War Syndrome [55,56], but not in ME/CFS.

In the broad group of neurological manifestations of ME/CFS, the component of generalized pain stands out, both in the context of ME/CFS and in the case of comorbid fibromyalgia [57]. In our study, the CoQ10 plus NADH supplementation induced an improvement on the bodily pain component of the SF-36 questionnaire at the 4-week treatment visit from baseline in the study participants. A previous study by our group to evaluate chronic pain using the McGill Pain questionnaire found no changes in pain from ME/CFS participants [28].

In patients with ME/CFS, nonrestorative sleep leads to a significant alteration in sleep quality [58]. Our results show that the CoQ10 plus NADH administration improved the perception of sleep quality, demonstrating new findings that differ from the aforementioned earlier study by our group [28], which also used the same validated PSQI questionnaire. On the contrary, a study in veterans with Gulf War Syndrome, which bears similarities to ME/CFS, found that only CoQ10 supplementation improved symptoms of physical function but had no beneficial effect on sleep quality [55].

Previous studies investigating the beneficial clinical effects of CoQ10 supplementation in heart failure (HF) have been conducted over the last few years. The findings have reported an improvement in bioenergetic and functional levels and endothelial function in these HF patients [59,60].

Previous reports have suggested that dietary supplements such as CoQ10 or NADH are safe and well-tolerated [18]. Our results confirm these observations and suggest that moderate doses of these molecules can be safely added to conventional therapy in ME/CFS.

Strengths and Limitations

This study has some limitations that must be considered. Firstly, the primary endpoint, the perception of fatigue recorded through the FIS-40 questionnaire, is a subjective parameter. In future work, objective physiological and biological parameters might be used, such as the maximum oxygen consumption and lactate/glucose levels during and after performing a cardiopulmonary challenge test (2-day consecutive CPET). Secondly, there were limitations associated with the study design, research setting, and participants' selection. The fact that all patients were Caucasian ME/CFS women and were recruited from a single tertiary referral center may have increased the proportion of seriously ill patients, and we must be cautious when generalizing these results to other populations in other healthcare settings such as primary care or the general population. Thirdly, the lack of statistical differences found between groups may have been due to the placebo effect (phosphatidylserine and vitamin C as excipients). Finally, the doses and follow-up timing of the intervention were pre-established, and so the dose–response effect could not be monitored and recorded among the study participants.

However, our study also has some important strengths: (1) the analysis of the combination of CoQ10 plus NADH as a nutritional supplement in ME/CFS, with the inclusion of a substantial number of participants, (2) the improvement in the perception of cognitive fatigue and health-related quality of life achieved by the combination of CoQ10 plus NADH, (3) the homogeneous inclusion criteria through the 1994 CDC/Fukuda definition, and (4) the consideration of gender with the inclusion only of women—the recruitment of age-and sex-matched participants is essential in mitochondrial function studies, due to age-related mitochondrial function decline (such as uncoupled mitochondrial respiration, citrate synthase activity and ATP levels)—and (5) the demonstration of the safety and good tolerance of the CoQ10 plus NADH administration among participants.

Multicenter trials are now required with homogeneous patient samples after carrying out the correct clinical phenotyping (through the establishment of well-defined subgroups, based on the diagnostic criteria, neurological symptoms, comorbid health conditions, and pharmacological and non-pharmacological treatments administered), and with recommendations to eat a balanced diet. We also support long-term follow-up studies including objective physiological and biological indicators, such as peak oxygen consumption (VO_2 as "gold standard" measure) and lactate/glucose ratio following an ergospirometry provocation test, and the assessment of information processing speed using computerized neuropsychological tests in order to verify the potential benefits of antioxidant therapy in people with ME/CFS.

5. Conclusions

To the best of our knowledge, this is the first study to assess the effects of oral CoQ10 plus NADH supplementation administered to a substantial number of ME/CFS patients ($n = 207$). Our findings suggest that, over a two-month period, this combination is potentially effective in reducing cognitive fatigue (also known as "brain fog") and overall fatigue perception, thus improving HRQoL in ME/CFS. The study shows that CoQ10 and NADH can be safely co-administered to ME/CFS patients and are generally well-tolerated at the dosages indicated. A therapeutic effect was also demonstrated on sleep quality within the experimental group. Long-term RCTs in larger ME/CFS cohorts should now be performed to confirm the effectiveness of CoQ10 and NADH co-supplementation in treating the hallmark symptom of post-exertional malaise using two-day consecutive cardiopulmonary exercise testing (2-day CPET).

Author Contributions: Conceptualization, J.C.-M., M.J.S., R.S.S. and J.A.-M.; methodology, J.C.-M., A.M.-M. and J.A.-M.; formal analysis, M.L.; investigation and resources, J.C.-M., M.J.S., R.S.S. and J.A.-M.; data curation, J.C.-M. and A.M.-M.; writing—original draft preparation, J.C.-M. and J.A.-M.; writing—review and editing, J.C.-M., M.J.S., A.M.-M. and J.A.-M.; visualization, J.C.-M. and J.A.-M.; supervision and project administration, J.C.-M., M.J.S., R.S.S. and J.A.-M.; funding acquisition, M.J.S. and J.A.-M. All authors have read and agreed to the published version of the manuscript to its submission.

Funding: J.C.-M. received financial support and honoraria from Vitae Health Innovation Co., S.L. (Montmeló, Barcelona, Spain). This study was partially supported by the Vall d'Hebron Hospital Research Institute (Barcelona, Spain). Vitae Health Innovation Co. supplied both treatments (Coenzyme Q10 and NADH supplement tablets and placebo).

Institutional Review Board Statement: All study procedures were reviewed and approved by the local Clinical Research Ethics Committee of the Vall d'Hebron University Hospital, Barcelona, Spain (protocol code: VITAE 2015, approved on 24 April 2015). The study was conducted according to the guidelines of the Declaration of Helsinki and the current Spanish regulations on clinical research and the standards of Good Clinical Practice of the European Union. It also followed the Consolidated Standards of Reporting Trials (CONSORT) guidelines.

Informed Consent Statement: Informed consent was obtained from all subjects involved in the study.

Data Availability Statement: All relevant data analyzed during the current trial are included in the article. Access to raw datasets may be provided upon reasonable request to the corresponding author.

Acknowledgments: The authors thank the patients who participated. The authors are grateful to Maria Cleofé Zaragoza for her help in writing and contributing to the paper. We also thank Michael Maudsley for editing and useful linguistic advice on the updated manuscript.

Conflicts of Interest: M.J.S. is an employee of Vitae Health Innovation, S.L. (Montmeló, Barcelona, Spain). As stated in the author contributions, the funders declare that they had no role in the design, execution, analysis and interpretation, and presentation of data. J.C.-M. received financial support from Vitae Health Innovation, S.L. to conduct this intervention study. The rest of the authors declare no conflict of interest.

References

1. Morris, G.; Puri, B.K.; Walker, A.; Maes, M.; Carvalho, A.F.; Walder, K.; Mazza, C.; Berk, M. Myalgic encephalomyelitis/chronic fatigue syndrome: From pathophysiological insights to novel therapeutic opportunities. *Pharmacol. Res.* **2019**, *148*, 104450. [CrossRef]
2. Lim, E.-J.; Ahn, Y.-C.; Jang, E.-S.; Lee, S.-W.; Lee, S.-H.; Son, C.-G. Systematic review and meta-analysis of the prevalence of chronic fatigue syndrome/myalgic encephalomyelitis (CFS/ME). *J. Transl. Med.* **2020**, *18*, 100. [CrossRef]
3. Castro-Marrero, J.; Faro, M.; Zaragozá, M.C.; Aliste, L.; De Sevilla, T.F.; Alegre, J. Unemployment and work disability in individuals with chronic fatigue syndrome/myalgic encephalomyelitis: A community-based cross-sectional study from Spain. *BMC Public Health* **2019**, *19*, 1–13. [CrossRef]
4. Fukuda, K.; Straus, S.E.; Hickie, I.; Sharpe, M.C.; Dobbins, J.G.; Komaroff, A. The Chronic Fatigue Syndrome: A Comprehensive Approach to Its Definition and Study. *Ann. Intern. Med.* **1994**, *121*, 953–959. [CrossRef]
5. Carruthers, B.M.; Jain, A.K.; De Meirleir, K.L.; Peterson, D.L.; Klimas, N.G.; Lerner, A.M.; Bested, A.C.; Flor-Henry, P.; Joshi, P.; Powles, A.C.P.; et al. Myalgic Encephalomyelitis/Chronic Fatigue Syndrome. *J. Chronic Fatigue Syndr.* **2003**, *11*, 7–115. [CrossRef]
6. Carruthers, B.M.; van de Sande, M.I.; de Meirleir, K.L.; Klimas, N.G.; Broderick, G.; Mitchell, T.; Staines, D.; Powles, A.C.P.; Speight, N.; Vallings, R.; et al. Myalgic encephalomyelitis: International Consensus Criteria. *J. Intern. Med.* **2011**, *270*, 327–338. [CrossRef]
7. Committee on the Diagnostic Criteria for Myalgic Encephalomyelitis/Chronic Fatigue Syndrome; Board on the Health of Select Populations; Institute of Medicine. *Beyond Myalgic Encephalomyelitis/Chronic Fatigue Syndrome: Redefining an Illness*; National Academies Press: Washington, DC, USA, 2015. [CrossRef]
8. Fisk, J.D.; Ritvo, P.G.; Ross, L.; Haase, D.A.; Marrie, T.J.; Schlech, W.F. Measuring the Functional Impact of Fatigue: Initial Validation of the Fatigue Impact Scale. *Clin. Infect. Dis.* **1994**, *18*, S79–S83. [CrossRef]
9. Buysse, D.J.; Reynolds, C.F., III; Monk, T.H.; Berman, S.R.; Kupfer, D.J. The Pittsburgh sleep quality index: A new instrument for psychiatric practice and research. *Psychiatry Res.* **1989**, *28*, 193–213. [CrossRef]
10. Alonso, J.; Prieto, L.; Antó, J.M. La versión española del SF-36 Health Survey (Cuestionario de Salud SF-36): Un instrumento para la medida de los resultados clínicos. *Med. Clin.* **1995**, *104*, 771–776.
11. Castro-Marrero, J.; Saez-Francàs, N.; Santillo, D.; Alegre, J. Treatment and management of chronic fatigue syndrome/myalgic encephalomyelitis: All roads lead to Rome. *Br. J. Pharmacol.* **2017**, *174*, 345–369. [CrossRef] [PubMed]
12. Anderson, G.; Maes, M. Mitochondria and immunity in chronic fatigue syndrome. *Prog. Neuro-Psychopharmacol. Biol. Psychiatry* **2020**, *103*, 109976. [CrossRef]
13. Filler, K.; Lyon, D.; Bennett, J.; McCain, N.; Elswick, R.; Lukkahatai, N.; Saligan, L.N. Association of mitochondrial dysfunction and fatigue: A review of the literature. *BBA Clin.* **2014**, *1*, 12–23. [CrossRef] [PubMed]
14. Hargreaves, I.; Heaton, R.A.; Mantle, D. Disorders of Human Coenzyme Q10 Metabolism: An Overview. *Int. J. Mol. Sci.* **2020**, *21*, 6695. [CrossRef]
15. Bjørklund, G.; Dadar, M.; Pen, J.J.; Chirumbolo, S.; Aaseth, J. Chronic fatigue syndrome (CFS): Suggestions for a nutritional treatment in the therapeutic approach. *Biomed. Pharmacother.* **2019**, *109*, 1000–1007. [CrossRef]
16. Campagnolo, N.; Johnston, S.; Collatz, A.; Staines, D.; Marshall-Gradisnik, S. Dietary and nutrition interventions for the therapeutic treatment of chronic fatigue syndrome/myalgic encephalomyelitis: A systematic review. *J. Hum. Nutr. Diet.* **2017**, *30*, 247–259. [CrossRef] [PubMed]

17. Maksoud, R.; Balinas, C.; Holden, S.; Cabanas, H.; Staines, D.; Marshall-Gradisnik, S. A systematic review of nutraceutical interventions for mitochondrial dysfunctions in myalgic encephalomyelitis/chronic fatigue syndrome. *J. Transl. Med.* **2021**, *19*, 1–11. [CrossRef] [PubMed]
18. Arenas-Jal, M.; Suñé-Negre, J.M.; García-Montoya, E. Coenzyme Q10 supplementation: Efficacy, safety, and formulation challenges. *Compr. Rev. Food Sci. Food Saf.* **2020**, *19*, 574–594. [CrossRef]
19. Testai, L.; Martelli, A.; Flori, L.; Cicero, A.; Colletti, A. Coenzyme Q_{10}: Clinical Applications beyond Cardiovascular Diseases. *Nutrients* **2021**, *13*, 1697. [CrossRef] [PubMed]
20. Chen, H.-C.; Huang, C.-C.; Lin, T.-J.; Hsu, M.-C.; Hsu, Y.-J. Ubiquinol Supplementation Alters Exercise Induced Fatigue by Increasing Lipid Utilization in Mice. *Nutrients* **2019**, *11*, 2550. [CrossRef] [PubMed]
21. Shimizu, K.; Kon, M.; Tanimura, Y.; Hanaoka, Y.; Kimura, F.; Akama, T.; Kono, I. Coenzyme Q10 supplementation downregulates the increase of monocytes expressing toll-like receptor 4 in response to 6-day intensive training in kendo athletes. *Appl. Physiol. Nutr. Metab.* **2015**, *40*, 575–581. [CrossRef] [PubMed]
22. Fukuda, S.; Koyama, H.; Kondo, K.; Fujii, H.; Hirayama, Y.; Tabata, T.; Okamura, M.; Yamakawa, T.; Okada, S.; Hirata, S.; et al. Effects of Nutritional Supplementation on Fatigue, and Autonomic and Immune Dysfunction in Patients with End-Stage Renal Disease: A Randomized, Double-Blind, Placebo-Controlled, Multicenter Trial. *PLoS ONE* **2015**, *10*, e0119578. [CrossRef]
23. Mancuso, M.; Angelini, C.; Bertini, E.; Carelli, V.; Comi, G.; Minetti, C.; Moggio, M.; Mongini, T.; Servidei, S.; Tonin, P.; et al. Fatigue and exercise intolerance in mitochondrial diseases. Literature revision and experience of the Italian Network of mitochondrial diseases. *Neuromuscul. Disord.* **2012**, *22*, S226–S229. [CrossRef] [PubMed]
24. Umanskaya, A.; Santulli, G.; Xie, W.; Andersson, D.; Reiken, S.R.; Marks, A.R. Genetically enhancing mitochondrial antioxidant activity improves muscle function in aging. *Proc. Natl. Acad. Sci. USA* **2014**, *111*, 15250–15255. [CrossRef]
25. Whitehead, N.P.; Kim, M.J.; Bible, K.L.; Adams, M.E.; Froehner, S.C. A new therapeutic effect of simvastatin revealed by functional improvement in muscular dystrophy. *Proc. Natl. Acad. Sci. USA* **2015**, *112*, 12864–12869. [CrossRef]
26. Castro-Marrero, J.; Cordero, M.D.; Saez-Francàs, N.; Jimenez-Gutierrez, C.; Aguilar-Montilla, F.J.; Aliste, L.; Alegre, J. Could Mitochondrial Dysfunction Be a Differentiating Marker Between Chronic Fatigue Syndrome and Fibromyalgia? *Antioxidants Redox Signal.* **2013**, *19*, 1855–1860. [CrossRef]
27. Castro-Marrero, J.; Cordero, M.D.; Segundo, M.J.; Saez-Francàs, N.; Calvo, N.; Román-Malo, L.; Aliste, L.; De Sevilla, T.F.; Alegre, J. Does Oral Coenzyme Q10 Plus NADH Supplementation Improve Fatigue and Biochemical Parameters in Chronic Fatigue Syndrome? *Antioxidants Redox Signal.* **2015**, *22*, 679–685. [CrossRef] [PubMed]
28. Castro-Marrero, J.; Saez-Francàs, N.; Segundo, M.J.; Calvo, N.; Faro, M.; Aliste, L.; de Sevilla, T.F.; Alegre, J. Effect of coenzyme Q10 plus nicotinamide adenine dinucleotide supplementation on maximum heart rate after exercise testing in chronic fatigue syndrome—A randomized, controlled, double-blind trial. *Clin. Nutr.* **2016**, *35*, 826–834. [CrossRef] [PubMed]
29. Tian, G.; Sawashita, J.; Kubo, H.; Nishio, S.-Y.; Hashimoto, S.; Suzuki, N.; Yoshimura, H.; Tsuruoka, M.; Wang, Y.; Liu, Y.; et al. Ubiquinol-10 supplementation activates mitochondria functions to decelerate senescence in senescence-accelerated mice. *Antioxid Redox Signal.* **2014**, *20*, 2606–2620. [CrossRef] [PubMed]
30. Morris, G.; Anderson, G.; Berk, M.; Maes, M. Coenzyme Q10 Depletion in Medical and Neuropsychiatric Disorders: Potential Repercussions and Therapeutic Implications. *Mol. Neurobiol.* **2013**, *48*, 883–903. [CrossRef]
31. Carmona, M.C.; Lefebvre, P.; Lefebvre, B.; Galinier, A.; Benani, A.; Jeanson, Y.; Louche, K.; Flajollet, S.; Ktorza, A.; Dacquet, C.; et al. Coadministration of coenzyme Q prevents rosiglitazone-induced adipogenesis in ob/ob mice. *Int. J. Obesity* **2009**, *33*, 204–211. [CrossRef]
32. Lee, S.K.; Lee, J.O.; Kim, J.H.; Kim, N.; You, G.Y.; Moon, J.W.; Sha, J.; Kim, S.J.; Lee, Y.W.; Kang, H.J.; et al. Coenzyme Q10 increases the fatty acid oxidation through AMPK-mediated PPAR-alpha induction in 3T3-L1 pre-adipocytes. *Cell Signal.* **2012**, *24*, 2329–2336. [CrossRef]
33. Huo, J.; Xu, Z.; Hosoe, K.; Kubo, H.; Miyahara, H.; Dai, J.; Mori, M.; Sawashita, J.; Higuchi, K. Coenzyme Q10 Prevents Senescence and Dysfunction Caused by Oxidative Stress in Vascular Endothelial Cells. *Oxidative Med. Cell. Longev.* **2018**, *2018*, 1–15. [CrossRef]
34. Tsai, K.-L.; Huang, Y.-H.; Kao, C.-L.; Yang, D.-M.; Lee, H.-C.; Chou, H.-Y.; Chen, Y.-C.; Chiou, G.-Y.; Chen, L.-H.; Yang, Y.-P.; et al. A novel mechanism of coenzyme Q10 protects against human endothelial cells from oxidative stress-induced injury by modulating NO-related pathways. *J. Nutr. Biochem.* **2012**, *23*, 458–468. [CrossRef]
35. Akbari, A.; Mobini, G.R.; Agah, S.; Morvaridzadeh, M.; Omidi, A.; Potter, E.; Fazelian, S.; Ardehali, S.H.; Daneshzad, E.; Dehghani, S. Coenzyme Q10 supplementation and oxidative stress parameters: A systematic review and meta-analysis of clinical trials. *Eur. J. Clin. Pharmacol.* **2020**, *76*, 1483–1499. [CrossRef] [PubMed]
36. Sangsefidi, Z.S.; Yaghoubi, F.; Hajiahmadi, S.; Hosseinzadeh, M. The effect of coenzyme Q10 supplementation on oxidative stress: A systematic review and meta-analysis of randomized controlled clinical trials. *Food Sci. Nutr.* **2020**, *8*, 1766–1776. [CrossRef]
37. Lee, B.-J.; Tseng, Y.-F.; Yen, C.-H.; Lin, P.-T. Effects of coenzyme Q10 supplementation (300 mg/day) on antioxidation and anti-inflammation in coronary artery disease patients during statins therapy: A randomized, placebo-controlled trial. *Nutr. J.* **2013**, *12*, 142. [CrossRef] [PubMed]
38. Moccia, M.; Capacchione, A.; Lanzillo, R.; Carbone, F.; Micillo, T.; Perna, F.; De Rosa, A.; Carotenuto, A.; Albero, R.; Matarese, G.; et al. Coenzyme Q10 supplementation reduces peripheral oxidative stress and inflammation in interferon-β1a-treated multiple sclerosis. *Ther. Adv. Neurol. Disord.* **2019**, *12*, 1–12. [CrossRef]

39. Arenas-Jal, M.; Suñé-Negre, J.; García-Montoya, E. Therapeutic potential of nicotinamide adenine dinucleotide (NAD). *Eur. J. Pharmacol.* **2020**, *879*, 173158. [CrossRef]
40. Santaella, M.L.; Font, I.; Disdier, O.M. Comparison of oral nicotinamide adenine dinucleotide (NADH) versus conventional therapy for chronic fatigue syndrome. *Puerto Rico Health Sci. J.* **2004**, *23*, 89–93.
41. Alegre, J.; Roses, J.M.; Javierre, C.; Ruiz Baques, A.; Segundo, M.J.; de Sevilla, T.F. Nicotinamida adenina dinucleotido (NADH) en pacientes con síndrome de fatiga crónica. *Rev. Clin. Esp.* **2010**, *210*, 284–288. [CrossRef]
42. Alcocer-Gómez, E.; Cano-García, F.J.; Cordero, M.D. Effect of coenzyme Q10 evaluated by 1990 and 2010 ACR Diagnostic Criteria for Fibromyalgia and SCL-90-R: Four case reports and literature review. *Nutrition* **2013**, *29*, 1422–1425. [CrossRef]
43. Forsyth, L.M.; Preuss, H.G.; MacDowell, A.L.; Chiazze, L.; Birkmayer, G.D.; Bellanti, J. Therapeutic effects of oral NADH on the symptoms of patients with chronic fatigue syndrome. *Ann. Allergy Asthma Immunol.* **1999**, *82*, 185–191. [CrossRef]
44. Fukuda, S.; Nojima, J.; Kajimoto, O.; Yamaguti, K.; Nakatomi, Y.; Kuratsune, H.; Watanabe, Y. Ubiquinol-10 supplementation improves autonomic nervous function and cognitive function in chronic fatigue syndrome. *BioFactors* **2016**, *42*, 431–440. [CrossRef] [PubMed]
45. Ostojic, S.M.; Stojanovic, M.; Drid, P.; Hoffman, J.R.; Sekulic, D.; Zenic, N. Supplementation with Guanidinoacetic Acid in Women with Chronic Fatigue Syndrome. *Nutrients* **2016**, *8*, 72. [CrossRef]
46. Montoya, J.G.; Anderson, J.N.; Adolphs, D.L.; Bateman, L.; Klimas, N.; Levine, S.M.; Garvert, D.W.; Kaiser, J.D. KPAX002 as a treatment for myalgic encephalomyelitis/chronic fatigue syndrome (ME/CFS): A prospective, randomized trial. *Int. J. Clin. Exp. Med.* **2018**, *11*, 2890–2900.
47. Vermeulen, R.C.W.; Scholte, H.R. Exploratory open label, randomized study of acetyl and propionyl-carnitine in chronic fa-tigue syndrome. *Psychosom. Med.* **2004**, *66*, 276–282. [CrossRef] [PubMed]
48. Menon, R.; Cribb, L.; Murphy, J.; Ashton, M.M.; Oliver, G.; Dowling, N.; Turner, A.; Dean, O.; Berk, M.; Ng, C.H.; et al. Mitochondrial modifying nutrients in treating chronic fatigue syndrome: A 16-week open-label pilot study. *Adv. Integr. Med.* **2017**, *4*, 109–114. [CrossRef]
49. Kaiser, J.D. A prospective, proof-of-concept investigation of KPAX002 in chronic fatigue syndrome. *Int. J. Clin. Exp. Med.* **2015**, *8*, 11064–11074.
50. Binukumar, B.K.; Gupta, N.; Sunkaria, A.; Kandimalla, R.; Wani, W.; Sharma, D.R.; Bal, A.; Gill, K.D. Protective Efficacy of Coenzyme Q10 Against DDVP-Induced Cognitive Impairments and Neurodegeneration in Rats. *Neurotox. Res.* **2011**, *21*, 345–357. [CrossRef] [PubMed]
51. Dumont, M.; Kipiani, K.; Yu, F.; Wille, E.; Katz, M.; Calingasan, N.Y.; Gouras, G.K.; Lin, M.T.; Beal, M.F. Coenzyme Q10 Decreases Amyloid Pathology and Improves Behavior in a Transgenic Mouse Model of Alzheimer's Disease. *J. Alzheimer's Dis.* **2011**, *27*, 211–223. [CrossRef] [PubMed]
52. Sanoobar, M.; Eghtesadi, S.; Azimi, A.; Khalili, M.; Khodadadi, B.; Jazayeri, S.; Gohari, M.R.; Aryaeian, N. Coenzyme Q10 supplementation ameliorates inflammatory markers in patients with multiple sclerosis: A double blind, placebo, controlled randomized clinical trial. *Nutr. Neurosci.* **2015**, *18*, 169–176. [CrossRef] [PubMed]
53. Sanoobar, M.; Dehghan, P.; Khalili, M.; Azimi, A.; Seifar, F. Coenzyme Q10 as a treatment for fatigue and depression in multiple sclerosis patients: A double blind randomized clinical trial. *Nutr. Neurosci.* **2015**, *19*, 138–143. [CrossRef] [PubMed]
54. Mehrabani, S.; Askari, G.; Miraghajani, M.; Tavakoly, R.; Arab, A. Effect of coenzyme Q10 supplementation on fatigue: A systematic review of interventional studies. *Complement. Ther. Med.* **2019**, *43*, 181–187. [CrossRef] [PubMed]
55. Golomb, B.A.; Allison, M.; Koperski, S.; Koslik, H.J.; Devaraj, S.; Ritchie, J.B. Coenzyme Q10 Benefits Symptoms in Gulf War Veterans: Results of a Randomized Double-Blind Study. *Neural Comput.* **2014**, *26*, 2594–2651. [CrossRef]
56. Sandler, C.X.; Lloyd, A.R. Chronic fatigue syndrome: Progress and possibilities. *Med. J. Aust.* **2020**, *212*, 428–433. [CrossRef] [PubMed]
57. Castro-Marrero, J.; Zaragozá, M.C.; González-Garcia, S.; Aliste, L.; Saez-Francàs, N.; Romero, O.; Ferré, A.; De Sevilla, T.F.; Alegre, J. Poor self-reported sleep quality and health-related quality of life in patients with chronic fatigue syndrome/myalgic encephalomyelitis. *J. Sleep Res.* **2018**, *27*, e12703. [CrossRef]
58. Silaidos, C.; Pilatus, U.; Grewal, R.; Matura, S.; Lienerth, B.; Pantel, J.; Eckert, G.P.; Silaidos, C.; Pilatus, U.; Grewal, R.; et al. Sex-associated differences in mitochondrial function in human peripheral blood mononuclear cells (PBMCs) and brain. *Biol. Sex Differ.* **2018**, *9*, 1–10. [CrossRef] [PubMed]
59. Di Lorenzo, A.; Iannuzzo, G.; Parlato, A.; Cuomo, G.; Testa, C.; Coppola, M.; D'Ambrosio, G.; Oliviero, D.A.; Sarullo, S.; Vitale, G.; et al. Clinical Evidence for Q10 Coenzyme Supplementation in Heart Failure: From Energetics to Functional Improvement. *J. Clin. Med.* **2020**, *9*, 1266. [CrossRef]
60. Kawashima, C.; Matsuzawa, Y.; Konishi, M.; Akiyama, E.; Suzuki, H.; Sato, R.; Nakahashi, H.; Kikuchi, S.; Kimura, Y.; Maejima, N.; et al. Ubiquinol Improves Endothelial Function in Patients with Heart Failure with Reduced Ejection Fraction: A Single-Center, Randomized Double-Blind Placebo-Controlled Crossover Pilot Study. *Am. J. Cardiovasc. Drugs* **2019**, *20*, 363–372. [CrossRef]

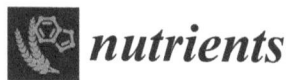

Article

Water-Soluble Tomato Concentrate, a Potential Antioxidant Supplement, Can Attenuate Platelet Apoptosis and Oxidative Stress in Healthy Middle-Aged and Elderly Adults: A Randomized, Double-Blinded, Crossover Clinical Trial

Zezhong Tian [1,2,3], Kongyao Li [1,2,3,4], Die Fan [5], Xiaoli Gao [6], Xilin Ma [1,2,3], Yimin Zhao [1,2,3], Dan Zhao [1,2,3], Ying Liang [1,2,3], Qiuhua Ji [1,2,3], Yiting Chen [1,2,3] and Yan Yang [1,2,3,*]

[1] School of Public Health (Shenzhen), Shenzhen Campus of Sun Yat-sen University, Sun Yat-sen University, Shenzhen 518107, China
[2] Guangdong Provincial Key Laboratory for Food, Nutrition and Health, Sun Yat-sen University, Guangzhou 510080, China
[3] Guangdong Engineering Technology Research Center of Nutrition Translation, Sun Yat-sen University, Guangzhou 510080, China
[4] Department of Non-Communicable Disease Prevention and Control, Shenzhen Nanshan Center for Chronic Disease Control, Shenzhen 518064, China
[5] Clinical Nutrition Department, The General Hospital of Western Theater Command, Chengdu 610000, China
[6] The Eighth Affiliated Hospital, Sun Yat-sen University, Shenzhen 518033, China
* Correspondence: yangyan3@mail.sysu.edu.cn

Abstract: Increased oxidative stress and platelet apoptotic in middle-aged and elderly adults are important risk factors for atherosclerotic cardiovascular disease (ASCVD). Therefore, it is of great significance to control the oxidative stress and platelet apoptosis in middle-aged and elderly adults. Previous acute clinical trials have shown that water-soluble tomato concentrate (WSTC) from fresh tomatoes could exert antiplatelet benefits after 3 h or 7 h, but its effects on platelet apoptosis and oxidative stress are still unknown, especially in healthy middle-aged and elderly adults. This current study aimed to examine the efficacies of WSTC on platelet apoptosis and oxidative stress in healthy middle-aged and elderly adults via a randomized double-blinded placebo-controlled crossover clinical trial (10 weeks in total). A total of 52 healthy middle-aged and elderly adults completed this trial. The results showed that WSTC could increase the serum total antioxidant capacity levels ($p < 0.05$) and decrease the serum malondialdehyde levels ($p < 0.05$) after a 4-week WSTC supplementation in healthy middle-aged and elderly adults. Platelet endogenous reactive oxygen species generation ($p < 0.05$), mitochondrial membrane potential dissipation ($p < 0.05$) and phosphatidylserine exposure ($p < 0.05$) were attenuated. In addition, our present study also found that WSTC could inhibit platelet aggregation and activation induced by collagen or ADP after intervention ($p < 0.05$), while having no effects on adverse events ($p > 0.05$). The results suggest that WSTC can inhibit oxidative stress and its related platelet apoptosis, which may provide a basis for the primary prevention of WSTC in ASCVD.

Keywords: water-soluble tomato concentrate; oxidative stress; platelet apoptosis; crossover clinical trial

Citation: Tian, Z.; Li, K.; Fan, D.; Gao, X.; Ma, X.; Zhao, Y.; Zhao, D.; Liang, Y.; Ji, Q.; Chen, Y.; et al. Water-Soluble Tomato Concentrate, a Potential Antioxidant Supplement, Can Attenuate Platelet Apoptosis and Oxidative Stress in Healthy Middle-Aged and Elderly Adults: A Randomized, Double-Blinded, Crossover Clinical Trial. *Nutrients* 2022, 14, 3374. https://doi.org/10.3390/nu14163374

Academic Editors: Bruno Trimarco and Gaetano Santulli

Received: 5 July 2022
Accepted: 15 August 2022
Published: 17 August 2022

Publisher's Note: MDPI stays neutral with regard to jurisdictional claims in published maps and institutional affiliations.

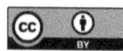

Copyright: © 2022 by the authors. Licensee MDPI, Basel, Switzerland. This article is an open access article distributed under the terms and conditions of the Creative Commons Attribution (CC BY) license (https://creativecommons.org/licenses/by/4.0/).

1. Introduction

Platelets, the most common anucleate blood cells, are essential for hemostasis, thrombosis, inflammation and atherosclerosis [1]. Animal experiments indicated that platelets are major contributors of vessel occlusion critical for cardiovascular events [2]. Accumulating evidence has shown that platelet apoptosis facilitated the progression of atherosclerotic cardiovascular disease (ASCVD) [3,4]. In different pathophysiological conditions (such as aging or dyslipidemia), the level of oxidative stress increases, thus further inducing the excessive apoptosis of platelets [5,6]. Oxidative stress and excessive apoptosis of platelets can exacerbate the risk of ASCVD [7–9].

A previous cross-sectional study [6] has shown that there was increased oxidative stress and platelet apoptotic markers in middle-aged and elderly adults, and further mice studies implicated a change in oxidative stress as the mechanism [6]. Mechanistic studies revealed that excessive reactive oxygen species (ROS) stimulated the expression and activation of pro-apoptosis proteins in the Bcl-2 family and promoted the translocation of pro-apoptosis proteins to the mitochondria [10–12]. Then, depolarization of the mitochondrial membrane potential ($\Delta\Psi m$) is initiated to form the mitochondrial permeability transition pore (mPTP), which leads to phosphatidylserine (PS) exposure and, ultimately, platelet apoptosis [10,11]. Excessive abnormal platelet apoptosis may increase the formation of PS-positive platelets and microparticles (MPs), which leads to increased procoagulant activity and thrombosis enhancement [13–15]. In addition, a cross-sectional study found that ROS production of platelets was strictly correlated with high platelet reactivity [16]. Therefore, controlling platelet apoptosis and oxidative stress can be applied for the early prevention of ASCVD in middle-aged and elderly adults.

A previous study has shown that a suitable diet, such as the Mediterranean diet, could attenuate platelet-related mortality in older adults at high cardiovascular risk [17]. Epidemiological studies suggested that tomato and tomato product consumption were associated with a reduced risk for ASCVD, which might be partly due to tomatoes containing substances with antiplatelet properties [18–20]. A large prospective study showed that there was little evidence for an overall association between dietary lycopene and the risk of ASCVD [21]. Another epidemiological study found there was no beneficial effect of higher plasma lycopene levels on myocardial infarction [22]. These indicated that other water-soluble ingredients in tomatoes might play an important role in decreasing the risk of ASCVDs. Water-soluble tomato concentrate (WSTC) is a concentrated tomato product via removing fat-soluble ingredients in tomatoes (Lycopersicon esculentum), which is primarily comprised of nucleoside derivatives, phenolic conjugates, flavonoid derivatives, and quercetin derivatives [23]. Previous studies in vitro have shown that WSTC exerted potent regulatory effects on the platelet function, such as platelet activation and aggregation inhibition [24,25]. In addition, our recent study also found that WSTC could inhibit platelet activation and aggregation in vitro [26]. Further acute randomized controlled trials (RCTs) in Britain have suggested that WSTC attenuated platelet aggregation and activation after a single dose of supplementation [25,27]. However, there has been no randomized controlled trial (RCT) exploring the effects of WSTC on platelet apoptosis. Whether it can inhibit oxidative stress is also unknown, especially in middle-aged and elderly adults.

Therefore, this present randomized placebo-controlled crossover trial aimed to examine the effects of WSTC on oxidative stress and platelet apoptosis in middle-aged and elderly adults.

2. Materials and Methods

2.1. Subject Recruitment for the Clinical Trial

Volunteers (35–70 years old) were from the health examination center of the First Affiliated Hospital of Sun Yat-sen University and three other community health centers in Guangzhou, Guangdong, China, from March to July 2019. Potential volunteers were interviewed by trained researchers using face-to-face structured screening questionnaires.

The following inclusion criteria were used: (1) men and women from 35 to 70 years old; (2) no serious vascular or hematological diseases; and (3) normal hematuria, liver or kidney function. The following exclusion criteria were used: (1) a history of hypertension, infectious disease, hemostatic disorders, diabetes mellitus or cardiovascular disease (CVD); (2) use of medications known to affect platelets in the past six months; (3) lactating or pregnant women; and (4) allergic to tomatoes or ingredients rich in tomatoes.

2.2. Study Design

The study followed a randomized, double-blinded, placebo-controlled crossover design with two 4-week interventions separated by a washout period of 2 weeks (10 weeks in total). In brief summary, the subjects in group 1 took a placebo tablet daily, while the subjects in the group 2 took 150 mg/day of WSTC for 4 weeks. Then, both groups entered a two-week washout period. After that, the two groups exchanged groups. Group 1 took 150 mg/day of WSTC, and group 2 took placebo tablets for 4 weeks (Figure 1).

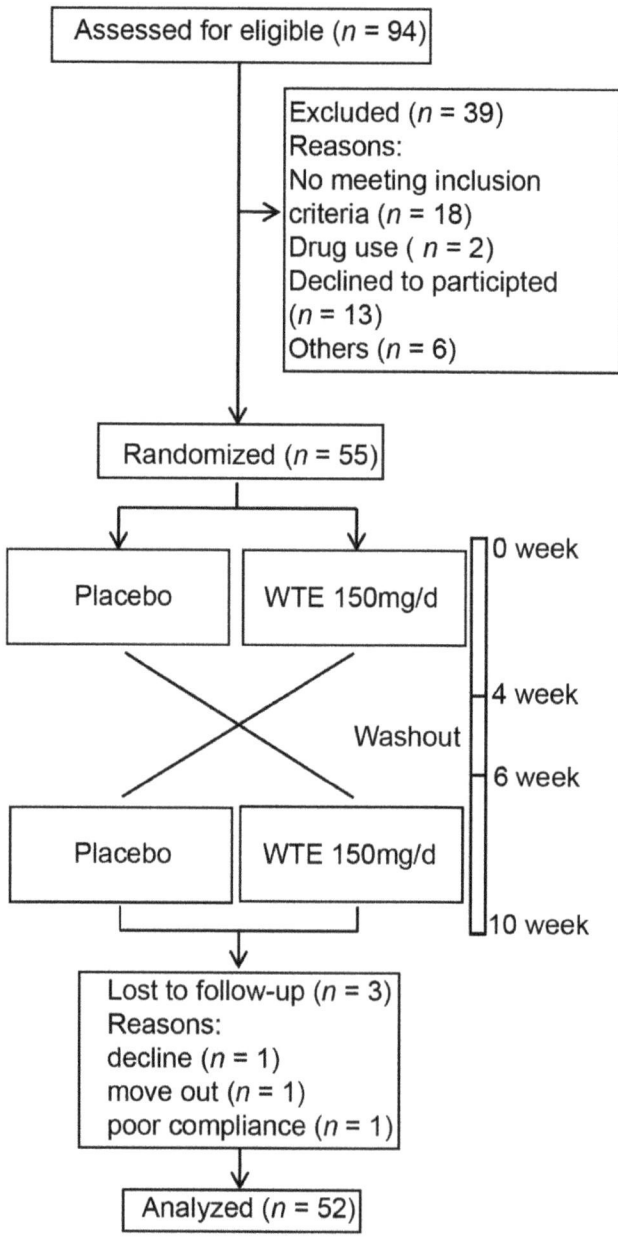

Figure 1. Flow diagram of the subject recruitment and participation procedure.

The volunteers in each gender group were randomly assigned to the two groups via hierarchical randomization. The subjects in both groups took one tablet daily during the two 4-week interventions. All subjects were followed up every two weeks, and the number of returned tablets was recorded to assess the compliance of the subjects. During the trial period, all subjects were instructed to maintain their usual diets and lifestyles but to refrain from the consumption of tomatoes and tomato products. A total of 52 subjects completed the trial (Figure 1). This current trial was conducted in accordance with the Declaration of Helsinki and was approved by the ethics committee of Sun Yat-Sen University (2016 No. 036). All of the subjects gave signed informed consent. This trial is registered at chictr.org as ChiCTR-POR-17012927.

2.3. Supplement Preparation

The placebo tablets and WSTC tablets were obtained from BY-HEALTH (Guangdong, China). The WSTC tablets contained 150 mg Fruitflow® II developed based on Fruitflow® I. Fruitflow® II primarily contained adenosine, chlorogenic acid and rutin (Supplemental Table S1) and was approved by the European Food Safety Authority as a cardioprotective functional ingredient [23]. The WSTC and placebo tablets also contained microcrystalline cellulose, lactose, croscarmellose sodium and silica. All WSTC and placebo tablets had the same weight, appearance and packaging.

2.4. Sample Size Planning for the Clinical Trial

Sample size estimation was performed via PASS software (version 15.0, NCSS Inc., Kaysville, UT, USA). A previous study reported that the changes (post-pre) of platelet aggregation after WSTC supplementation were $-9.7 \pm 4.1\%$ and $-3.1 \pm 3.9\%$ in the WSTC group and the control group, respectively [27]. Based on a two-tailed α level of 0.05 and β level of 0.10, we performed the two-sample t-tests assuming equal variance and determined that 40 subjects should be recruited. Allowing for a 20% dropout rate, at least 50 subjects were required. Since previous studies only explored the effects of WSTC on platelet-related functions, there was no data on the effects of WSTC on oxidative stress for sample size calculations. Based on this, we also performed a post hoc power analysis to extrapolate the sample size according to our current results, as previously described [28]. In summary, our current study found that the MDA levels after WSTC supplementation were 2.83 ± 0.50 nmol/mL and 3.41 ± 0.89 nmol/mL in the intervention group and control group, respectively. According to a two-tailed α level of 0.05 and β level of 0.10, we performed the two-sample t-tests assuming equal variance and determined that 34 subjects should be recruited. Allowing for a 20% dropout rate, at least 43 subjects were required. The sample size in our current study was close to the sample size estimation.

2.5. Basic Information and Anthropometric Measurement

Basic information and anthropometric measurements were collected as previously described [29]. Basic information was collected via a structured questionnaire by a trained investigator in face-to-face interviews. Height, weight, neck circumference, hip circumference, waist circumference and blood pressure were recorded at weeks 0, 4, 6 and 10. Heart rate and blood pressure (BP) were detected using oscillation monitoring technology (Omron U30 Intellisense, JPN). All measurements were performed under standardized procedures, and the mean value of two measurements was recorded. A 24-h diet record on 3 consecutive days and an international physical activity questionnaire were used to monitor the volunteers' eating habits and physical activities during the trial. The physical activity data were converted into metabolic equivalents [30], and dietary nutrient intake was calculated according to the Chinese Food Composition Table [31].

2.6. Laboratory Measurement

The volunteers fasted for 10–12 h overnight, and venous blood was collected from 8:00–9:00 a.m. on the following day on weeks 0, 4, 6 and 10. The electrical impedance method was used for the routine blood examination. The concentrations of low-density lipoprotein cholesterol (LDL-C), total cholesterol (TC), triglyceride (TG) and creatinine were measured using enzymatic methods. The concentration of serum alanine aminotransferase was determined using the rate method. Serum malonaldehyde (MDA) was determined by the TBA method using commercial kits (catalog no. A003-1-2, Jiancheng, Nanjing, China), and the serum total antioxidant capacity (TAC) was determined by the FRAP method using commercial kits (catalog no. A015-3-1, Jiancheng, Nanjing, China).

The thrombin clotting time (TT), prothrombin time (PT), activated partial thromboplastin time (APTT), and plasma fibrinogen (Fib) estimations were detected by a Sysmex CS-5100 System (Siemens Healthineers, Erlangen, Germany).

2.7. Detection of Platelet Aggregation and Activation

As previously described [25,27,32], platelet aggregation was analyzed via the CHRONO-LOG aggregometer (Chrono-log, Havertown, PA, USA). Briefly, 500 μL of fresh platelet-rich plasma (PRP) from citrated blood was incubated at 37 °C for 5 min. Then, PRP (3.0×10^8 platelets/mL) was stimulated by 5 μmol/L ADP or 2 μg/mL collagen on the Chronolog aggregometer at 37 °C with a sample stir speed of 1000 rpm. The maximum reversible platelet aggregation was monitored and recorded.

The expression of P-selectin and PAC-1 on platelets was measured using a CytoFLEX flow cytometer (Beckman Coulter, Brea, CA, USA) as previously described [32,33]. Fresh PRP (5×10^6 platelets/mL) from citrated blood were labeled with FITC-conjugated anti-human CD62P antibody or FITC-conjugated anti-human PAC-1 antibody for 20 min with the stimulation of ADP or collagen. Then, the samples were fixed with 1% paraformaldehyde and analyzed using a CytoFLEX flow cytometer with CytExpert 2.0 (Beckman Coulter, Brea, CA, USA).

2.8. Measurement of ROS, $\Delta\Psi m$ and PS Exposure in Human Platelets

Endogenous ROS was measured using DCFH-DA (Sigma-Aldrich, Burlington, MA, USA). Briefly, the platelets were preincubated with DCFH-DA (10 μM) at 37 °C in the dark for 30 min and washed with PIPES. The preincubated platelets in the clinical trial were incubated with or without thrombin (2 unit) for 30 min and detected using flow cytometry. The cells were collected and detected using a Spark® multimode microplate reader (TECAN, Canton of Zurich, Switzerland) at an excitation wavelength of 488 nm and emission wavelength of 525 nm.

Platelet $\Delta\Psi m$ was measured using tetramethylrhodamine methyl ester (TMRM; Abcam, Cambridge, UK). Washed platelets (5×10^6/mL) were preincubated with or without thrombin for 30 min. All of the samples were incubated with TMRM (400 nM) for 20 min at 37 °C in the dark and measured using flow cytometry.

PS exposure was measured using PE-annexin V (Becton Dickinson, Franklin Lakes, NJ, USA) according to the manufacturer's instructions. Prepared samples were incubated with PE-annexin V for 15 min at room temperature, and then, PS was measured by flow cytometry within 30 min.

2.9. Statistical Analysis

The data were analyzed using SPSS 20.0 statistical software and GraphPad Prism 5.01 software. The data analysis of the individuals in this study followed the intention-to-treat (ITT) principle, as in previous studies [33,34]. All data were presented as the means ± standard errors of the means (SEMs). The data from week 0 and week 6 (after washout) were combined as pretrial (baseline) data, and the data from weeks 4 and 10 were combined as posttrial data in the clinical trial. The comparability of the two groups at baseline was assessed by one-way analysis of variance (ANOVA). ANOVA was also used to determine the significance of the differences between the placebo and WSTC supplementation groups after 4 weeks of intervention. To further determine the effect of WSTC supplementation on oxidative stress and platelet apoptosis, Student's t-tests for paired data were used to examine significant differences before and after WSTC or placebo supplementation in all volunteers, as in previous studies [28,35]. The differences were considered significant at $p < 0.05$.

3. Results

3.1. Subsection

The mean age of the subjects was 56 years old (44–68 years old), and 30.77% were males. Baseline data were collected before distribution, including sociodemographic data, medical histories, drug use information and anthropometric characteristics (Table 1). There was no significant difference in the anthropometric characteristics, blood lipids or blood glucose between the two groups of volunteers at baseline or during the intervention period (Supplementary Table S2). In addition, there was no significant difference in energy, intake of nutrients or physical activity between the two groups at baseline or after the 4-week intervention (Supplementary Table S3).

Table 1. Baseline characteristics.

	N = 52
Age, (years)	56.13 ± 1.01 [a]
Gender (male/female)	16/36
Education attainment	
Primary school	2(3.85%)
Middle school	23(44.23%)
College	27(51.92%)
Occupations	
Sales/workers/farmers	18(34.61%)
Professionals/technicians	29(55.76%)
Others	5(9.62%)
Anthropometrics	
Weight (kg)	64.17 ± 1.70
BMI (kg/m^2)	24.57 ± 0.46
NC (cm)	34.40 ± 1.08
WC (cm)	84.99 ± 1.59
WHR	0.88 ± 0.01
SBP (mmHg)	118.32 ± 2.19
DBP (mmHg)	77.19 ± 1.47
Lifestyle factors	
Current smoking	2(3.8%)
Regular alcohol drinking	11(21%)

[a] The results are presented as the mean ± standard error of the mean for continuous variables and n (%) for categorical variables. Abbreviation: BMI, body mass index, WC, waist circumference, NC, neck circumference, WHR, waist-to-hip ratio, DBP, diastolic blood pressure and SBP, systolic blood pressure.

3.2. Effects of WSTC Supplementation on TAC and MDA in Healthy Middle-Aged and Elderly Adults

There were no significant differences in the serum TAC or MDA levels between the placebo and WSTC groups at baseline. After the 4-week intervention, WSTC supplementation significantly increased the serum TAC levels ($p < 0.05$) and reduced the serum MDA levels ($p < 0.05$) in healthy middle-aged and elderly adults (Figure 2A,B). There were also significant differences in the serum TAC levels ($p < 0.01$) and MDA levels ($p < 0.01$) between the placebo and WSTC groups after intervention. However, there was no significant difference in the serum TAC levels and MDA levels in the placebo group before vs. after the intervention (Figure 2A,B).

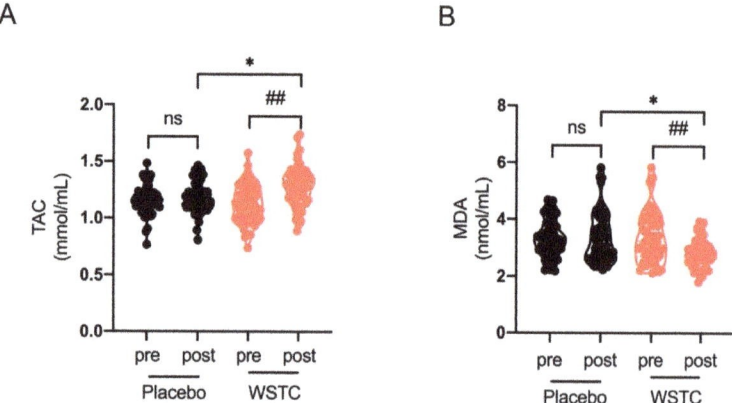

Figure 2. Effects of WSTC supplementation on the serum TAC and MDA levels in healthy middle-aged and elderly adults. (**A**,**B**) Serum TAC and MDA levels. The values are presented as the means ± SEMs. At baseline, there was no significant difference for the TAC and MDA levels between the two groups. * $p < 0.05$, one-way analysis of variance for independent data is used for comparison between the two groups after 4 weeks of intervention. ## $p < 0.01$ vs. baseline in the WSTC group, assessed by a paired Student's *t*-test. Abbreviations: TAC, total antioxidant capacity, MDA, malonaldehyde, WSTC, water-soluble tomato concentrate and ns, no significance.

3.3. WSTC Supplementation Attenuated Platelet ROS Generation in Healthy Middle-Aged and Elderly Adults

As shown in Figure 3, there was no significant difference in circulating platelet endogenous ROS between the two groups at baseline. Circulating platelet endogenous ROS generation in healthy middle-aged and elderly adults was significantly lower in the WSTC supplementation group after 4 weeks of supplementation compared to the placebo group ($p < 0.05$). WSTC supplementation for 4 weeks significantly reduced platelet endogenous ROS generation in healthy middle-aged and elderly adults ($p < 0.01$). In the placebo group, there was no significant change before or after the intervention ($p > 0.05$) (Figure 3).

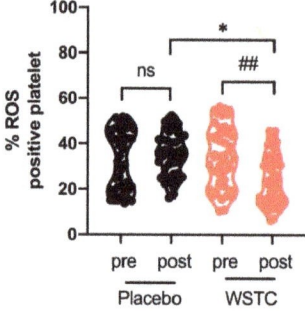

Figure 3. Effect of WSTC supplementation on ROS generation in healthy middle-aged and elderly adults. Human wash platelets were prepared from volunteers before (pre) and after (post) 4 weeks of WSTC or placebo consumption. The washed platelets were pretreated with H2DCF-DA, and ROS was measured by flow cytometry. At baseline, there is no significant difference in the ROS generation between the two groups. * $p < 0.05$, one-way analysis of variance for independent data, is used for comparison between the two groups after 4 weeks of intervention. ## $p < 0.01$ vs. baseline in the WSTC group, assessed by a paired Student's *t*-test. Abbreviations: ROS, reactive oxygen species, WSTC, water-soluble tomato concentrate and ns, no significance.

3.4. WSTC Supplementation Attenuated Platelet ΔΨm Dissipation and PS Exposure in Healthy Middle-Aged and Elderly Adults

At baseline, there were no significant differences in platelet ΔΨm dissipation and PS exposure between the placebo and WSTC groups. Increased circulating platelet ΔΨm has been observed in healthy middle-aged and elderly adults ($p < 0.05$) after 4 weeks of WSTC supplementation ($p < 0.05$) (Figure 4A). Additionally, after WSTC supplementation, WSTC supplementation also markedly attenuated the platelet PS exposure in healthy middle-aged and elderly adults ($p < 0.05$) (Figure 4B). Compared with the placebo group, the platelet ΔΨm in the WSTC group was significantly higher ($p < 0.05$) and platelet PS exposure was significantly lower ($p < 0.01$). However, there was no significant difference in the platelet ΔΨm dissipation and PS exposure in the placebo group before vs. after the intervention (Figure 4A,B).

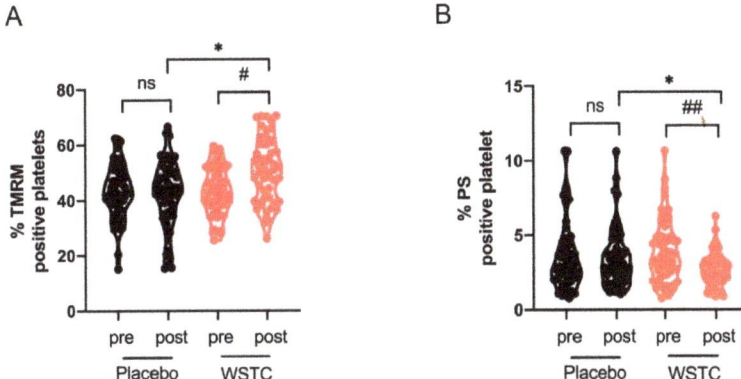

Figure 4. Effect of WSTC supplementation on ΔΨm dissipation and PS exposure in healthy middle-aged and elderly adults. Human wash platelets were prepared from volunteers before (pre) and after (post) 4 weeks of WSTC or placebo consumption. (**A**) Platelet ΔΨm dissipation was measured using TMRM by flow cytometry. (**B**) Annexin V-PE was used to assess platelet PS exposure by flow cytometry. At baseline, there was no significant difference in any variable for ΔΨm dissipation and PS exposure between the two groups. * $p < 0.05$, one-way analysis of variance for independent data was used for comparison between the two groups after 4 weeks of intervention. # $p < 0.05$ and ## $p < 0.01$ vs. baseline in the WSTC group, assessed by a paired Student's t-test. Abbreviations: PS, phosphatidylserine and WSTC, water-soluble tomato concentrate.

3.5. WSTC Supplementation Attenuated ROS Generation and ΔΨm Dissipation in Thrombin-Treated Platelets

Previous studies have shown that thrombin induced platelet apoptotic events via ROS generation. Therefore, we identified a possible association between ROS and platelet apoptosis using thrombin in the context of WSTC supplementation [36]. At the baseline, the platelet ROS generation and ΔΨm dissipation in the two groups were comparable ($p > 0.05$). WSTC significantly attenuated platelet ROS generation and ΔΨm dissipation in response to thrombin (2 unit) after 4 weeks of supplementation ($p < 0.05$) (Figure 5A,B). Additionally, the platelet ΔΨm in the WSTC group was significantly higher ($p < 0.01$) than that in the placebo group ($p < 0.01$), and platelet ROS generation in the WSTC group was significantly lower than that in the placebo group ($p < 0.001$). There was no significant difference between baseline and the 4-week intervention of the placebo group ($p > 0.05$) (Figure 5A,B).

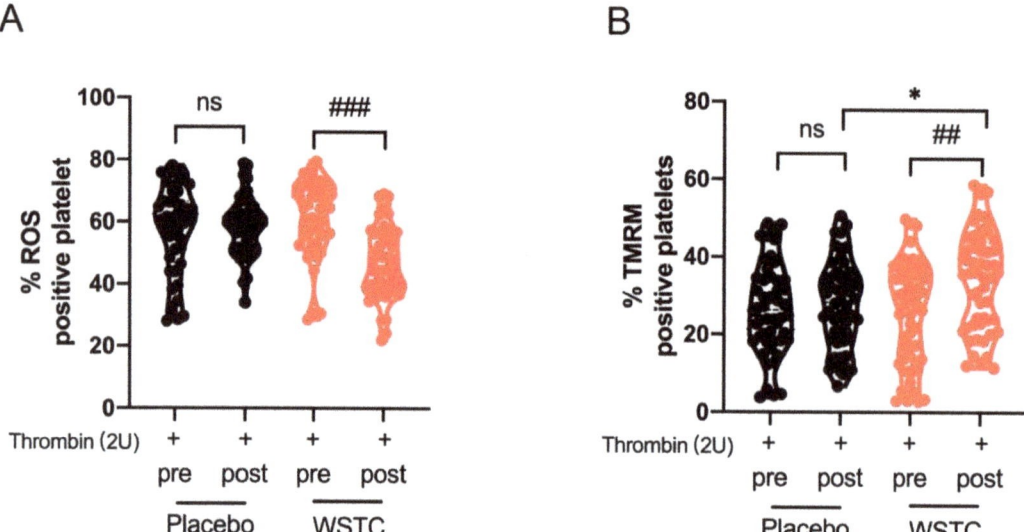

Figure 5. Effects of WSTC supplementation on ΔΨm dissipation and ROS in response to thrombin. Human wash platelets were prepared from volunteers before (pre) and after (post) 4 weeks of WSTC or placebo consumption. (**A**) H2DCF-DA-treated platelets were incubated with thrombin (2 unit), and ROS were measured by flow cytometry. (**B**) The wash platelets were incubated with thrombin (2 unit), and TMRM was used to detect ΔΨm measured by flow cytometry. At baseline, there was no significant difference in any variable about ΔΨm dissipation and ROS between the two groups. * $p < 0.05$, one-way analysis of variance for independent data was used for comparison between the two groups after 4 weeks of intervention. ## $p < 0.01$ and ### $p < 0.001$ vs. baseline in the WSTC group, assessed by a paired Student's *t*-test. Abbreviations: ROS, reactive oxygen species and WSTC, water-soluble tomato concentrate.

3.6. WSTC Supplementation Inhibited Platelet Aggregation and Activation in Healthy Middle-Aged and Elderly Adults

Previous acute studies in Britain have found that WSTC significantly inhibited collagen- and ADP-induced platelet aggregation [25,27]. Therefore, we also measured platelet activation and aggregation stimulated by collagen and ADP in healthy middle-aged and elderly adults. We found that four weeks of WSTC supplementation effectively reduced the platelet aggregation induced by ADP or collagen ($p < 0.05$) (Figure 6A,B). WSTC supplementation in healthy middle-aged and elderly adults markedly attenuated platelet surface P-selectin expression and glycoprotein IIb IIIa activation (PAC-1) induced by ADP or collagen ($p < 0.05$) (Figure 6C–E). There were also significant differences in platelet aggregation induced by ADP or collagen between the placebo and WSTC groups after the intervention ($p < 0.05$) (Figure 6A,B). Compared with the placebo group, platelet surface P-selectin expression and glycoprotein IIb IIIa activation (PAC-1) induced by ADP or collagen in the WSTC group were significantly lower after a 4-week supplementation ($p < 0.05$) (Figure 6C–E).

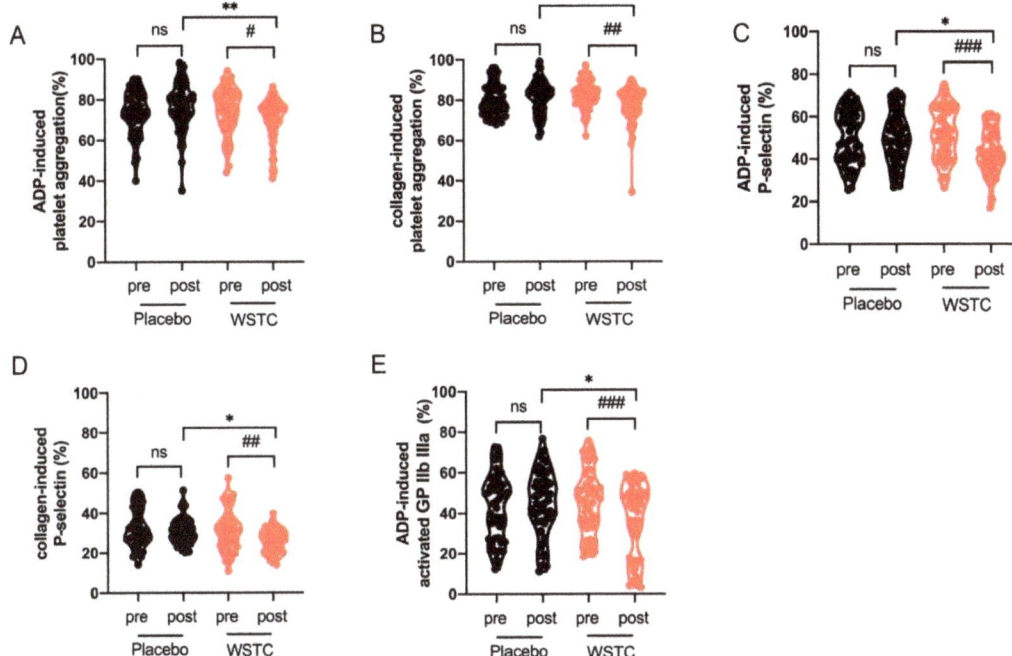

Figure 6. WSTC supplementation inhibited platelet aggregation and activation in healthy middle-aged and elderly adults. Human PRP was prepared from volunteers before (pre) and after (post) 4 weeks of WSTC or placebo consumption. (**A,B**) Platelet aggregation was stimulated by ADP or collagen. PRP was stimulated with ADP or collagen. The platelet surface expression of (**C,D**) P-selectin and (**E**) PAC-1 was analyzed by flow cytometry. The values are presented as the means ± SEMs. At baseline, there was no significant difference for platelet aggregation and activation between the two groups. * $p < 0.05$ and ** $p < 0.01$, one-way analysis of variance for independent data was used for a comparison between the two groups after 4 weeks of intervention. # $p < 0.05$, ## $p < 0.01$ and ### $p < 0.001$ vs. baseline in the WSTC group, assessed by a paired Student's *t*-test. Abbreviations: PRP, platelet-rich plasma and WSTC, water-soluble tomato concentrate.

3.7. Safety Evaluation

Previous studies did not observe clinical side effects after 0–7 days of WSTC intervention [27]. We performed 4 weeks of WSTC supplementation for the first time and found that no adverse event was reported during the whole intervention period. In addition, considering the antiplatelet effects of WSTC, we carefully determined whether the clotting pathways were affected by WSTC alongside the antiplatelet effects. We examined the coagulation function of the subjects and found that a 4-week intervention of WSTC did not affect APTT, TT, PT, PT-INR, Fib and PT-R in healthy middle-aged and elderly adults ($p > 0.05$, Table 2). There was no significant difference in the platelet parameters, coagulation function or liver and kidney function in the WSTC group compared to the placebo group ($p > 0.05$, Table 2).

Table 2. Blood chemistry and plasma clotting times at baseline and after the 4-week treatment [b].

	Placebo (n = 52)		150mg WSTC (n = 52)	
	Baseline	4 Weeks	Baseline	4 Weeks
Liver function				
ALT (U/L)	21.08 ± 1.57 [a]	21.27 ± 2.03	21.75 ± 1.97	20.55 ± 1.51
Total protein (g/L)	74.19 ± 0.50	73.37 ± 0.45	73.58 ± 0.56	73.16 ± 0.53
Albumin (g/L)	47.05 ± 0.32	45.97 ± 0.33	46.63 ± 0.36	45.55 ± 0.35
Albumin/Globulin	1.77 ± 0.04	1.69 ± 0.03	1.76 ± 0.03	1.68 ± 0.03
Renal function				
Urea (mmol/L)	4.86 ± 1.42	4.97 ± 0.15	5.01 ± 0.17	4.82 ± 0.14
Creatinine (μmol/L)	78.35 ± 2.44	78.29 ± 2.30	79.21 ± 2.36	78.44 ± 2.38
Plasma clotting times				
Prothrombin time (s)	10.81 ± 0.73	11.26 ± 0.81	10.90 ± 0.71	11.16 ± 0.73
APTT (s)	28.75 ± 0.24	28.64 ± 0.28	28.68 ± 0.28	28.48 ± 0.25
Thrombin time (s)	18.76 ± 0.09	18.76 ± 0.13	18.77 ± 0.10	18.91 ± 0.11
Fibrinogen (g/L)	2.98 ± 0.06	3.03 ± 0.08	3.01 ± 0.07	2.92 ± 0.08
Platelet parameters				
PLT (10^9/L)	244.20 ± 9.05	253.53 ± 9.90	244.12 ± 8.71	250.69 ± 9.27
MPV (fl)	10.20 ± 0.15	10.18 ± 0.13	10.17 ± 0.15	10.22 ± 0.15

[a] Mean ± SEM (all such values). [b] A one-way analysis of variance for independent data was used for comparison between the two groups at baseline and after 4 weeks of intervention. There was no significant difference for any variable concerning the blood chemistry and plasma clotting times between the two groups at baseline and after the 4-week intervention. Abbreviations: ALT, alanine aminotransferase, PT-R, prothrombin time ratio, PLT, plaque level test, MPV, medial plaque volume and APTT, activated partial thromboplastin time.

4. Discussion

An increasing number of studies now suggest broad protective effects of functional foods against CVD [23,37,38]. The present study used a randomized placebo-controlled clinical trial and showed that 4 weeks of supplementation with WSTC (150 mg/day) increased the antioxidative capacity in serum (e.g., increased TAC and decreased MDA levels) and attenuated circulating platelet ROS generation and apoptosis (e.g., attenuated ΔΨm decrease and PS exposure) in healthy middle-aged and elderly adults. Additionally, the 4 weeks of WSTC supplementation also inhibited platelet activation and aggregation, which was consistent with previous studies [25,27]. Our results suggest that WSTC is a promising agent for ASCVD prevention that exerts its beneficial effects via the control of oxidative stress and platelet apoptosis.

Mitochondrial alterations contribute to the pathogenesis of CVD [39]. Mitochondria also play a central role in platelet metabolism, and mitochondrial membrane depolarization is the initial step of mitochondrial-mediated apoptosis [40]. WSTC supplementation significantly attenuated platelet ΔΨm dissipation in our present study, which suggests that WSTC plays a vital role in reducing early damage to platelet function. Negatively charged PS is exposed to the outer membrane of apoptotic platelets, and it is a central procoagulant factor that accelerates the progression of thrombosis [4,41,42]. PS-positive apoptotic platelets are enhanced in patients with prothrombotic states [43]. Notably, our results also showed that supplementation with WSTC attenuated platelet PS exposure on circulating platelets, which may contribute to thrombotic disease inhibition. In addition, our previous in vitro study support as well that WSTC could modulate platelet ΔΨm dissipation and inhibit Cytochrome c release, caspase activation and PS exposure in H_2O_2-treated platelets [44]. These results indicated that WSTC might inhibit mitochondria-dependent platelet apoptosis. These findings are consistent with Xiao et al., who revealed that quercetin, one component of WSTC, inhibited stored platelet apoptosis by increasing the Bcl-2/Bax ratio in a concentration-dependent manner [45]. Notably, nutrients promote apoptosis in cancer cells, but chlorogenic acid, rutin and polyphenols (e.g., resveratrol and curcumin) have to exert an antiapoptotic effect by inhibiting oxidative stress in normal cell lines [46,47]. Whether one or more components of WSTC or only the mixture contribute to protecting platelet apoptosis is worthy of further study. Overall, our data suggest that

WSTC supplementation may alleviate the risks of atherothrombosis via attenuating platelet apoptosis in healthy middle-aged and older people.

Oxidative stress is a central pathological mechanism in ASCVD that induces hypertrophic signaling, apoptosis and necrosis [48]. Antioxidant administration reduces oxidative stress-related apoptosis in the pathogenesis of lots of diseases [49,50]. The present study showed that WSTC supplementation effectively increased TAC while decreasing the MDA levels and platelet endogenous ROS generation, which is consistent with other studies showing that the main bioactive components of WSTC possessed antioxidant properties [51–53]. Under certain thrombotic conditions, the levels of oxidative stress (e.g., ROS) are enhanced, and platelet redox homeostasis is disrupted; these changes have many important proatherogenic effects, including the stimulation of platelet hyperreactivity and apoptosis [36]. Whether WSTC attenuates oxidative stress-related platelet apoptosis under disease conditions merits further investigation. Our present study shows that WSTC may exert its beneficial effects on ASCVD prevention via the control of oxidative stress in healthy middle-aged and elderly adults.

Superoxide anion and H_2O_2 are the main ROS. The superoxide anion may be converted into H_2O_2 to modulate intraplatelet redox physiological signaling and stimulate platelet apoptosis [12,54]. Previous studies revealed that H_2O_2-induced ROS production was consistent with the changes observed in apoptosis [49]. Our previous in vitro study showed that pretreatment with WSTC dose-dependently attenuated ROS generation in H_2O_2-treated platelets, and a combined treatment with WSTC and NAC did not result in significant differences in the apoptosis levels compared with the WSTC treatment alone [44]. A further in vitro study showed that WSTC could increase the expression level of LC3II/I in H_2O_2-treated platelets. Furthermore, the effect of WSTC on decreasing $\Delta\Psi m$ depolarization in H_2O_2-treated platelets was reversed by an autophagy inhibitor (3-MA) [44]. These indicated that WSTC can significantly reduce the H_2O_2-induced platelet oxidative damage by promoting autophagy in vitro. Therefore, oxidative stress could potentially be essential in inhibiting platelet apoptosis by WSTC. The attenuation of ROS-scavenging activity only partially reflects the antioxidant potential, and the antioxidant properties of WSTC may also contribute to its antiapoptotic benefits, which are worthy of further investigation.

WSTC, authorized by the European Food Safety Agency, is approved to take 150 mg/day in the format of powder, tablet or capsule [23]. Therefore, the dose of 150 mg/day was used in this clinical trial. WSTC was first found to have antiplatelet functions (e.g., anti-activation and anti-aggregation effects) in Britain. Previous acute clinical trials found that WSTC supplementation could attenuate platelet activation and aggregation after 3 h or 7 h [27,55]. To further verify the accuracy of this result, we also explored the effect of WSTC on platelet function in this study. Notably, our study found that 150 mg/day of WSTC has remarkably inhibited platelet activation and aggregation induced by collagen or ADP after a 4-week intervention in healthy middle-aged and elderly adults. These are consistent with previous studies in Britain. Taking antiplatelet drugs such as aspirin and warfarin can reduce the risk of cardiovascular events, but it may also increase the risk of bleeding [56]. Due to the antiplatelet effects of WSTC, we also explored whether WSTC could affect the coagulation function. In our clinical trial, WSTC does not affect the coagulation function related to the prothrombin system after 4 weeks of WSTC supplementation. Our previous animal experiment also found that WSTC could not prolong the bleeding time of mice [26]. Interestingly, our previous study found that the inhibitory effect of 4 weeks of WSTC on platelet aggregation and activation can be eliminated after a 2-week washout period [57]. In addition, we also found that a 4-week intervention of WSTC had no effect on the liver function or kidney function in healthy middle-aged and elderly adults, and this was consistent with previous studies [23,58]. Although whether there is a risk of bleeding after long-term use still needs to be confirmed by further studies with larger sample sizes and longer intervention durations, the current results suggest that WSTC may be used as a potentially safe and reliable nutrient supplement for regulating platelet function.

Strengths and Limitations

There are some strengths and certain limitations in this study. The major strength of this study is the design of a double-blinded, randomized, placebo-controlled, crossover trial. Another strength is that we tested the platelet ROS generation, PS exposure and $\Delta\Psi m$ at baseline and during follow-up, which should be completed in two hours after blood collection. For the first time, we explored the effect of WSTC on oxidative stress and platelet apoptosis in healthy middle-aged and elderly adults. This could be another advantage. As in previous studies [28,34], we also maintain all usual dietary intake and physical activities via questionnaires to control the effects of a confounding bias. Nevertheless, there are still some limitations present in this study. One of the limitations is that, due to the complex composition of WSTC, it is unlikely for us to measure the serum levels of WSTC or its metabolites. The results of this study only indicated a potential benefit of WSTC on the early prevention of CVDs in healthy middle-aged and elderly adults, and the prevention of WSTC in individuals with metabolic diseases merits further clinical study. This may be another limitation of our study.

5. Conclusions

The results showed that four weeks of WSTC supplementation could attenuate oxidative stress and platelet apoptosis in healthy middle-aged and elderly adults. In addition, our study further added evidence that WSTC could safely and effectively reduce platelet aggregation and activation in healthy middle-aged and elderly adults. Therefore, our current results indicate that the beneficial effects of WSTC may have a potential role in the early prevention of ASCVD.

Supplementary Materials: The following supporting information can be downloaded at https://www.mdpi.com/article/10.3390/nu14163374/s1: Table S1: The composition of water-soluble tomato extract, Table S2: Anthropometric measurements, lipid profiles and glucose at baseline and 4 weeks after treatment, Table S3: Daily dietary intakes and physical activity at baseline and 4 weeks after treatment.

Author Contributions: Z.T. and K.L. contributed equally to this work. Y.Y. designed this study. Z.T. and K.L. performed all the experiments and analyzed the data with assistance from D.F., X.G., X.M. and Y.Z. Z.T. and K.L. wrote a draft of the manuscript. D.F., X.G., X.M., Y.Z., D.Z., Y.L., Q.J. and Y.C. revised this draft manuscript. Y.Y. was the principal investigator who designed this study and had primary responsibility for the final manuscript. All authors have read and agreed to the published version of the manuscript.

Funding: This work was supported by the National Natural Science Foundation of China (No. 82030098, 81872617 and 81730090); the Shenzhen Science and Technology Innovation Commission (JCYJ20180307153228190) and the By-health Research Foundation.

Institutional Review Board Statement: The study complied with the Declaration of Helsinki and was approved by the Ethics Committee of Sun Yat-Sen University (2016 No. 036).

Informed Consent Statement: All subjects in this study have read and gave signed informed consent.

Data Availability Statement: Data, protocol of this study, plan of statistical analysis and informed consent will be made available upon reasonable request via email to the corresponding author.

Acknowledgments: The authors acknowledge the assistance of all the volunteers for their participation and the help of the American journal experts and Yidi Wu in editing this manuscript.

Conflicts of Interest: The authors declare no conflict of interest.

References

1. Xu, X.R.; Zhang, D.; Oswald, B.E.; Carrim, N.; Wang, X.; Hou, Y.; Zhang, Q.; Lavalle, C.; McKeown, T.; Marshall, A.H.; et al. Platelets are versatile cells: New discoveries in hemostasis, thrombosis, immune responses, tumor metastasis and beyond. *Crit. Rev. Clin. Lab. Sci.* **2016**, *53*, 409–430. [CrossRef] [PubMed]
2. Gowert, N.S.; Donner, L.; Chatterjee, M.; Eisele, Y.S.; Towhid, S.T.; Munzer, P.; Walker, B.; Ogorek, I.; Borst, O.; Grandoch, M.; et al. Blood platelets in the progression of Alzheimer's disease. *PLoS ONE* **2014**, *9*, e90523. [CrossRef] [PubMed]
3. Burnouf, T.; Goubran, H.A.; Chou, M.L.; Devos, D.; Radosevic, M. Platelet microparticles: Detection and assessment of their paradoxical functional roles in disease and regenerative medicine. *Blood Rev.* **2014**, *28*, 155–166. [CrossRef] [PubMed]
4. Thushara, R.M.; Hemshekhar, M.; Basappa; Kemparaju, K.; Rangappa, K.S.; Girish, K.S. Biologicals, platelet apoptosis and human diseases: An outlook. *Crit. Rev. Oncol. Hematol.* **2015**, *93*, 149–158. [CrossRef] [PubMed]
5. Han, F.; Liu, H.; Wang, K.; Yang, J.; Yang, L.; Liu, J.; Zhang, M.; Dun, W. Correlation Between Thalamus-Related Functional Connectivity and Serum BDNF Levels During the Periovulatory Phase of Primary Dysmenorrhea. *Front. Hum. Neurosci.* **2019**, *13*, 333. [CrossRef]
6. Jain, K.; Tyagi, T.; Patell, K.; Xie, Y.; Kadado, A.J.; Lee, S.H.; Yarovinsky, T.; Du, J.; Hwang, J.; Martin, K.A.; et al. Age associated non-linear regulation of redox homeostasis in the anucleate platelet: Implications for CVD risk patients. *EBioMedicine* **2019**, *44*, 28–40. [CrossRef]
7. Förstermann, U.; Xia, N.; Li, H. Roles of Vascular Oxidative Stress and Nitric Oxide in the Pathogenesis of Atherosclerosis. *Circ. Res.* **2017**, *120*, 713–735. [CrossRef]
8. Mone, P.; Varzideh, F.; Jankauskas, S.S.; Pansini, A.; Lombardi, A.; Frullone, S.; Santulli, G. SGLT2 Inhibition via Empagliflozin Improves Endothelial Function and Reduces Mitochondrial Oxidative Stress: Insights from Frail Hypertensive and Diabetic Patients. *Hypertension* **2022**, *79*, 1633–1643. [CrossRef]
9. Ijsselmuiden, A.J.; Musters, R.J.; de Ruiter, G.; van Heerebeek, L.; Alderse-Baas, F.; van Schilfgaarde, M.; Leyte, A.; Tangelder, G.J.; Laarman, G.J.; Paulus, W.J. Circulating white blood cells and platelets amplify oxidative stress in heart failure. *Nat. Clin. Pract. Cardiovasc. Med.* **2008**, *5*, 811–820. [CrossRef]
10. Lopez, J.J.; Salido, G.M.; Gomez-Arteta, E.; Rosado, J.A.; Pariente, J.A. Thrombin induces apoptotic events through the generation of reactive oxygen species in human platelets. *J. Thromb. Haemost.* **2007**, *5*, 1283–1291. [CrossRef]
11. Leytin, V. Apoptosis in the anucleate platelet. *Blood Rev.* **2012**, *26*, 51–63. [CrossRef] [PubMed]
12. Pietraforte, D.; Vona, R.; Marchesi, A.; de Jacobis, I.T.; Villani, A.; Del Principe, D.; Straface, E. Redox control of platelet functions in physiology and pathophysiology. *Antioxid. Redox Signal.* **2014**, *21*, 177–193. [CrossRef] [PubMed]
13. Bae, O.N.; Lim, K.M.; Noh, J.Y.; Chung, S.M.; Kim, S.H.; Chung, J.H. Trivalent methylated arsenical-induced phosphatidylserine exposure and apoptosis in platelets may lead to increased thrombus formation. *Toxicol. Appl. Pharmacol.* **2009**, *239*, 144–153. [CrossRef]
14. Rautou, P.E.; Vion, A.C.; Amabile, N.; Chironi, G.; Simon, A.; Tedgui, A.; Boulanger, C.M. Microparticles, vascular function, and atherothrombosis. *Circ. Res.* **2011**, *109*, 593–606. [CrossRef] [PubMed]
15. Melki, I.; Tessandier, N.; Zufferey, A.; Boilard, E. Platelet microvesicles in health and disease. *Platelets* **2017**, *28*, 214–221. [CrossRef]
16. Becatti, M.; Fiorillo, C.; Gori, A.M.; Marcucci, R.; Paniccia, R.; Giusti, B.; Violi, F.; Pignatelli, P.; Gensini, G.F.; Abbate, R. Platelet and leukocyte ROS production and lipoperoxidation are associated with high platelet reactivity in Non-ST elevation myocardial infarction (NSTEMI) patients on dual antiplatelet treatment. *Atherosclerosis* **2013**, *231*, 392–400. [CrossRef]
17. Hernaez, A.; Lassale, C.; Castro-Barquero, S.; Ros, E.; Tresserra-Rimbau, A.; Castaner, O.; Pinto, X.; Vazquez-Ruiz, Z.; Sorli, J.V.; Salas-Salvado, J.; et al. Mediterranean Diet Maintained Platelet Count within a Healthy Range and Decreased Thrombocytopenia-Related Mortality Risk: A Randomized Controlled Trial. *Nutrients* **2021**, *13*, 559. [CrossRef]
18. Cheng, H.M.; Koutsidis, G.; Lodge, J.K.; Ashor, A.; Siervo, M.; Lara, J. Tomato and lycopene supplementation and cardiovascular risk factors: A systematic review and meta-analysis. *Atherosclerosis* **2017**, *257*, 100–108. [CrossRef]
19. Cámara, M.; Fernández-Ruiz, V.; Sánchez-Mata, M.C.; Domínguez Díaz, L.; Kardinaal, A.; van Lieshout, M. Evidence of antiplatelet aggregation effects from the consumption of tomato products, according to EFSA health claim requirements. *Crit. Rev. Food Sci. Nutr.* **2020**, *60*, 1515–1522. [CrossRef]
20. Olas, B. Anti-Aggregatory Potential of Selected Vegetables-Promising Dietary Components for the Prevention and Treatment of Cardiovascular Disease. *Adv. Nutr.* **2019**, *10*, 280–290. [CrossRef]
21. Sesso, H.D.; Liu, S.; Gaziano, J.M.; Buring, J.E. Dietary lycopene, tomato-based food products and cardiovascular disease in women. *J. Nutr.* **2003**, *133*, 2336–2341. [CrossRef] [PubMed]
22. Hak, A.E.; Stampfer, M.J.; Campos, H.; Sesso, H.D.; Gaziano, J.M.; Willett, W.; Ma, J. Plasma carotenoids and tocopherols and risk of myocardial infarction in a low-risk population of US male physicians. *Circulation* **2003**, *108*, 802–807. [CrossRef] [PubMed]
23. O'Kennedy, N.; Raederstorff, D.; Duttaroy, A.K. Fruitflow®: The first European Food Safety Authority-approved natural cardio-protective functional ingredient. *Eur. J. Nutr.* **2017**, *56*, 461–482. [CrossRef] [PubMed]
24. Dutta-Roy, A.K.; Crosbie, L.; Gordon, M.J. Effects of tomato extract on human platelet aggregation in vitro. *Platelets* **2001**, *12*, 218–227. [CrossRef]
25. O'Kennedy, N.; Crosbie, L.; van Lieshout, M.; Broom, J.I.; Webb, D.J.; Duttaroy, A.K. Effects of antiplatelet components of tomato extract on platelet function in vitro and ex vivo: A time-course cannulation study in healthy humans. *Am. J. Clin. Nutr.* **2006**, *84*, 570–579. [CrossRef]

26. Fan, D.; Tian, Z.Z.; Zuo, X.; Ya, F.L.; Yang, Y. Fruitflow, a Water-soluble Tomato Concentrate, Inhibits Platelet Activation, Aggregation and Thrombosis by Regulating the Signaling Pathway of PI3K/Akt and MAPKs. *J. Sun Yat-Sen Univ. (Med. Sci.)* **2020**, *41*, 243–250. [CrossRef]
27. O'Kennedy, N.; Crosbie, L.; Song, H.J.; Zhang, X.; Horgan, G.; Duttaroy, A.K. A randomised controlled trial comparing a dietary antiplatelet, the water-soluble tomato extract Fruitflow, with 75 mg aspirin in healthy subjects. *Eur. J. Clin. Nutr.* **2017**, *71*, 723–730. [CrossRef]
28. Tian, Z.; Li, K.; Fan, D.; Zhao, Y.; Gao, X.; Ma, X.; Xu, L.; Shi, Y.; Ya, F.; Zou, J.; et al. Dose-dependent effects of anthocyanin supplementation on platelet function in subjects with dyslipidemia: A randomized clinical trial. *EBioMedicine* **2021**, *70*, 103533. [CrossRef]
29. Xu, Z.; Xie, J.; Zhang, H.; Pang, J.; Li, Q.; Wang, X.; Xu, H.; Sun, X.; Zhao, H.; Yang, Y.; et al. Anthocyanin supplementation at different doses improves cholesterol efflux capacity in subjects with dyslipidemia—A randomized controlled trial. *Eur. J. Clin. Nutr.* **2021**, *75*, 345–354. [CrossRef]
30. Craig, C.L.; Marshall, A.L.; Sjostrom, M.; Bauman, A.E.; Booth, M.L.; Ainsworth, B.E.; Pratt, M.; Ekelund, U.; Yngve, A.; Sallis, J.F.; et al. International physical activity questionnaire: 12-country reliability and validity. *Med. Sci. Sports Exerc.* **2003**, *35*, 1381–1395. [CrossRef]
31. Ju, L.; Yu, D.; Fang, H.; Guo, Q.; Xu, X.; Li, S.; Zhao, L. Trends and food sources composition of energy, protein and fat in Chinese residents, 1992-2012. *Wei Sheng Yan Jiu = J. Hyg. Res.* **2018**, *47*, 689–704.
32. Yang, Y.; Shi, Z.; Reheman, A.; Jin, J.W.; Li, C.; Wang, Y.; Andrews, M.C.; Chen, P.; Zhu, G.; Ling, W.; et al. Plant food delphinidin-3-glucoside significantly inhibits platelet activation and thrombosis: Novel protective roles against cardiovascular diseases. *PLoS ONE* **2012**, *7*, e37323. [CrossRef]
33. Ya, F.L.; Xu, X.R.; Shi, Y.L.; Gallant, R.C.; Song, F.L.; Zuo, X.; Zhao, Y.M.; Tian, Z.Z.; Zhang, C.; Xu, X.P.; et al. Coenzyme Q10 Upregulates Platelet cAMP/PKA Pathway and Attenuates Integrin alpha IIb beta 3 Signaling and Thrombus Growth. *Mol. Nutr. Food Res.* **2019**, *63*, e1900662. [CrossRef] [PubMed]
34. Zou, J.; Tian, Z.; Zhao, Y.; Qiu, X.; Mao, Y.; Li, K.; Shi, Y.; Zhao, D.; Liang, Y.; Ji, Q.; et al. Coenzyme Q10 supplementation improves cholesterol efflux capacity and antiinflammatory properties of high-density lipoprotein in Chinese adults with dyslipidemia. *Nutrition* **2022**, *101*, 111703. [CrossRef]
35. Zhang, H.; Xu, Z.; Zhao, H.; Wang, X.; Pang, J.; Li, Q.; Yang, Y.; Ling, W. Anthocyanin supplementation improves anti-oxidative and anti-inflammatory capacity in a dose-response manner in subjects with dyslipidemia. *Redox Biol.* **2020**, *32*, 101474. [CrossRef]
36. Lopez, J.J.; Salido, G.M.; Pariente, J.A.; Rosado, J.A. Thrombin induces activation and translocation of Bid, Bax and Bak to the mitochondria in human platelets. *J. Thromb. Haemost.* **2008**, *6*, 1780–1788. [CrossRef]
37. Parohan, M.; Anjom-Shoae, J.; Nasiri, M.; Khodadost, M.; Khatibi, S.R.; Sadeghi, O. Dietary total antioxidant capacity and mortality from all causes, cardiovascular disease and cancer: A systematic review and dose-response meta-analysis of prospective cohort studies. *Eur. J. Nutr.* **2019**, *58*, 2175–2189. [CrossRef]
38. Burton-Freeman, B.; Sesso, H.D. Whole food versus supplement: Comparing the clinical evidence of tomato intake and lycopene supplementation on cardiovascular risk factors. *Adv. Nutr.* **2014**, *5*, 457–485. [CrossRef]
39. Sorrentino, V.; Menzies, K.J.; Auwerx, J. Repairing Mitochondrial Dysfunction in Disease. *Annu. Rev. Pharmacol. Toxicol.* **2018**, *58*, 353–389. [CrossRef]
40. Leytin, V.; Allen, D.J.; Mutlu, A.; Gyulkhandanyan, A.V.; Mykhaylov, S.; Freedman, J. Mitochondrial control of platelet apoptosis: Effect of cyclosporin A, an inhibitor of the mitochondrial permeability transition pore. *Lab. Investig.* **2009**, *89*, 374–384. [CrossRef]
41. Pang, A.; Cui, Y.; Chen, Y.; Cheng, N.; Delaney, M.K.; Gu, M.; Stojanovic-Terpo, A.; Zhu, C.; Du, X. Shear-induced integrin signaling in platelet phosphatidylserine exposure, microvesicle release, and coagulation. *Blood* **2018**, *132*, 533–543. [CrossRef] [PubMed]
42. Gyulkhandanyan, A.V.; Mutlu, A.; Freedman, J.; Leytin, V. Markers of platelet apoptosis: Methodology and applications. *J. Thromb. Thrombolysis* **2012**, *33*, 397–411. [CrossRef] [PubMed]
43. Sener, A.; Ozsavci, D.; Oba, R.; Demirel, G.Y.; Uras, F.; Yardimci, K.T. Do platelet apoptosis, activation, aggregation, lipid peroxidation and platelet-leukocyte aggregate formation occur simultaneously in hyperlipidemia? *Clin. Biochem.* **2005**, *38*, 1081–1087. [CrossRef] [PubMed]
44. Li, K.-Y.; Shi, Y.-L.; Ma, X.-L.; Tian, Z.-Z.; Zou, J.-C.; Wang, R.-J.; Mao, Y.-H.; Yang, Y. Fruitflow, a Water-soluble Tomato Extract, Regulates Platelet Oxidative Damage via Autophagy in Vitro. *J. Sun Yat-Sen Univ. (Med. Sci.)* **2021**, *42*, 321–327. [CrossRef]
45. Xiao, Q.; Chen, X.Y.; Ouyang, Q.; Jiang, L.X.; Wu, Y.Q.; Jiang, Y.F. Effect of Quercetin on Apoptosis of Platelets and Its Mechanism. *Zhongguo Shi Yan Xue Ye Xue Za Zhi* **2019**, *27*, 1612–1616. [CrossRef]
46. Ma, J.Q.; Liu, C.M.; Yang, W. Protective effect of rutin against carbon tetrachloride-induced oxidative stress, inflammation and apoptosis in mouse kidney associated with the ceramide, MAPKs, p53 and calpain activities. *Chem. Biol. Interact.* **2018**, *286*, 26–33. [CrossRef]
47. Hada, Y.; Uchida, H.A.; Otaka, N.; Onishi, Y.; Okamoto, S.; Nishiwaki, M.; Takemoto, R.; Takeuchi, H.; Wada, J. The Protective Effect of Chlorogenic Acid on Vascular Senescence via the Nrf2/HO-1 Pathway. *Int. J. Mol. Sci.* **2020**, *21*, 4527. [CrossRef]
48. Cervantes Gracia, K.; Llanas-Cornejo, D.; Husi, H. CVD and Oxidative Stress. *J. Clin. Med.* **2017**, *6*, 22. [CrossRef]
49. Lee, S.H.; Du, J.; Stitham, J.; Atteya, G.; Lee, S.; Xiang, Y.; Wang, D.; Jin, Y.; Leslie, K.L.; Spollett, G.; et al. Inducing mitophagy in diabetic platelets protects against severe oxidative stress. *EMBO Mol. Med.* **2016**, *8*, 779–795. [CrossRef]

50. Tang, W.H.; Stitham, J.; Jin, Y.; Liu, R.; Lee, S.H.; Du, J.; Atteya, G.; Gleim, S.; Spollett, G.; Martin, K.; et al. Aldose reductase-mediated phosphorylation of p53 leads to mitochondrial dysfunction and damage in diabetic platelets. *Circulation* **2014**, *129*, 1598–1609. [CrossRef]
51. Hussain, T.; Tan, B.; Yin, Y.; Blachier, F.; Tossou, M.C.; Rahu, N. Oxidative Stress and Inflammation: What Polyphenols Can Do for Us? *Oxid. Med. Cell. Longev.* **2016**, *2016*, 7432797. [CrossRef] [PubMed]
52. Zaidun, N.H.; Thent, Z.C.; Latiff, A.A. Combating oxidative stress disorders with citrus flavonoid: Naringenin. *Life Sci.* **2018**, *208*, 111–122. [CrossRef] [PubMed]
53. Duarte, J.; Francisco, V.; Perez-Vizcaino, F. Modulation of nitric oxide by flavonoids. *Food Funct.* **2014**, *5*, 1653–1668. [CrossRef] [PubMed]
54. Freedman, J.E. Oxidative stress and platelets. *Arterioscler. Thromb. Vasc. Biol.* **2008**, *28*, s11–s16. [CrossRef]
55. O'Kennedy, N.; Crosbie, L.; Whelan, S.; Luther, V.; Horgan, G.; Broom, J.I.; Webb, D.J.; Duttaroy, A.K. Effects of tomato extract on platelet function: A double-blinded crossover study in healthy humans. *Am. J. Clin. Nutr.* **2006**, *84*, 561–569. [CrossRef]
56. Mone, P.; Trimarco, B.; Santulli, G. Aspirin, NOACs, warfarin: Which is the best choice to tackle cognitive decline in elderly patients? Insights from the GIRAF and ASCEND-Dementia trials presented at the AHA 2021. *Eur. Heart J. Cardiovasc. Pharmacother.* **2022**, *8*, E7–E8. [CrossRef] [PubMed]
57. Tian, Z.; Fan, D.; Li, K.; Zhao, D.; Liang, Y.; Ji, Q.; Gao, X.; Ma, X.; Zhao, Y.; Mao, Y.; et al. Four-Week Supplementation of Water-Soluble Tomato Extract Attenuates Platelet Function in Chinese Healthy Middle-Aged and Older Individuals: A Randomized, Double-Blinded, and Crossover Clinical Trial. *Front. Nutr.* **2022**, *9*, 891241. [CrossRef]
58. Uddin, M.; Biswas, D.; Ghosh, A.; O'Kennedy, N.; Duttaroy, A.K. Consumption of Fruitflow® lowers blood pressure in pre-hypertensive males: A randomised, placebo controlled, double blind, cross-over study. *Int. J. Food Sci. Nutr.* **2018**, *69*, 494–502. [CrossRef]

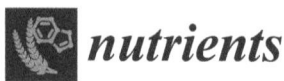

Article

Effect of Dietary Supplementation with Eufortyn® Colesterolo Plus on Serum Lipids, Endothelial Reactivity, Indexes of Non-Alcoholic Fatty Liver Disease and Systemic Inflammation in Healthy Subjects with Polygenic Hypercholesterolemia: The ANEMONE Study

Federica Fogacci [1,2,3], Elisabetta Rizzoli [1,2], Marina Giovannini [1,2], Marilisa Bove [1,2], Sergio D'Addato [1,2], Claudio Borghi [1,2] and Arrigo F. G. Cicero [1,2,3,*]

[1] Hypertension and Cardiovascular Risk Research Center, Medical and Surgical Sciences Department, Sant'Orsola-Malpighi University Hospital, 40138 Bologna, Italy; federicafogacci@gmail.com (F.F.); elisabetta.rizzoli@unibo.it (E.R.); marina.giovannini3@unibo.it (M.G.); marilisa.bove@aosp.bo.it (M.B.); sergio.daddato@unibo.it (S.D.); claudio.borghi@unibo.it (C.B.)
[2] IRCCS Policlinico S. Orsola—Malpighi di Bologna, 40138 Bologna, Italy
[3] Italian Nutraceutical Society (SINut), 40138 Bologna, Italy
* Correspondence: arrigo.cicero@unibo.it

Citation: Fogacci, F.; Rizzoli, E.; Giovannini, M.; Bove, M.; D'Addato, S.; Borghi, C.; Cicero, A.F.G. Effect of Dietary Supplementation with Eufortyn® Colesterolo Plus on Serum Lipids, Endothelial Reactivity, Indexes of Non-Alcoholic Fatty Liver Disease and Systemic Inflammation in Healthy Subjects with Polygenic Hypercholesterolemia: The ANEMONE Study. *Nutrients* 2022, 14, 2099. https://doi.org/10.3390/nu14102099

Academic Editors: Bruno Trimarco and Gaetano Santulli

Received: 10 April 2022
Accepted: 17 May 2022
Published: 18 May 2022

Publisher's Note: MDPI stays neutral with regard to jurisdictional claims in published maps and institutional affiliations.

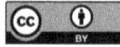

Copyright: © 2022 by the authors. Licensee MDPI, Basel, Switzerland. This article is an open access article distributed under the terms and conditions of the Creative Commons Attribution (CC BY) license (https://creativecommons.org/licenses/by/4.0/).

Abstract: We aimed to evaluate if dietary supplementation with a nutraceutical compound (Eufortyn® Colesterolo Plus) containing standardized bergamot polyphenolic fraction phytosome (Vazguard®), artichoke extract (Pycrinil®), artichoke dry extract. (*Cynara scolymus* L.), Q10 phytosome(Ubiqosome®) and zinc, could positively affect serum lipids concentration, systemic inflammation and indexes of non-alcoholic fatty liver disease (NAFLD) in 60 healthy subjects with polygenic hypercholesterolemia. Participants were adhering to a low-fat, low-sodium Mediterranean diet for a month before being randomly allocated to 8-week treatment with 1 pill each day of either Eufortyn® Colesterolo Plus or placebo. Dietary supplementation with Eufortyn® Colesterolo Plus was associated with significant improvement in total cholesterol (TC), low-density lipoprotein cholesterol (LDL-C), non-high-density lipoprotein cholesterol (non-HDL-C), high-sensitivity C-reactive protein (hs-CRP) and endothelial reactivity (ER) in comparison with baseline, and with significant reductions in waist circumference, TC, LDL-C, LDL-C/HDL-C, lipid accumulation product and fatty liver index compared to placebo. The study shows that dietary supplementation with standardized bergamot polyphenolic fraction phytosome, artichoke extracts, Q10 phytosome and zinc safely exerts significant improvements in serum lipids, systemic inflammation, indexes of NAFLD and endothelial reactivity in healthy subjects with moderate hypercholesterolemia.

Keywords: dietary supplement; nutraceutical compound; cholesterol; artichoke; bergamot

1. Introduction

Polyphenols are secondary plant metabolites and bioactive compounds naturally occurring in plants and plant-derived products [1].

Pooling data from several epidemiological and clinical studies, total flavonoids and specific subclasses have been associated with a reduced incidence of cardiovascular (CV) diseases (CVD), diabetes mellitus and all-cause mortality [2].

Flavonoids have been shown to act as free radical scavenging, and exert antioxidant, hepatoprotective and anti-inflammatory activities [3]. Actually, flavonoids' biological activities reflect their chemical and biochemical properties, including the ability to regulate gene expression in chronic diseases and modulate several molecular pathways [4].

Recently, artichoke and bergamot standardized flavonoid extracts have been suggested as safe lipid-lowering nutraceuticals [5]. Based on this evidence, we aimed to evaluate if dietary supplementation with a nutraceutical compound containing standardized bergamot polyphenolic fraction phytosome® and artichoke extracts could positively affect serum lipids concentration and, secondly, insulin sensitivity, systemic inflammation and indexes of non-alcoholic fatty liver disease (NAFLD) in healthy subjects with moderate hypercholesterolemia.

2. Materials and Methods

2.1. Study Design and Participants

This was a randomized, double-blind, placebo-controlled, parallel-group clinical study that enrolled a sample of Italian free-living subjects with polygenic hypercholesterolemia recruited from the Lipid Clinic of the S. Orsola Malpighi University Hospital, Bologna, Italy.

Participants were required to be aged between 18 and 70 years, with moderately high levels of LDL-C (LDL-C > 115 mg/dL and < 190 mg/dL) and an estimated 10-year cardiovascular risk < 5% according to the SCORE (Systematic COronary Risk Evaluation) risk charts, not requiring lipid-lowering treatments [6]. Exclusion criteria included the following: TG < 400 mg/dL; previous history of CVD; obesity (body mass index (BMI) > 30 Kg/m^2); diabetes mellitus; uncontrolled hypertension (i.e., systolic and diastolic blood pressures > 190/100 mmHg); a positive test for human immunodeficiency virus or hepatitis B/C/E; uncontrolled thyroid diseases; history of malignancies; use of medication or nutritional supplement that altered blood pressure levels or serum lipids (e.g., statins, ezetimibe, fibrates, omega-3 fatty acids and bile acid resins); use of anticoagulants; alcoholism; pregnancy; and breastfeeding.

Enrolled subjects were adhering to a low-fat, low-sodium Mediterranean diet for four weeks before randomization and during the study. The intervention period lasted 8 weeks. Before and after treatment, patients were evaluated for clinical status, and by the execution of a physical examination and laboratory and hemodynamic analyses. The study timeline is described in detail in Figure 1.

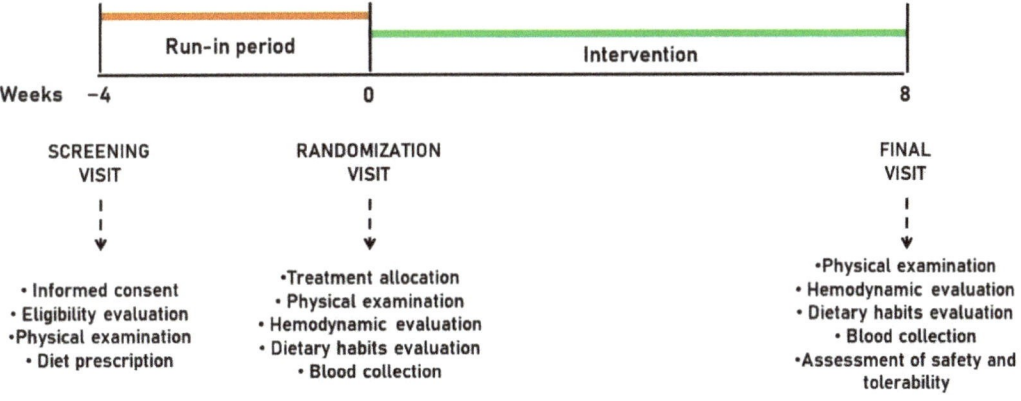

Figure 1. Study timeline.

The study fully complied with the ethical guidelines of the Declaration of Helsinki and with The International Council for Harmonization of Technical Requirements for Registration of Pharmaceuticals for Human Use (ICH) Harmonized Tripartite Guideline for Good Clinical Practice (GCP). The study protocol was approved by the Ethical Committee of the University of Bologna and registered in ClinicalTrials.gov (accessed on 1 May 2020) (ID: NCT04574505). All patients provided written informed consent to participate.

2.2. Treatment

After the 1-month period of diet standardization, enrolled subjects were randomized to receive daily either an indistinguishable pill of placebo orEufortyn® Colesterolo Plus containing Vazguard® (caffeoylquinic acids ≥ 20.0%, total flavonoids ≥ 5.0% and Cynaropicrin ≥ 5.0%), Pycrinil® (total flavanones 11.0–19.0%), artichoke (*Cynara scolymus* L.) dry extract, Ubiqsome® and zinc (Table 1).

Table 1. Quantitative composition of the active treatment, namely Eufortyn® Colesterolo Plus, tested in the clinical study.

Ingredients	Quantity per Tablet
Vazguard® (Phytosome Bergamot Polyphenolic fraction)	1000 mg
Pycrinil® artichoke d.e. (*Cynara cardunculus* L.)	100 mg
Artichoke d.e. (*Cynara scolymus* L.)	20 mg
Ubiqsome® (Coenzyme Q10 phytosome)	25 mg
equivalent to Coenzyme Q10	5 mg
Zinc	5 mg

d.e. = dry extract.

The study products were manufactured and packaged by Scharper S.p.A. (Milan, Italy), in accordance with Quality Management System ISO 9001:2008 and the European Good Manufacturing Practices (GMP), satisfying requirements in the "Code Of Federal Regulation" title 21,volume 2, part 111.

At the time of randomization, each patient was provided with boxes containing 60 tablets (either active ingredients or placebo).

Randomization was performed centrally, by computer-generated codes. Participants and investigators were blinded to the group assignment. Randomization codes were kept in a sealed envelope that was opened after study completion and data analysis.

For the entire duration of the study, patients were instructed to take a pill of the assigned treatment once daily, at about the same time each day, preferably during the evening meal.

At the end of the clinical trial, all unused pills were retrieved for inventory. Participants' compliance was assessed by counting the number of returned pills.

2.3. Assessments

2.3.1. Clinical Data and Anthropometric Measurements

Information gathered in the patients' history included presence of ASCVD and other systemic diseases, allergies and medications. Validated semi-quantitative questionnaires including a Food Frequency Questionnaire (FFQ) were used to assess demographic variables, recreational physical activity and dietary and smoking habits [7].

Analysis of diet composition was performed using the MètaDieta® software (INRAN/IEO 2008 revision/ADI). Data were handled in compliance with the company procedure IOA87.

Waist circumference (WC) was measured in a horizontal plane at the end of a normal expiration, at the midpoint between the inferior margin of the last rib and the superior iliac crest. Height and weight were respectively measured to the nearest 0.1 cm and 0.1 Kg, with subjects standing erect with eyes directed straight, wearing light clothes and with bare feet. BMI was calculated as body weight in kilograms, divided by height squared in meters (Kg/m^2).

2.3.2. Laboratory Analyses

Biochemical analyses were carried out on venous blood withdrawn after overnight fasting (at least 12 h). Serum was obtained by addition of disodium ethylenediaminetetraacetate (Na_2EDTA) (1 mg/mL) and blood centrifugation at 3000 RPM for 15 min at 25 °C.

Immediately after centrifugation, trained personnel performed laboratory analyses according to standardized methods [8]. The following parameters were directly assessed: Total cholesterol (TC), triglycerides (TG), high-density lipoprotein cholesterol (HDL-C), apolipoprotein B-100 (Apo B-100), apolipoprotein AI (Apo AI), fasting plasma glucose (FPG), creatinine, high-sensitivity C-reactive protein (hs-CRP), creatine phosphokinase (CPK), gamma-glutamyl transferase (GGT), alanine transaminase (ALT) and aspartate transaminase (AST).

LDL-C was obtained by the Friedewald formula. Non-HDL cholesterol (Non-HDL-C) resulted from the difference between TC and HDL-C. The glomerular filtration rate (eGFR) was estimated by the Chronic Kidney Disease Epidemiology Collaboration (CKD-epi) equation [9].

Lipid accumulation product (LAP) was calculated as (WC − 65) × TG (expressed in mmol/L) for men and (WC − 58) × TG (expressed in mmol/L) for women [10]. Hepatic steatosis index (HSI) resulted from 8 × AST/ALT ratio + BMI (+2 for women) [11]. Finally, fatty liver index (FLI) was calculated as follows: $[e^{0.953 \times \ln(TG) + 0.139 \times BMI + 0.718 \times \ln(GGT) + 0.053 \times WC - 15.745} / (1 + e^{0.953 \times \ln(TG) + 0.139 \times BMI + 0.718 \times \ln(GGT) + 0.053 \times WC - 15.745})] \times 100$ [12].

2.3.3. Blood Pressure Measurements

Blood pressure (BP) was measured in accordance with the recommendations of the International Guidelines for the management of arterial hypertension [13]. Resting systolic (SBP) and diastolic BP (DBP) were measured with a validated oscillometric device and a cuff of the appropriate size applied on the right upper arm. To improve detection accuracy, three BP readings were sequentially obtained at 1-minute intervals. The first reading was discarded, and the average between the second and the third reading was recorded as the study variable.

2.3.4. Endothelial Reactivity

Endothelial function of the arterial vasculature is an important early marker of atherosclerosis, reflecting the ability of the endothelial layer to release nitric oxide (NO), modulating smooth muscle tone in the arterial wall of the conduit arteries [14].

Following the current guidelines [15], during the clinical study endothelial function was evaluated through Endocheck® (BC Biomedical Laboratories Ltd., Vancouver, BC, Canada), a method embedded within the Vicorder® device that guarantees very good intra- and inter-operator reliability [16]. The measurement was carried out with patients in supine position and in abstinence from cigarette smoking and caffeinated beverages for at least 12 h. After a 10-minute rest, the brachial pulse volume (PV) waveforms were recorded at baseline for 10 s and during reactive hyperemia. The BP cuff was inflated to 200 mmHg for 5 min and PV waveforms were recorded for 3 min after the cuff was released. Endothelial reactivity (ER) was calculated as change in the PV waveform area, comparing waveforms before and during hyperemia through the equation $\sqrt{PV2/PV1}$, where PV1 represents PV at the baseline and PV2 represents PV during hyperemia [17].

2.3.5. Assessment of Safety and Tolerability

Safety and tolerability were evaluated through continuous monitoring during the study in order to detect any adverse event, clinical safety, laboratory findings, vital sign measurements and physical examinations. A blinded, independent expert clinical event committee was appointed by the principal investigator in order to categorize the adverse events that could possibly be experienced during the trial as not related, unlikely related, possibly related, probably related, or definitely related to the tested treatment [18].

2.4. Statistical Analysis

Data were analyzed using intention to treat by means of the Statistical Package for Social Science (SPSS) 25.0, version for Windows.

Sample size was calculated for the change in LDL-C. A total of 28 subjects per group were needed to detect a mean change in LDL-C at 8 weeks of 12 mg/dL with a power of 0.90 and an alpha error of 0.05. A total sample size of 60 patients (30 patients/arm) was included in the study to allow for a dropout rate of 10%.

The Kolmogorov–Smirnov test was used to test the normality distribution of the studied variables. Non-normally distribute variables were log-transformed before further statistical testing. Baseline characteristics of the population were compared using Levene's test followed by the independent Student's T test and by the χ^2 test followed by Fisher's exact test. Between-group differences were assessed by repeated-measures ANOVA followed by Tukey's post hoc test. All data were expressed as means and related standard deviations. All tests were two-sided. A p level of <0.05 was considered significant for all tests.

3. Results

3.1. Efficacy Analysis

A total of 94 volunteers was screened, and 60 subjects underwent randomization from November 2020 through November 2021. Sixty enrolled subjects successfully completed the trial according to the study design (Figure 2).

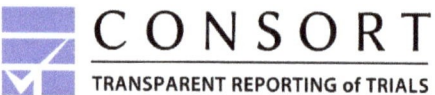

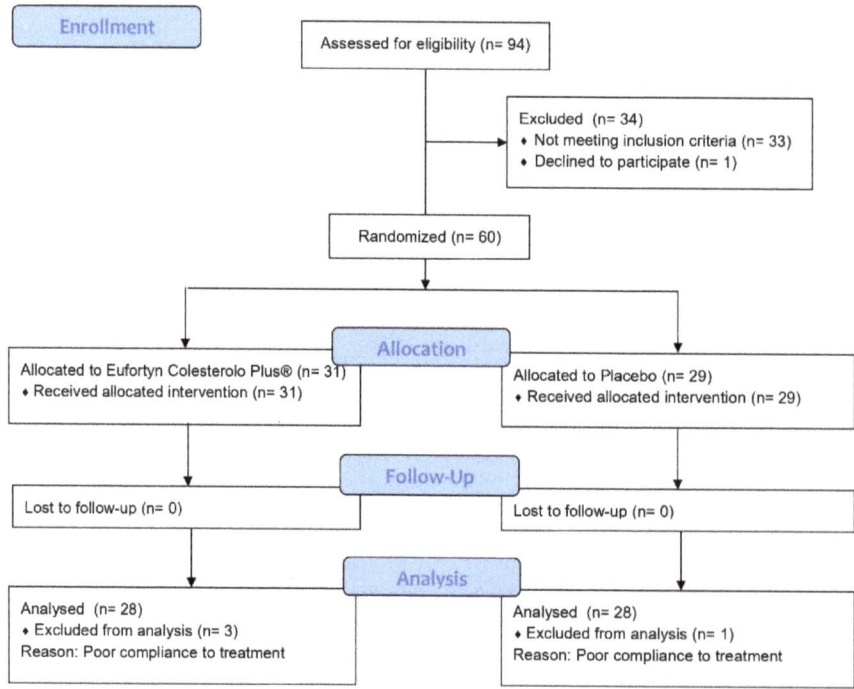

Figure 2. CONSORT flow diagram of the progress through the phases of the clinical study.

The mean compliance to the treatment was 91 ± 2% in the active treatment group and 89 ± 2% in the placebo group. Three individuals allocated to treatment with Eufortyn® Colesterolo Plus and one individual in the placebo group were excluded from analysis because of poor compliance to treatment.

The final distribution by sex did not show any significant differences between groups ($p > 0.05$), with 14 women allocated to placebo and 16 women allocated to Eufortyn® Colesterolo Plus and no detectable interaction effect.

During the run-in period a non-statistically significant trend toward body weight decrease was observed in both considered groups. No statistically significant changes were recorded in the dietary habits of the enrolled individuals from randomization until the end of the study, with any changes in total energy and macronutrient intake (Table 2).

Table 2. Diet composition (g/day) at enrollment and at the end of the clinical trial. Values are reported as mean ± SD.

Parameters	Placebo (n. 28)		Eufortyn® Colesterolo Plus (n. 28)	
	Baseline	Week 8	Baseline	Week 8
Total energy (Kcal/day)	1629 ± 110	1611 ± 105	1591 ± 99	1586 ± 116
Carbohydrates (% of total energy)	54.4 ± 2.3	53.2 ± 2.5	54.5 ± 2.1	54.4 ± 2.4
Proteins (% of total energy)	18.2 ± 1.4	18.4 ± 1.6	17.8 ± 1.5	18.1 ± 1.3
Animal protein (% of total energy)	10.5 ± 0.9	9.9 ± 0.9	10.6 ± 0.7	10.9 ± 0.8
Vegetal protein (% of total energy)	7.3 ± 0.6	7.5 ± 0.8	6.7 ± 0.6	6.8 ± 0.7
Total fats (% of total energy)	27.7 ± 2.0	27.5 ± 2.3	27.2 ± 1.7	28.0 ± 2.1
Saturated fatty acids (% of total energy)	8.0 ± 0.8	8.2 ± 0.7	8.3 ± 0.7	7.8 ± 0.9
MUFA (% of total energy)	12.6 ± 1.1	12.2 ± 1.0	12.8 ± 1.0	12.3 ± 1.1
PUFA (% of total energy)	6.7 ± 0.6	6.2 ± 0.7	6.5 ± 0.5	6.7 ± 0.6
Total dietary fibers (g/day)	18.9 ± 2.5	19.1 ± 2.8	19.3 ± 2.5	18.7 ± 2.4
Cholesterol (mg/day)	191.2 ± 13.3	187.2 ± 12.3	192.8 ± 11.5	194.8 ± 10.7

MUFA = Monounsaturated fatty acids; n = Number of individuals; PUFA = Polyunsaturated fatty acids.

The study groups were well matched for all the considered variables at baseline, except for heart rate, which was significantly higher in the active treatment group (Table 3). At the end of the trial, dietary supplementation with Eufortyn® Colesterolo Plus was associated with significant improvement in TC, LDL-C, non-HDL-C, hsCRP and ER in comparison with baseline, and with significant reductions in WC, TC, LDL-C, LDL-C/HDL-C, LAP, and FLI compared to placebo (Table 3). TC and LDL-C improved with Eufortyn® Colesterolo Plus versus both baseline and placebo.

3.2. Safety Analysis

All participants completed the clinical trial according to the study design (dropout rate = 0%). No treatment-emergent adverse events were reported and no laboratory abnormalities occurred during the study.

Table 3. Anthropometric, hemodynamic and blood chemistry parameters from the baseline to the end of the clinical trial, expressed as mean ± SD.

Parameters	Placebo (n. 28)		Eufortyn® Colesterolo Plus (n. 28)	
	Baseline	Week 8	Baseline	Week 8
Age (years)	54 ± 3	-	54 ± 4	-
Body Mass Index (Kg/m^2)	24.3 ± 3.9	24.4 ± 3.7	23.9 ± 2.9	23.7 ± 2.7
Waist Circumference (cm)	87.1 ± 14.0	87.1 ± 13.8	85.8 ± 12.4	84.8 ± 11.4 §
SBP (mmHg)	135.4 ± 16.1	131.6 ± 17.7	133.8 ± 16.5	130.9 ± 17.9
DBP (mmHg)	73.5 ± 12.5	72.8 ± 10.3	73.8 ± 10.7	75.7 ± 12.8
Heart Rate (bpm)	65.5 ± 11.2	69.1 ± 12.3	73.3 ± 13.3 §	71.0 ± 13.0
Total Cholesterol (mg/dL)	223.7 ± 24.7	227.7 ± 22.3	229.2 ± 20.8	214.5 ± 22.9 §,*
LDL-C (mg/dL)	141.9 ± 20.1	144.9 ± 20.2	143.3 ± 17.3	131.2 ± 19.8 §,*
HDL-C (mg/dL)	57.4 ± 17.6	56.5 ± 14.9	64.9 ± 18.9 §	61.8 ± 18.0
Non-HDL-C (mg/dL)	166.4 ± 23.6	159.5 ± 29.0	165.3 ± 20.1	158.7 ± 23.1 *
LDL-C/HDL-C	2.7 ± 0.8	2.7 ± 0.8	2.5 ± 0.8	2.4 ± 0.8 §
Triglycerides (mg/dL)	117.3 ± 70.2	126.3 ± 59.5	109.7 ± 54.3	112.9 ± 47.3 §
Apolipoprotein B-100 (mg/dL)	122.0 ± 16.2	126.2 ± 17.6	118.0 ± 14.6	121.4 ± 16.9
Apolipoprotein AI (mg/dL)	154.2 ± 26.3	154.4 ± 24.2	160.4 ± 27.9	155.9 ± 28.8
FPG (mg/dL)	90.1 ± 8.5	91.4 ± 7.1	88.2 ± 11.3	89.2 ± 10.5
AST (U/L)	21.2 ± 7.2	21.2 ± 4.6	22.3 ± 4.6	22.8 ± 4.6
ALT (U/L)	22.7 ± 14.4	20.6 ± 10.3	19.2 ± 6.9 §	19.0 ± 6.9
gGT (U/L)	25.2 ± 20.5	25.2 ± 17.9	21.9 ± 13.3 §	22.4 ± 13.6
Lipid Accumulation Product	34.9 ± 16.4	38.1 ± 19.1	33.4 ± 16.3	32.9 ± 13.3 §
Hepatic Steatosis Index	33.4 ± 5.2	32.8 ± 4.9	32.1 ± 4.1	31.7 ± 3.8
Fatty Liver Index	31.4 ± 15.9	29.5 ± 17.6	26.4 ± 14.5	26.2 ± 13.9 §
CPK (U/L)	102.3 ± 74.8	108.4 ± 104.1	114.1 ± 67.8	99.2 ± 51.0
eGFR (mL/min)	85.9 ± 15.8	85.9 ± 16.1	85.6 ± 15.9	83.0 ± 16.7
hs-CRP (mg/L)	0.15 ± 0.15	0.12 ± 0.10	0.17 ± 0.24	0.13 ± 0.15 *
Endothelial reactivity	1.37 ± 0.31	1.38 ± 0.17	1.33 ± 0.27	1.43 ± 0.22 *

* $p < 0.05$ versus baseline; § $p < 0.05$ versus placebo. ALT = Alanine aminotransferase; AST = Aspartate aminotransferase; CPK = Creatine phosphokinase; DBP = Diastolic blood pressure; eGFR = Estimated glomerular filtration rate; FPG = Fasting plasma glucose; gGT = Gamma-glutamyl transferase; HDL-C = High-density lipoprotein cholesterol; hs-CRP = High sensitivity C reactive protein; LDL-C = Low-density lipoprotein cholesterol; SBP = Systolic blood pressure.

4. Discussion

In the last decades, there has been a growing interest in the usefulness of natural compounds targeting multiple biochemical pathways [19]. In this context, dietary polyphenols have gained particular attention [20]. A growing body of evidence suggest that artichoke and bergamot standardized flavonoid extracts improve the lipid pattern in moderately hypercholesterolemic individuals, such that their use has been promoted as safe lipid-lowering agents [21,22]. Moreover, artichoke extracts and bergamot polyphenolic fraction have anti-inflammatory and antioxidant properties [23,24].

In animal models, artichoke flavonoids hinder cholesterol biosynthesis from 14-C-acetate, probably through the inhibition of 3-hydroxy-3-methylglutaryl-Coenzyme A (HMG-CoA) reductase [25]. Furthermore, artichoke flavonoids interact with liver sterol regulatory element-binding proteins (SREPBs) and acetyl-CoA C-acetyltransferase (ACAT) and increase bile acids fecal excretion [26].

In the present study, dietary supplementation with bergamot polyphenolic fraction phytosome, artichoke extracts, Q10 phytosome and zinc was effective in lowering a number of serum lipoprotein fractions, with an additional statistically significant effect on fasting plasma glucose, systemic inflammation and indexes of NAFLD. Moreover, dietary supplementation with Eufortyn® Colesterolo Plus resulted in a significant improvement in ER after as early as 8 weeks. Particular attention should be paid to the prognostic meaning of this latest finding, since endothelial function is an important early marker of atherosclerosis, reflecting the ability of the endothelial layer to release nitric oxide (NO) and modulate smooth muscle tone in the arterial wall [27]. Such improvements in endothelial function have been previously found to be associated with a significant reduction in CVD risk [28].

Based on evidence from preclinical studies, artichoke's polyphenols, such as caffeoylquinic acids, regulate the expression of a variety of genes, including vascular endothelial growth factor (VEGF), endothelin 1 (ET-1) and endothelial NO synthase (eNOS), which promote the vasodilation mediated by the endothelial cells. Moreover, luteolin andcynaroside stimulate NOS messenger ribonucleic acid (mRNA) in human endothelial cells, with consequent NO production and potential beneficial activity in the prevention of CVD [29]. Finally, coenzyme Q10 and zinc potentially have a synergistic effect with the antioxidant properties of polyphenol compounds, also improving the plasma levels of metalloenzymes (including superoxide dismutase) [30,31].

As originally reported by the CTT (Cholesterol Treatment Trialists') meta-analyses of the statin trials, there is a linear association between LDL-C reduction and decrease in atherosclerotic CVD (ASCVD) events [32]. Robust and growing evidence highlights that this linear association is observed regardless of the LDL-C lowering approach adopted (i.e., low-fat diet, anion exchange resins, ezetimibe, etc.) [33]. In this context, the improvement in LDL-C during treatment with Eufortyn® Colesterolo Plus has a clinical relevance, especially considering the concerns that have been recently raised by the European Food and Safety Agency (EFSA) regarding the safety of red yeast rice-based food supplements [34]. Moreover, unlike the other nutraceuticals specifically inhibiting cholesterol synthesis or absorption [35], bergamot polyphenolic fraction and artichoke extracts have an impact on both lipid and glucose metabolism [33,36]. For these reasons and according to our observations, Eufortyn® Colesterolo Plus could have a role in the management and prevention of multifactorial metabolic disorders such as metabolic syndrome and NAFLD [37,38].

Despite the relevant findings and the practical implications, this study is not without limitations. We acknowledge the relatively small sample size, even though the study was powered for the primary outcomes and to detect between-groups differences in safety and tolerability. Moreover, the relatively short follow-up means it is not possible to assess the possible occurrence of adaptation phenomena; however, these have never been documented for polyphenols before. We also acknowledge that some investigated parameters improved in a way that was not mirrored in previous clinical studies testing bergamot polyphenolic fraction and artichoke extracts with more impressive results [39,40]. The reason might be found in the stringent eligibility criteria of the present study, which did, however, ensure high internal validity and reliability of the results. Another limitation of the study is the lack of ultrasound evaluation or transient elastography (fibroscan) of liver stiffness.

More research is needed that focuses on the underlying reasons and mechanisms of the effects observed during the study. For instance, the effect on serum lipids and inflammation is likely to be partially mediated by modification of the gut microbiota induced by polyphenols supplementation. Available experimental data suggest that supplementation with bergamot and artichoke polyphenolic fractionsis able to exert a beneficial effect on the composition of the gut microbiota [4,41]. However, to date, thereis no specific evidence related to simultaneous supplementation with these nutraceutical compounds. Finally, it is critically important that further longer-term clinical studies clarify whether the treatment-dependent changes in liver function tests reflect a significant improvement in liver stiffness.

5. Conclusions

In conclusion, the study shows that dietary supplementation with standardized bergamot polyphenolic fraction phytosome, artichoke extracts, Q10 phytosome and zinc safely exerts significant improvements in serum lipids, systemic inflammation, indexes of NAFLD and endothelial function in healthy subjects with moderate hypercholesterolemia.

Author Contributions: Conceptualization, A.F.G.C.; methodology, A.F.G.C.; formal analysis, A.F.G.C.; investigation, F.F., E.R., M.G., M.B. and S.D.; data curation, A.F.G.C., F.F., E.R. and C.B.; writing—original draft preparation, A.F.G.C. and F.F.; writing—review and editing, E.R., M.G., M.B., S.D. and C.B.; supervision, A.F.G.C.; project administration, A.F.G.C.; funding acquisition, A.F.G.C. All authors have read and agreed to the published version of the manuscript.

Funding: Products were manufactured and provided by Scharper S.p.A. (Milano, MI, Italy), who also fully funded the study.

Institutional Review Board Statement: The study was conducted according to the guidelines of the Declaration of Helsinki, and approved by the Ethics Committee of the University of Bologna (ComitatoEtico di Area Vasta Emilia Centro dellaRegione Emilia Romagna-Protocol code: 448/2020/Sper/AOUBo; Date of approval: 21 May 2020).

Informed Consent Statement: Informed consent was obtained from all individuals involved in the study.

Data Availability Statement: Data supporting study's findings are available from the Corresponding Author with the permission of the University of Bologna and the sponsor.

Acknowledgments: The authors are sincerely grateful to all the subjects who agreed to participate in the clinical trial.

Conflicts of Interest: The authors declare no conflict of interest. Scharper S.p.A. (Milano, MI, Italy) had no role in the design of the study; in the collection, analyses, and interpretation of data; in writing of the manuscript; or in the decision to publish the results.

References

1. Tangney, C.C.; Rasmussen, H.E. Polyphenols, inflammation, and cardiovascular disease. *Curr. Atheroscler. Rep.* **2013**, *15*, 324. [CrossRef] [PubMed]
2. Di Lorenzo, C.; Colombo, F.; Biella, S.; Stockley, C.; Restani, P. Polyphenols and human health: The role of bioavailability. *Nutrients* **2021**, *13*, 273. [CrossRef] [PubMed]
3. Kumar, S.; Pandey, A.K. Chemistry and biological activities of flavonoids: An overview. *Sci. World J.* **2013**, *2013*, 162750. [CrossRef] [PubMed]
4. Martín, M.Á.; Ramos, S. Impact of dietary flavanols on microbiota, immunity and inflammation in metabolic diseases. *Nutrients* **2021**, *13*, 850. [CrossRef]
5. Cicero, A.F.G.; Colletti, A.; Bajraktari, G.; Descamps, O.; Djuric, D.M.; Ezhov, M.; Fras, Z.; Katsiki, N.; Langlois, M.; Latkovskis, G.; et al. Lipid lowering nutraceuticals in clinical practice: Position paper from an International Lipid Expert Panel. *Nutr. Res. Rev.* **2020**, *33*, 155–179. [CrossRef] [PubMed]
6. Authors/Task Force Members; ESC Committee for Practice Guidelines (CPG); ESC National Cardiac Societies. 2019 ESC/EAS guidelines for the management of dyslipidaemias: Lipid modification to reduce cardiovascular risk. *Atherosclerosis* **2019**, *290*, 140–205. [CrossRef]
7. Cicero, A.F.G.; Caliceti, C.; Fogacci, F.; Giovannini, M.; Calabria, D.; Colletti, A.; Veronesi, M.; Roda, A.; Borghi, C. Effect of apple polyphenols on vascular oxidative stress and endothelium function: A translational study. *Mol. Nutr. Food Res.* **2017**, *61*, 1700373. [CrossRef]
8. Cicero, A.F.G.; Fogacci, F.; Bove, M.; Giovannini, M.; Borghi, C. Impact of a short-term synbiotic supplementation on metabolic syndrome and systemic inflammation in elderly patients: A randomized placebo-controlled clinical trial. *Eur. J. Nutr.* **2021**, *60*, 655–663. [CrossRef]
9. Levey, A.S.; Stevens, L.A.; Schmid, C.H.; Zhang, Y.L.; Castro, A.F., 3rd; Feldman, H.I.; Kusek, J.W.; Eggers, P.; Van Lente, F.; Greene, T.; et al. A new equation to estimate glomerular filtration rate. *Ann. Intern. Med.* **2009**, *150*, 604–612. [CrossRef]
10. Bedogni, G.; Kahn, H.S.; Bellentani, S.; Tiribelli, C. A simple index of lipid overaccumulation is a good marker of liver steatosis. *BMC Gastroenterol.* **2010**, *10*, 98. [CrossRef]
11. Lee, J.H.; Kim, D.; Kim, H.J.; Lee, C.H.; Yang, J.I.; Kim, W.; Kim, Y.J.; Yoon, J.H.; Cho, S.H.; Sung, M.W.; et al. Hepatic steatosis index: A simple screening tool reflecting nonalcoholic fatty liver disease. *Dig. Liver Dis.* **2010**, *42*, 503–508. [CrossRef] [PubMed]
12. Cicero, A.F.G.; Gitto, S.; Fogacci, F.; Rosticci, M.; Giovannini, M.; D'Addato, S.; Andreone, P.; Borghi, C.; Brisighella Heart Study Group Medical and Surgical Sciences Department, University of Bologna. Fatty liver index is associated to pulse wave velocity in healthy subjects: Data from the Brisighella Heart Study. *Eur. J. Intern. Med.* **2018**, *53*, 29–33. [CrossRef] [PubMed]
13. Williams, B.; Mancia, G.; Spiering, W.; AgabitiRosei, E.; Azizi, M.; Burnier, M.; Clement, D.L.; Coca, A.; de Simone, G.; Dominiczak, A.; et al. Authors/Task Force Members. 2018 ESC/ESH Guidelines for the management of arterial hypertension: The Task Force for the management of arterial hypertension of the European Society of Cardiology and the European Society of Hypertension. *J. Hypertens.* **2018**, *36*, 1953–2041. [CrossRef]

14. Thijssen, D.H.J.; Bruno, R.M.; van Mil, A.C.C.M.; Holder, S.M.; Faita, F.; Greyling, A.; Zock, P.L.; Taddei, S.; Deanfield, J.E.; Luscher, T.; et al. Expert consensus and evidence-based recommendations for the assessment of flow-mediated dilation in humans. *Eur. Heart J.* 2019, *40*, 2534–2547. [CrossRef] [PubMed]
15. Corretti, M.C.; Anderson, T.J.; Benjamin, E.J.; Celermajer, D.; Charbonneau, F.; Creager, M.A.; Deanfield, J.; Drexler, H.; Gerhard-Herman, M.; Herrington, D.; et al. Guidelines for the ultrasound assessment of endothelial—dependent flow—mediated vasodilation of the brachial artery: A report of the International Brachial Artery Reactivity Task Force. *J. Am. Coll. Cardiol.* 2002, *39*, 257–265. [CrossRef]
16. McGreevy, C.; Barry, M.; Bennett, K.; Williams, D. Repeatability of the measurement of aortic pulse wave velocity (aPWV) in the clinical assessment of arterial stiffness in community-dwelling older patients using the Vicorder(®) device. *Scand. J. Clin. Lab. Investig.* 2013, *73*, 269–273. [CrossRef]
17. Day, L.M.; Maki-Petaja, K.M.; Wilkinson, I.B.; McEniery, C.M. Assessment of brachial artery reactivity using the endocheck: Repeatability, reproducibility and preliminary comparison with ultrasound. *Artery Res.* 2013, *7*, 119–120. [CrossRef]
18. Cicero, A.F.G.; Fogacci, F.; Veronesi, M.; Strocchi, E.; Grandi, E.; Rizzoli, E.; Poli, A.; Marangoni, F.; Borghi, C. A randomized placebo-controlled clinical trial to evaluate the medium-term effects of oat fibers on human health: The beta-glucan effects on lipid profile, glycemia and intestinal health (BELT) study. *Nutrients* 2020, *12*, 686. [CrossRef]
19. Cicero, A.F.G.; Fogacci, F.; Colletti, A. Food and plant bioactives for reducing cardiometabolic disease risk: An evidence based approach. *Food Funct.* 2017, *8*, 2076–2088. [CrossRef]
20. Feldman, F.; Koudoufio, M.; Desjardins, Y.; Spahis, S.; Delvin, E.; Levy, E. Efficacy of polyphenols in the management of dyslipidemia: A focus on clinical studies. *Nutrients* 2021, *13*, 672. [CrossRef]
21. Cicero, A.F.G.; Fogacci, F.; Bove, M.; Giovannini, M.; Borghi, C. Three-arm, placebo-controlled, randomized clinical trial evaluating the metabolic effect of a combined nutraceutical containing a bergamot standardized flavonoid extract in dyslipidemic overweight subjects. *Phytother. Res.* 2019, *33*, 2094–2101. [CrossRef] [PubMed]
22. Cicero, A.F.G.; Fogacci, F.; Bove, M.; Giovannini, M.; Veronesi, M.; Borghi, C. Short-term effects of dry extracts of artichoke and berberis in hypercholesterolemic patients without cardiovascular disease. *Am. J. Cardiol.* 2019, *123*, 588–591. [CrossRef] [PubMed]
23. Gliozzi, M.; Walker, R.; Mollace, V. Bergamot polyphenols: Pleiotropic players in the treatment of metabolic syndrome. *J. Metab. Syndr.* 2014, *3*, 143.
24. Santos, H.O.; Bueno, A.A.; Mota, J.F. The effect of artichoke on lipid profile: A review of possible mechanisms of action. *Pharmacol. Res.* 2018, *137*, 170–178. [CrossRef]
25. Gebhardt, R. Inhibition of cholesterol biosynthesis in primary cultured rat hepatocytes by artichoke (*Cynara scolymus* L.) extracts. *J. Pharmacol. Exp. Ther.* 1998, *286*, 1122–1128.
26. Sahebkar, A.; Pirro, M.; Banach, M.; Mikhailidis, D.P.; Atkin, S.L.; Cicero, A.F.G. Lipid-lowering activity of artichoke extracts: A systematic review and meta-analysis. *Crit. Rev. Food Sci. Nutr.* 2018, *58*, 2549–2556. [CrossRef]
27. Tousoulis, D.; Kampoli, A.M.; Tentolouris, C.; Papageorgiou, N.; Stefanadis, C. The role of nitric oxide on endothelial function. *Curr. Vasc. Pharmacol.* 2012, *10*, 4–18. [CrossRef]
28. Matsuzawa, Y.; Kwon, T.G.; Lennon, R.J.; Lerman, L.O.; Lerman, A. Prognostic value of flow-mediated vasodilation in brachial artery and fingertip artery for cardiovascular events: A systematic review and meta-analysis. *J. Am. Heart Assoc.* 2015, *4*, e002270. [CrossRef]
29. Li, H.; Xia, N.; Brausch, I.; Yao, Y.; Förstermann, U. Flavonoids from artichoke (*Cynara scolymus* L.) up-regulate endothelial-type nitric-oxide synthase gene expression in human endothelial cells. *J. Pharmacol. Exp. Ther.* 2004, *310*, 926–932. [CrossRef]
30. Lee, B.J.; Huang, Y.C.; Chen, S.J.; Lin, P.T. Coenzyme Q10 supplementation reduces oxidative stress and increases antioxidant enzyme activity in patients with coronary artery disease. *Nutrition* 2012, *28*, 250–255. [CrossRef]
31. Vázquez-Lorente, H.; Molina-López, J.; Herrera-Quintana, L.; Gamarra-Morales, Y.; Quintero-Osso, B.; López-González, B.; Planells, E. Erythrocyte Zn concentration and antioxidant response after supplementation with Zn in a postmenopausal population. A double-blind randomized trial. *Exp. Gerontol.* 2022, *162*, 111766. [CrossRef] [PubMed]
32. Baigent, C.; Keech, A.; Kearney, P.M.; Blackwell, L.; Buck, G.; Pollicino, C.; Kirby, A.; Sourjina, T.; Peto, R.; Collins, R.; et al. Efficacy and safety of cholesterol-lowering treatment: Prospective meta-analysis of data from 90,056 participants in 14 randomised trials of statins. *Lancet* 2005, *366*, 1267–1278. [CrossRef] [PubMed]
33. Silverman, M.G.; Ference, B.A.; Im, K.; Wiviott, S.D.; Giugliano, R.P.; Grundy, S.M.; Braunwald, E.; Sabatine, M.S. Association between lowering LDL-C and cardiovascular risk reduction among different therapeutic interventions: A systematic review and meta-analysis. *JAMA* 2016, *316*, 1289–1297. [CrossRef] [PubMed]
34. EFSA ANS Panel (EFSA Panel Food Additives and Nutrient Sources added to Food); Younes, M.; Aggett, P.; Aguilar, F.; Crebelli, R.; Dusemund, B.; Filipi, C.M.; Frutos, M.J.; Galtier, P.; Gott, D.; et al. Scientific opinion on the safety of monacolins in red yeast rice. *EFSA J.* 2018, *16*, 5368. [CrossRef]
35. Cicero, A.F.G.; Fogacci, F.; Stoian, A.P.; Vrablik, M.; Al Rasadi, K.; Banach, M.; Toth, P.P.; Rizzo, M. Nutraceuticals in the management of dyslipidemia: Which, when, and for whom? Could nutraceuticals help low-risk individuals with non-optimal lipid levels? *Curr. Atheroscler. Rep.* 2021, *23*, 57. [CrossRef] [PubMed]
36. Ballistreri, G.; Amenta, M.; Fabroni, S.; Consoli, V.; Grosso, S.; Vanella, L.; Sorrenti, V.; Rapisarda, P. Evaluation of lipid and cholesterol-lowering effect of bioflavonoids from bergamot extract. *Nat. Prod. Res.* 2020, *35*, 5378–5383. [CrossRef]

37. Cicero, A.F.; Colletti, A. Role of phytochemicals in the management of metabolic syndrome. *Phytomedicine* **2016**, *23*, 1134–1144. [CrossRef]
38. Cicero, A.F.; Colletti, A.; Bellentani, S. Nutraceutical approach to non-alcoholic fatty liver disease (NAFLD): The available clinical evidence. *Nutrients* **2018**, *10*, 1153. [CrossRef]
39. Lamiquiz-Moneo, I.; Giné-González, J.; Alisente, S.; Bea, A.M.; Pérez-Calahorra, S.; Marco-Benedí, V.; Baila-Rueda, L.; Jarauta, E.; Cenarro, A.; Civeira, F.; et al. Effect of bergamot on lipid profile in humans: A systematic review. *Crit. Rev. Food Sci. Nutr.* **2020**, *60*, 3133–3143. [CrossRef]
40. Riva, A.; Petrangolini, G.; Allegrini, P.; Perna, S.; Giacosa, A.; Peroni, G.; Faliva, M.A.; Naso, M.; Rondanelli, M. Artichoke and bergamot phytosome alliance: A randomized double blind clinical trial in mild hypercholesterolemia. *Nutrients* **2021**, *14*, 108. [CrossRef]
41. Domínguez-Fernández, M.; Ludwig, I.A.; De Peña, M.P.; Cid, C. Bioaccessibility of Tudela artichoke (*Cynara scolymus* cv. Blanca de Tudela) (poly)phenols: The effects of heat treatment, simulated gastrointestinal digestion and human colonic microbiota. *Food Funct.* **2021**, *12*, 1996–2011. [CrossRef] [PubMed]

MDPI
St. Alban-Anlage 66
4052 Basel
Switzerland
www.mdpi.com

Nutrients Editorial Office
E-mail: nutrients@mdpi.com
www.mdpi.com/journal/nutrients

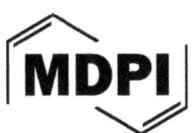

Disclaimer/Publisher's Note: The statements, opinions and data contained in all publications are solely those of the individual author(s) and contributor(s) and not of MDPI and/or the editor(s). MDPI and/or the editor(s) disclaim responsibility for any injury to people or property resulting from any ideas, methods, instructions or products referred to in the content.

www.ingramcontent.com/pod-product-compliance
Lightning Source LLC
LaVergne TN
LVHW070155120526
838202LV00013BA/1148